In: Health and Human Development Series

COMPLEMENTARY MEDICINE SYSTEMS: COMPARISON AND INTEGRATION

HEALTH AND HUMAN DEVELOPMENT SERIES

Joav Merrick (editor)

Disability from a Humanistic Perspective: Towards a Better Quality of Life
Shunit Reiter
2008 ISBN 978-1-60456-412-9

Complementary Medicine Systems: Comparison and Integration
Karl W. Kratky
2008 ISBN 978-1-60456-475-4

In: Health and Human Development Series

COMPLEMENTARY MEDICINE SYSTEMS: COMPARISON AND INTEGRATION

KARL W. KRATKY

Nova Science
New York

MT

Library of Congress Cataloging-in-Publication Data

Kratky, Karl W. [Komplementäre Medizinsysteme. English]
Complementary medicine systems : comparison and integration / Karl W. Kratky (author).
    p. ; cm.
Originally published in German as: Komplementäre Medizinsysteme / Karl W. Kratky. c2003.
Includes bibliographical references and index.
ISBN 978-1-60456-475-4 (hardcover)
1. Alternative medicine. 2. Medicine, Comparative. I. Title.
[DNLM: 1. Complementary Therapies. WB 890 K891c 2008a]
R733.K66413   2008
610--dc22   2008010948

Published by Nova Science Publishers, Inc.   +   New York

3/9/09

For Uschi &
Angelika Richard
Fabian Katja Felix

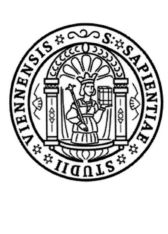

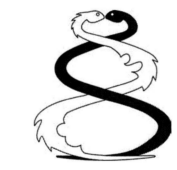

BRIEF CONTENTS

---

[*] The chapter marked with an asterisk is meant for more in-depth knowledge in a particular subject for those interested and can otherwise be skipped.

DETAILED CONTENTS

---

[*] The chapter marked with an asterisk is meant for more in-depth knowledge in a particular subject for those interested and can otherwise be skipped.

---

* The subchapters marked with an asterisk are meant for more in-depth knowledge in a particular subject for those interested and can otherwise be skipped.

---

* The chapter and subchapters marked with an asterisk are meant for more in-depth knowledge in a particular subject for those interested and can otherwise be skipped.

Prologue

This book is a result of the lecture 'Similarities of Complementary Medical Methods', which I have been giving since 1997 at the University of Vienna. The corresponding research had begun 10 years previously and will probably not conclude in the near future. This interdisciplinary and intercultural lecture plays a special role at the university, where usually subject-specific topics are the central focus. On the other hand, cross-connections to two curricula have resulted, where I have been engaged as an instructor in the meantime:

i) European Master's Degree Programme for Integrated Health Sciences at the Interuniversity College for Health and Development, Graz / Castle of Seggau, Austria (www.inter-uni.net, director: Peter Christian Endler). It was also Chris Endler who inspired me to put down my thoughts on paper, for which I am very grateful. The English translation was supported by the Leonardo da Vinci programme, project no. LdV A/02/B/F/PP-124.205. Meanwhile I belong to the official team of the Interuniversity College.

ii) the course 'Ancient Oriental Music Therapy' at the Institute for Ethno-Music Therapy (www.ethnomusik.com, Rosenau, Austria, director: Gerhard Tucek).

In addition, many conversations took place, in which particular points were discussed. In some cases, the book directly points to statements made by my conversation partners (under 'personal communication'). As to the figures, Werner Gruber helped me a lot and in this way contributed greatly to the better understanding of this book.

My wife, Ursula, created the proper surroundings and setting, which enabled me to let my thoughts mature over a longer period. Thank you very much!

The present book is based on a German one (Kratky 2003a). Before translation, I corrected the errors in the German version, actualised the literature and improved several subchapters. Chapter 7, the key chapter that links parts I and II of the book, was rewritten in appreciable parts. The translation itself then was a formidable task. Several persons were engaged in the first step: Vera Marquardt, Evelyn Kohout, Marc Elliott and Eva Maria Spitzer. The main job was done by Ruth Kidson (assisted by her husband John Kidson in Chs.5 and 12), who did not only improve the quality of translation considerably, but also made content-related suggestions. In the final stage, Eva Maria Spitzer was again very helpful.

I am very grateful to Nova Science Publishers (Frank and Maya Columbus as well as Donna Dennis) and to Joav Merrick, the editor of the series "health and human development". I am happy that the book is published within this series.

Some comments regarding the structure of the book: The introduction and the subsequent summary of chapters serve to orient the reader to the contents. Then two parts with seven chapters each follow. Part I addresses basic considerations and introduces selected complementary medicine systems. Building on this, Part II develops an intercultural model, which forms a common basis for interpretation, comparison and integration of complementary medicine systems. References and an index round off the book.

Actually, it is *two books in one*, and that with differing degrees of difficulty. The last subchapter of some chapters is marked with an asterisk (within the book and in the table of contents) to denote a deepening of the subject matter. If the reader just wants an overview of the topic, he/she can safely skip these sections. If, however, the reader wants to know more, he/she is invited to deepen his/her knowledge accordingly. Subchapters are marked in the text as follows: for example Ch.8.4, or simply 8.4.

One more word regarding the language: The expressions used are to be understood without reference to sex (when, for example, we talk about a *physician* or a *patient*); exceptions will be pointed out.

Introduction: Navigating the Book

A work like this is practically never done,
one has to declare it done
after one has spent enough time
and has done what is possible.

Goethe

Complementary medical methods are related among each other as well as to Western scientific medicine (so-called orthodox medicine) and in comparing them, similarities and differences are addressed. It is of course impossible to consider everything. Only a few typical examples can be selected. It is important in this process to bring the entire topic into one *system*. Behind this seemingly harmless word, however, two very different meanings are hidden, which are reflected in the adjectives *systematic* and *systemic*. *Systematics* concerns itself with ordering or classification, such as Linné's work with regard to plants. Every species, for example, is characterised by the corresponding genus and the specific difference. Emphasising the differences leads to a hierarchical classification. Everything has its order and place; this approach forms a rather static picture of separate units, in other words a compilation of structures. With regard to organisms, this method then corresponds particularly to anatomy. Analogously, diseases, diagnoses and therapies can be classified. On a higher level, this is also the case for the medical methods themselves. This approach largely corresponds to modern Western thought and thus to orthodox medicine.

System, in the sense of *systemic,* points to a very different direction. In systemic family therapy, systemic management or ecosystems, for example, the interconnection of parts plays a central role – it is the interplay that turns the collection of parts into a system. Western orthodox medicine speaks of a systemic phenomenon when an effect is felt in an area of the body different from the origin of the stimulus. Linked interactions result in a confusing picture, which is shaped by dynamics, rhythms, cycles and evolution. For instance, many medicine systems have historically evolved in connection with other ones. Tibetan medicine, for example, is rooted in itself but also incorporates Indian, Chinese and Greek/Arabic influences. Within the scope of considering the organism – for example in physiology, where the focus is more on functions and processes than structures – the opportunity presents itself to use a systemic approach. A characteristic in this area is the *feedback loop*, through which every action feeds back to (and affects) the place of origin. This is how biofeedback allows processes not accessible to conscious will to be controlled via fed-back signals on a monitor: e.g. heart rate or electrical skin conductance. Diagnosis and therapy can sometimes no longer be separated in view of such feedback loops.

Antique Greek medicine, which had a great influence over many centuries, was committed to this systemic approach (*the theory of the four humours*). In modern times, this viewpoint has lost its appeal more and more. In current developments like in psychoneuroimmunology or in chronomedicine, systemic thought enjoys a comeback in Western medicine, and will probably become more and more popular. The side effects of therapies play a central role here. For example, Western orthodox medicine utilises many effective medications in accord with the systematic approach, which emphasises *effectiveness*. These medications, however, often also have severe *side* effects, because of insufficient observations of *re*actions and *inter*actions as they would correspond to systemic thought. Asiatic herb mixtures have the lead in this regard, but these on the other hand do not fulfil our demands for consistent composition – an exciting field.

The *systematic* approach can be seen as pointing out differences, while the *systemic* approach emphasises similarities. From a different point of view, however, the two approaches are complementary and mutually interdependent. Similarities can only be determined if one has presumed differences and vice versa – one mirrors the other. The viewpoint of analogy and of (mutual) mirroring also corresponds to the statement that a patient's inner attitude is mirrored in his/her illness. Talking about signs, correspondences, sequences by analogy, symbols or rituals denotes a *symbolic* approach, which has little to do with our Western way of thinking – or does it? Every word written or spoken stands for something different, existing in the 'external world', which at first has absolutely nothing to do with the combination of sounds or letters. This assignment has to be learned, which usually happens in childhood. Since this period is more or less far in the past for us, we no longer recognise the lack of immediacy of speech and writing. This only happens in the case of graphics, tables and formulae, which primarily are used in natural sciences and which we are no longer able to learn with ease as teenagers or adults. For this reason, this book is designed on several levels. Along with the text, there will be illustrations and tables, sometimes formulae. Do not worry about the latter; you will get enough information via the other paths of communication to understand the connections.

Ancient ways of healing and a large part of ethnotherapies and even some forms of modern psychotherapy, which work with visualisations and rituals, use the symbolic approach. The placebo phenomenon often suggests a symbolic approach, and consequently Western orthodox medicine has a hard time with it. It is not about *side* effects (systemic approach) but about something which should not have any effect at all. It is no wonder, then, that the placebo effect is devalued, but it is a pity that the possibilities to utilise this effect for Western orthodox medicine are therefore being neglected. The doctor's charisma, the right word at the right time and confidence transferred to the patient can have a miraculous effect; all it takes is allowing.

In the following text, systematic, systemic and symbolic approaches will also be called *views* or *perspectives*, which correspond to different *world views*. Under this aspect, several medicine systems will be considered in this book without evaluation or devaluation. If you would like to tackle a particular method presented in this book, you will have to find out for yourself if it suits you or not. Finally, in the last chapter another perspective only hinted at previously will come into play, the *symbiotic* approach. It is connected with transpersonal and spiritual phenomena and corresponds to a world view that assumes a basic unity in all things. With that, it diametrically opposes the Western idea of division and specialisation. However, as is explained in the last chapter, there are also similarities.

When reading the chapters, the various perspectives or world views underlying the particular medicine systems can be used as navigational aids. The chapters are generally linked with each other and the medical disciplines are united under the common aspect of an integrative and intercultural model, which is developed primarily in Chapters 8 and 9. The aim of this model is to find a common language to allow a translation from one medicine system to the other. These have their respective advantages, which can be translated and utilised in other medicine systems. By the way, the terms *medicine system*, *medical discipline* and *medical method* are used synonymously.

By a medical discipline, we do not mean in general a closed, unified system but a multitude of branches and possibilities of interpretation. Within traditional schools, it is usually a matter of various phases of development including modern variations. There is, for example, not ONE Traditional Chinese Medicine but several traditions varying in time and place. In the West, a 'modern' version, which fits in better with Western thought, has been adopted: the philosophical background is neglected, the technique of acupuncture brought into the foreground. In China acupuncture is only one of many forms of therapy, and not even the most important. This book stresses intercultural connections of medicine systems, not Western thought. As it turns out, the old Chinese tradition with six phases of transformation (elements) is more suitable for this endeavour than the nowadays predominantly used five-element system. In this respect, the approach chosen here offers an opportunity to characterise the various versions of medicine systems from another point of view.

This book is the result of reflections and research over many years. It is not a completed work, however, and remains open for further development. Comments, suggestions for improvement, further examples and references are welcome; please send these per e-mail to karl.kratky@univie.ac.at.

Summary of Chapters

1. Field of Tension between Orthodox and Complementary Medicine

Medicine systems differ in thought, language and world views. Is the *patient* or the *illness* in the foreground? Is it about understanding the symptoms or finding the actual cause of illness? Some of these questions are listed and addressed with examples. Afterwards terms will be discussed, with which medicine systems are characterised. What exactly is, for example, *complementary, alternative and orthodox medicine*? Especially the term 'conventional medicine' proves to be rather complex. Finally, facets of holistic medicine and the Western need for scientific confirmation are addressed.

2. Understanding between Ages and Cultures

First various aspects of language and communication are addressed. In this connection, the word 'healing' is examined in more detail. Then we will look into world views and scientific theories, which will lead us to three ways of thinking. With the aid of the Hawaiian tradition, this approach is extended to four perspectives or views, with which we can look at the world: the *systematic, systemic, symbolic and symbiotic view*. These reflect four different world views. In our Western society, especially the logical / systematic perspective is common, but also cybernetic / systemic and constructivist / symbolic perspectives can be found. The holistic / symbiotic view on the other hand fits in better with the spiritual realm and traditional societies. In the course of millennia, however, a lot has changed. In this connection, we will deal with classical Antiquity and take a closer look at *Greek medicine* (theory of the four humours and temperaments). Then we will draw an arc to the beginning of modern times and then further to today's Western medicine, which is hardly 200 years old.

3. Systemic View I: Chaos and Fractals

The systemic view is addressed here in detail. It leaves behind one-way thinking and includes cycles or *feedback loops* – thus the connection to cybernetics. Cycles reflect effects back to their starting point, which makes the dynamics difficult to follow. Networks and cycles occur frequently in nature, but man tries to neglect these feedback loops whenever possible. This, for instance, carries the danger of underestimating *drug interactions*. Another simplification, from which the systemic view departs, is the assumption of linear relationships ('double cause – double effect'). *Non-linear relationships*, which in general lead to complex system behaviour, are more realistic. The so-called logistic map, which describes generational successions in animal populations, is given as an illustrative example. Thereby periodic fluctuations in the number of animals can result. Depending on the growth rate, the fluctuations can even become non-periodical. Therefore, chaotic processes not predictable in the long run can occur. Complex systems can show not only *chaos* (in terms of chaos research) but can also form *fractal patterns*. Essentially these are formations whose structure remains constant in the process of zooming in. By the way, self-similarity (over several levels) is rather common in nature; just look at a tree with its branches or the human blood vessel system.

4. Systemic View II:
Self-Organisation and Chaos Control

The computer's role was critical for the investigation of chaos. Especially *computer graphics* make it possible to recognise *self-organisation* amid chaos. Behind seemingly coincidental processes we find order. For illustrative purposes, we will look at an example from meteorology. When a layer of air has a higher temperature at its lower edge, a collective circular motion in form of air coils develops once a critical temperature difference has been reached. This process can be described with formulae for a particular coil. Further increase of temperature difference results in another transition, which then leads to a chaotic alternation of rotational direction. The coil rotates clockwise for a while and then again counter-clockwise. If, however, one changes the illustration and looks at the process in the so-called phase space, a fractal results – thus hidden behind the chaos we find order.

Chaotic processes react to disturbances with much sensitivity, for this reason they are more difficult to predict. On the other hand, these systems can be influenced, even controlled, with minimal interventions. A method for chaos control is introduced briefly. A further aspect of complex systems is *stochastic resonance*. It concerns the fact that noise at a suitable loudness can improve signal recognition (example: the human ear). So if the noise level is too low, it is beneficial to increase it – in contrast to the common practice of suppressing the noise as much as possible at all cost.

5. Homoeopathy and Related Methods

Homoeopathy is the first complementary medicine system addressed in detail. To begin with, we will look at *time- and dose-dependent reverse effects*, then the central simile principle of homoeopathy is dealt with, and from there we will suggest a generalisation. Hahnemann rediscovered this principle, which can already be found among others in Homer's *Iliad* in the form of the saying 'the one who hit you will heal you'. Accordingly, remedies have an opposite effect on healthy and on ill persons. This can be used for *drug proving* on healthy individuals in order to predict for which patients the tested remedy will have an effect. Another important aspect in producing homoeopathic remedies is the *potentisation*, a procedure that Hahnemann developed in elaborate tests. It is a matter of diluting as well as shaking (or triturating), since through a simple dilution the effect of the remedy would keep being reduced and finally disappear. As a result of the process of potentisation the question arises which potency is optimal in a specific case.

At the end of the chapter, questions of constitution and *illness dynamics* are asked from the homoeopathic viewpoint. Hahnemann kept developing homoeopathy up to old age by questing for the deeper causes of diseases. The resulting *system of miasms* is controversial among homoeopaths, but will play an important role in later chapters – in comparison to other medicine systems and also concerning dynamics of diseases. In this chapter, we will look at Hering's Law in regard to dynamics. Among other things, this law states that during recovery the sequence of symptoms occurs in reversed order to that during the progression of illness.

6. Feedback Diagnoses and Feedback Therapies

The effects of feedback loops, which were only just mentioned in Chapter 5, are now investigated in detail. While in general feedback processes tend to occur in diagnosis as well as in therapy, this fact can be utilised on purpose as diagnosis and therapy itself can be fed back. As an example, we will look at *electro-acupuncture* according to Voll and will also discuss difficulties arising from this method. The same turns out to be true for muscle testing in kinesiology. Another example is *biofeedback*. After some practice, one learns via monitor-feedback how to consciously 'direct' (bodily) functions that are normally controlled by the autonomic nervous system (e.g. like the skin-temperature of the left little finger). In this case, not only systemic but also symbolic aspects come into play. If the skin temperature for instance is represented by a certain colour on the monitor, the user merely needs to desire a change in colour (e.g. toward blue) – well, it usually proves to work! In order to succeed one has to suppress one's will to render things somehow 'differently' – apparently via slightly *altered states of consciousness*, which are well known in ethnomedicine. This soon brings us back to the question of different medical concepts.

In a strict sense, *bioresonance therapy* is also a feedback therapy since signals of the organism are being fed back to it in altered form. A connection with chaos control, which was introduced in Chapter 4, can be made. Finally, *autologous therapies* are mentioned which feed back the body's own substances (instead of signals).

7. Traditional Chinese Medicine and its Roots

Traditional Chinese Medicine (TCM) is much more than mere acupuncture, although the latter is the best-known technique in the West. An important foundation for Chinese thought is the polar pair *yin and yang*. Combined with vacuity / deficiency and repletion / excess, three basic types and six elements result, which are arranged in a circle. Five of those are identified with the conventional Chinese *elements* wood, fire, earth, metal and water while in ancient times a sixth element used to be applied. A few years ago, I reconsidered this element and called it *flora*. This process will be discussed in detail in Chapter 7 and keeps coming up while comparing other medicine systems in the subsequent chapters. Pertaining to tradition each of the five conventional elements is assigned to two of the twelve *meridians*; the two meridians for flora thus result automatically. Afterwards the relationship of the six elements to each other will be explained, as well as their relationship concerning the four views introduced in Chapter 2. The characteristics of the elements (e.g. the tastes) will also be listed and complemented.

The energy, *qi*, circulates in the twelve meridians, namely in the so-called large energy cycle, which is divided into three revolutions that in turn are subdivided into four meridians (or two elements). Traditionally, each meridian is assigned to two hours, while the cycle ('*meridian clock*') ends after 24 hours and then starts anew. This will be readdressed in Chapter 11, where the meridian or organ clock will be reconfirmed on a scientific basis. However, the location of meridians and acupuncture points now needs to be confirmed. For this purpose, two methods are discussed. Afterwards the Chinese pulse diagnosis will be described, which serves as an assessment of the energetic state of the meridians. Finally, we will compare the Chinese to the Tibetan as well as to the French forms of pulse diagnosis.

8. Ayurveda and Tibetan Medicine

In this chapter the *second part of the book* begins, i.e. the integration of medicine systems into a complete picture. Thereby we will utilise and expand the circle representation introduced in Chapter 7. To accomplish this, *Ayurveda* will be introduced with its three regulatory types (doshas) and six subtypes (two-dosha regions) that will be related to Traditional Chinese Medicine, while at the same time *Tibetan medicine* will be helpful to serve as a bridge. The same method will be employed for comparing pulse diagnoses, elements and tastes. Therefore, the sixth Indian flavour, 'sour', which has been missing within conventional TCM, can be attributed to flora. Simple diet guidelines can also be deduced from the tastes.

Finally, we will look at the Ayurvedic cycles of digestion and life, which leads from the circle representation to the *health disc*. There the life cycle can easily be represented as a '*life spiral'* that starts and ends with flora. Besides, it is now possible to sketch the path from falling ill to recovery and to build a bridge to Hering's Law (Chapter 5).

9. Advancement of the Cross-Cultural Model

The geometric model developed in Chapters 7 and 8 will be studied a little closer, starting with the *circle representation*. The two axes will be identified with yin and yang, or respectively, humidity and temperature. Moreover, mathematical expressions for yin and yang energies will be suggested: The sum or difference indicates the total energy, respectively a yin or yang surplus, which turn can be used to make statements about the metabolism (bridge to Ayurveda). Characteristic values can be brought into connection with the six Chinese elements. The next step brings a scrutiny of the *health disc* and the life spiral. In this process, a seventh area is added to the six two-dosha areas: the three-dosha type, which is situated around the centre of the disc. Therefore, the question arises how the circle of the circle representation might ideally be embedded into the health disc. The answer to this question leads us to a small area on the disc, which corresponds to the yin repletion / excess, the fourth Chinese type, which was missing on the circle. Finally, a transition from the health disc to a *cone* is considered and explained.

A point's movement on the circle, the disc or the cone corresponds to a more and more detailed description of a person's changing *state of health*. A point near the boundary on the health disc corresponds to an imbalanced dosha distribution (tendency toward illness), a point near the middle to a well-balanced distribution (healthiness). The proportion of the doshas can now be depicted through additive mixtures of the *three primary colours* red, green and blue. While the circle only allows a change in hue, the disc also permits change of intensity; as for the cone, brightness can be varied in addition.

10. Western Type Assignments

Several Western typologies will now be linked to the health disc. For this purpose we will begin with the three- and four-part structuring of the organism as proposed by *Anthroposophical medicine*; a relation to the various brain waves (EEG) will also be suggested. The three or respectively six *dispositions by Huter* follow, which correspond well with the Chinese elements. We will also build a bridge to the views introduced in Chapter 2. Furthermore, we will address the question which type of person invents a certain kind of therapy or benefits from it.

A comparison to *cybernetic types of control* follows, which prove to be astoundingly similar to the doshas, the Ayurvedic regulatory principles. Statements of Ayurveda can thus be specified. Finally, comparisons will be made with psychological or psychotherapeutic typologies, which describe basic feelings and characters.

11. Chronobiology and Chronomedicine

First, daily and seasonal fluctuations are addressed from the Eastern point of view, the Chinese organ clock playing a central role. Then we will look at the corresponding Western chronomedicine in terms of daily rhythms, where especially the results by Hildebrandt come into play. There are far-reaching parallels between Eastern and Western results. Afterwards we will be looking at the *pulse-respiration quotient*, i.e. the frequency ratio of pulse and respiration, while the significance of Hildebrandt's data (regarding not only the doshas, but also the Chinese elements) will be established.

The physiological dynamics can be compared with the dynamics of illness. For this purpose a model with six levels of illness exists in Traditional Chinese Medicine as well as in Ayurveda, although the Chinese model proves to be more concrete and can be depicted on the health disc. By the aid of the extended miasms, a *second illness dynamics* with three stages can be integrated into the disc. Thereby TCM also provides vague indications, whereas ones that are more definite stem from the so-called enneagram, a system of nine characters, which resolves into a six- and three-fold dynamics.

12. Recent Developments around Homoeopathy

There are several interesting recent developments in the area of homoeopathy, which can be easily related to the previous subject matter. Firstly, we will discuss *homotoxicology* according to Reckeweg, interpreting illness as a progressive battle against toxicity. Six levels of illness will be differentiated, which are closely related to the six levels in Traditional Chinese Medicine. Next, we will discuss expansions of conventional and homoeopathic principles as to *healing through harmonising* and will consider several ideas of regulative medicine. Subsequently there will be a detailed discussion of the already mentioned *extended miasms* by Gienow, which allow cross-linking to Ayurveda, to Anthroposophical medicine as well as to the 'complex theory' of C.G. Jung. We will also take a closer look at Scholten's *homoeopathy of the elements*. This new field deals with homoeopathic effects of the chemical elements, which ultimately form the building blocks for all basic homoeopathic substances. It turns out that the structure of the Periodic Table of the Chemical Elements corresponds conspicuously well to the systematics of their homoeopathic effects. Finally, we will look at the consideration of kingdoms by Rosenthal and Sankaran.

13.* A Deeper Understanding of Falling Ill and Recovering

The results achieved so far, especially the conformity of various medicine systems, as seen in terms of the *health disc*, can now be tied together. For each position of the disc, we will therefore define a simple landscape model whose lowest point will specify the organism's most probable state in each case (the precise position where an imagined ball would come to rest). Now the health disc can be divided into zones according to the various landscape characteristics, which will be interpreted. There are *one, two or three valleys*. Furthermore, the depth and width of the valleys play a specific role, because depending on their values a ball that has been brought into motion again and again (by 'noise') could possibly roll into a neighbouring valley. Therewith, stability, flexibility and the *organism's capacity for regulation* as a function of locality on the health disc will be shaped. Now Ayurvedic, homoeopathic and miasmatic assertions can follow freely. The distinctive ambivalence of the model will give rise to a new interpretation of *homoeopathy's* mode of action, where the stochastic resonance (introduced in Chapter 4) will play a role.

14. Unity in Diversity: Ethnological and Spiritual Aspects

In this chapter – at least on rudimentary levels – spiritual aspects will be addressed, first of all from *Indian and Tibetan perspectives*. The three doshas can be found again in the three poisons of delusion, the six types in terms of the six states of existence. Later on the *Jewish tradition* will be mentioned, whose interpretation (three axes of tension and their six poles) can be depicted usefully on the circle. These statements particularly address the special role of flora, i.e. the sixth Chinese element. The Jewish tradition will now be contrasted to the Germanic tradition (runes), whereby astounding parallels subsequently result. Here, the relationship to flora will also receive special attention. Then the enneagram, which was already mentioned in Chapter 11, will be discussed in detail. The 6+3=9 types of the enneagram will actually be assigned to the health disc. Finally, we will return to Europe, posing the question of today's spirituality and mysticism. In doing so we will be addressing transpersonal psychology, which allows a Western approach to those kinds of phenomena which otherwise only occur in ethnic realms.

Part I:
Facets of Complementary Medicine

Chapter 1

Field of Tension between Orthodox and Complementary Medicine

1.1. Approaches in the Treatment of Ill People

In the first two chapters, we will address fundamental questions concerning world views and the concept of man. Table 1.1 offers an introductory comparison of different ways of thinking by means of polar pairs. In this table, the left hand column relates more to complementary medicine and the right hand column to a more orthodox medical view. We will select a few examples from the four groups of pairs listed in this table.

Individual versus General (Beginning of Group 1)

Does a particular medicine system primarily consider the individual who has fallen ill, or is it more concerned with general statements about disease? For example, how do certain medications affect certain diseases, and what conclusions can be drawn from this for particular individuals? Many complementary medicine systems claim to set themselves apart from orthodox Western medicine by treating patients on an individual basis. But one has to ask whether this is, in fact, possible. Every medicine system is based on fundamentals and principles of treatment. These principles, however, go beyond individual considerations. If every case were truly different from every other case, then we would not be able to learn from former cases and apply this knowledge to the one currently being treated.

Non-recurring versus Reproducible

The existence of cases of spontaneous healing, for example, is not disputed by orthodox Western medicine. It can be argued, however, that they occur so infrequently that orthodox Western medicine cannot use them in order to develop a particular method. Orthodox Western medicine relies on reproducibility of outcomes and their statistical significance.

Table 1.1. Criteria for distinguishing medicine systems

Subjective Individual Non-recurring (individual fate) Well-being / malaise	Objective General Reproducible (statistics) Diagnostic findings

Over-interpreting, inventing
False hopes
Utilising chance and placebo
 	
Symptom, syndrome, patterns of
                disharmony
Analogous, parallel
	Neglecting indications ('hard facts')
	False despair
	Negating or eliminating chance and
	                placebo
	Actual cause
	
	Causal, sequential (effective agent)

Ill person Internal focus (immune system) Patient responsibility Self-healing powers, self-regulation	Illness External focus ('enemy') Doctor's responsibility Physician in control
Waiting, letting happen … passive Essentially unchanged medicine Humoral pathology, 'theory of the four humours' Energy	Doing, handling … active Rapid progress of methods Cellular pathology, solidism Matter

Well-being / Malaise versus Diagnostic Findings

What happens when the patient's subjective sense of well-being or of malaise does not agree with the objective findings? In this case, the doctor may say "The patient must be imagining it. His blood tests are perfect; he cannot possibly be ill." The patient on the other hand thinks *"I don't care about my blood tests. I feel ill and I want the way I feel to be acknowledged."* Often a sense of malaise arises long before a clinical condition can be detected. Therefore, the question needs to be asked: Where does illness begin for me? At which point do I intervene in order to avoid illness? Orthodox Western medicine tends not to jump into action until objective findings are to hand. From the perspective of Ayurveda (Indian medicine, see Ch. 8) orthodox Western medicine reacts too late. For this reason, substantial interventions are then necessary. The Ayurvedic physician attempts to intercept illness at a very early stage. From the Western perspective, however, the patient is not yet ill at that point. Thus, orthodox Western medicine argues that the effectiveness of Ayurveda cannot be tested, since therapy begins at a time when the patient is not yet ill. The Ayurvedic physician answers that it is exactly that which constitutes the wisdom of this medicine system: the intervention is timely enough to prevent the manifestation of illness. In this way, we can shine a light on one view from the perspective of another.

Over-interpretation versus Neglecting Indications (Beginning of Group 2)

If you take the smallest indications and all possible connections into consideration, you can quasi hear the grass grow. This poses a risk that you may just invent or at least over-interpret something. On the other hand, those who only believe in 'hard facts' might neglect or even overlook important indications.

False Hope versus False Despair

Alternative therapists who treat patients with cancer are often accused of arousing false hopes. This is a very touchy point, since not every person has the same chance of recovery from the same condition. Just telling a patient that he is likely to die in the near future in-creases the probability that he will, in fact, die (unless he is a fighter or someone who likes to prove others wrong). However, if the doctor tells a patient that he treated someone last year who had a similar condition and who is now doing well, one can argue that the doctor will arouse false hopes in his patient. However, this presumes that everything is objective and that there is a clear distinction between true and false hope. In this respect, one could accuse orthodox Western medicine of producing false despair.

Symptom, Syndrome, Patterns of Disharmony versus Actual Cause

This is a matter of perspective: are we fighting the causes or just treating symptoms? Orthodox Western medicine frequently finds itself in the peculiar position of being accused of not attacking the deeper causes of illness. However, since this medicine system in partic-ular is based on causal-analytical science, it should be *the* medicine system that fights causes. On the other hand, there are complementary forms of therapy, such as Traditional Chinese Medicine, which look at illness from the perspective of patterns of disharmony and treat them accordingly – as symptoms or syndromes. This is a difficult issue because the concept of cause has changed during the course of the centuries and is perceived in different ways in different cultures. We shall come back to this in Ch. 2.

The Ill Person versus the Illness (and the Other Pairs of Group 3)

The third group concerns the role of the patient and that of the therapist. Does the thera-pist see the ill *person* or the *illness* he wishes to heal? Is it the ill person with his or her abilities and internal defence mechanisms who is in the foreground, or is it an external enemy which has invaded the patient and must be combated – possibly by bypassing the immune system. Some therapies, such as chemotherapy, are harmful to the immune system. Nevertheless, one proceeds on the assumption that the benefit outweighs the damage caused. In addition, one needs to look at the question of responsibility. Does the doctor delegate plenty of responsibility to the patient or does he try to carry it all himself? The approach of *auto-regulative medicine* (as in the subtitle of the book by Melchart & Wagner 1993) points out that the patient recovers by himself or at least contributes greatly to his own recovery. In orthodox Western medicine, responsibility is primarily placed on the doctor's shoulders. Interestingly, this does not happen in psychotherapy, which, in this respect, is different from psychiatry. The psychiatrist takes responsibility for prescribing the correct medication, while the psychotherapist generally attempts to activate the patient's sense of self-responsibility. There are advantages and disadvantages to both approaches. Giving the patient a lot of responsibility sounds good, but how many patients can bear it? There is a thin line between self-responsibility and feelings of guilt.

Awaiting, Letting Happen versus Doing, Handling (Beginning of Group 4)

A homoeopath I once consulted was, during our meeting, twice called to the telephone to give advice. Both times he said: *"Don't do anything. It is a reaction to the medication. If it has not improved by tomorrow, please let me know."* Waiting and allowing things to happen naturally both require trust, which is one issue orthodox Western medicine cannot grasp. Its practitioners are also often accused of still engaging in interventions at the end of a person's life, when it is obvious that they can no longer be of any use. Orthodox Western medicine also tends to exhaust all possibilities from a legal perspective and thus may be guilty of over-treating. Waiting and allowing things to happen, with its concomitant advantages and disadvantages, is found primarily in complementary medicine systems.

Essentially Unchanged Medicine versus Rapid Progress of Methods

Is the rapid progress in orthodox Western medicine a good or a bad thing? There are very ancient medicine systems (such as Far Eastern methods of healing) that have remained largely unchanged over the centuries. These systems are based on a wealth of experience – and man has changed very little during the course of time. Orthodox Western medicine, on the other hand, keeps fighting new diseases and accordingly continues to develop rapidly. Yesterday's lecture is already partly out-dated today.

Humoral Pathology versus Cellular Pathology and Solidism

Different people hold different ideas of what constitutes health and illness. If your first thoughts head in the direction of something being disturbed at a certain site (a bone fracture would be a typical case), then you are taking the view of orthodox Western medicine. More precisely, this is the doctrine of *solidism* [which is defined by the Shorter Oxford English dictionary (Trumble et al. 2003) as "The doctrine or theory which refers all diseases to the state of, or to morbid changes in, the solid parts of the body."] In this respect, there has been a development from organs to cells to the level of genes. *Humoral pathology* on the other hand is based on disturbances in the organism's dynamics, an example being the theory of the four humours in Ancient Greece (Ch.2). According to Traditional Chinese Medicine, illness arises when qi cannot flow freely. These contrasts addressed here, admittedly, are being softened nowadays – the keyword here is *psychoneuroimmunology*. Paradoxically, genetic research could lead to an integration of a small part (one gene) into the whole (the organism), since important genes exist which are responsible for the (self-)regulative processes of the entire body.

1.2. The Terminology of Medicine Systems

Now we shall look at the terms by which medicine systems are characterised (Table 1.2). The various expressions in each column are related to one another but are not identical. As in Table 1.1, the left hand column contains a list of terms that are primarily associated with complementary medicine systems while those in the right hand column are more related to orthodox medicine. This type of arrangement corresponds to that used in Table 1.1. However, usually we read from left to right. If we accept orthodox medicine as the standard, we would thus expect to find it on the *left* and that which is complementary to it on the *right* hand side. The representation chosen here corresponds to "strangification", the distancing method/technique used by the philosophy of science, which is often helpful in overcoming habitual thought patterns. In addition, evaluations and devaluations are to be avoided as much as possible in all comparisons.

Table 1.2. Expressions for characterising complementary and orthodox medicine (based on Stacher 1996). Connecting both sides leads to *holistic* or *integrative* medicine – see Ch. 1.3

Complementary medicine Alternative medicine Unconventional medicine	Orthodox medicine Academic medicine Conventional medicine
Medicine based on experience Naturopathy Empirical medicine	Textbook medicine Scientific medicine Experimental medicine
Biological medicine Gentle medicine Regulative medicine	Technocratic medicine Laboratory medicine Organ medicine

The First Group of Terms in Each Column

On the left hand side, we find *complementary, alternative* and *unconventional*. Complementary and alternative do not have the same meaning. Alternative means *either ... or*. One chooses between alternatives and decides for one or the other. An extreme follower of a certain alternative medicine system is not interested in any other method, not even orthodox Western medicine. *Complementary*, on the other hand, means a mutual supplement (*both ... and*), but not necessarily at the same time. It is also possible to move back and forth between two therapy methods. The complementary approach has much to do with polarity and can be compared to the Chinese yin and yang. It is not about opposites but about a flowing transition and mutual dependence. For example, a complementary practitioner might only work with one particular method, but he does not disregard other methods and will refer a patient to a therapist from a different school if he believes the latter's methods will be more effective for that patient. As far as *conventional* and *unconventional* are concerned, orthodox Western medicine is normally considered to be conventional. The word *convention*, however, also implies agreement, freedom of choice and tradition. In China, then, Traditional Chinese Medicine should be considered conventional – as long as China sees it this way. This term is certainly tricky.

The Second Group of Terms in Each Column

The following three pairs of terms pose some surprising problems. On the left hand side, we have *medicine based on experience, naturopathy* and *empirical medicine*. These refer to all that can be experienced, to that which nature has to offer in whatever form. It is strange that this is not listed on the side of orthodox medicine. Does orthodox medicine have no experience? Does it not have anything to do with nature? Is its approach not empirical? Let us look at the terms on the right hand side. Experience is paired up with *teaching* (textbook), nature with (*natural*) *science* and empiricism with *experiment*. This results in the following association: Some people go into the forest and look around to see what is there (e.g. medicinal herbs), while others go to the university and listen to lectures. But what is the difference between *empiricism* and *experiment*? First, let me point out that natural sciences do not concern themselves with nature in its entirety but only with a very narrow aspect – and that rather successfully. Experience and empiricism distinguish themselves from science and experiment (for example, the experiments with falling bodies done by Galileo) by being nature-oriented. We may take as an analogy a mountain farmer who knows, by looking at the sky, that climbing a certain mountain is perilous at present. A city dweller, however, will not listen to his advice, for he is well trained and carries the best equipment – and the farmer is just a farmer. The consequence is that the city dweller is caught in a snow shower and has a fall. The mountain farmer had the advantage of experience over him – something which requires lengthy observation, namely the observation of nature as it is. *Naturopathy*, too, is based on this.

This is much too complicated for the natural sciences. Instead, models representing a small aspect of 'artificial nature' are constructed and theories developed, which then, of course, are only valid in a correspondingly limited area. As long as the researchers are aware of this limitation, no objections can really be brought forward. Many useful discoveries have been made in modern natural science and technology by focusing on a particular area rather than on nature as a *whole*. Of course, natural science has developed more and more over the course of the centuries and has expanded its scope to match. Nevertheless, it should take note that there is still a large surrounding area that remains in the dark – just as with an area illuminated by floodlight.

What should orthodox Western medicine do in this situation? Should it wait until the sciences have progressed further in their research? Should it decline to work with the discoveries of the 'inanimate' sciences, physics and chemistry, since they are only partly applicable to the complex system of a human being? Should a trained physician, who has spent seven years studying and learning, tell some of his patients: *"I'm sorry, but what you need wasn't covered in my training. I can't help you"?* This would hardly be helpful for the patient, who must be taken seriously in his hour of need. The question posed at the beginning of this paragraph, of course, applies just as well to complementary medicine. How holism comes into play will be discussed below.

The Third Group of Terms in Each Column

The last group shows how difficult it is to find expressions that do not evaluate or de-valuate. The terms biological, gentle and *regulative* medicine on the left hand side make a rather positive impression; the terms *technocratic, laboratory* and *organ* medicine on the right hand side are more negative. The remarks that were made on naturopathy and natural sciences (second group) also apply to biological versus technocratic. *Gentle* versus *laboratory* medicine is closely connected to *letting happen* versus *doing* in Table 1.1. Do as little as possible and only intervene when necessary – this is the gentle approach. *Laboratory* medicine on the other hand tends to utilise the equipment already in place – at the risk of doing too much. *Regulative* medicine versus *organ* medicine is closely connected to the comparison of humoral to cellular pathology (Table 1.1).

1.3. Facets of Integrative and Holistic Medicine

We have discussed many terms in connection with complementary and orthodox medicine and now the question arises: what about *integrative* and *holistic* medicine (which will subsequently be treated as synonymous)? First of all, the word holistic medicine has many different facets. The *first* relates to taking into account the whole person – in other words, not "the gall bladder in bed 10" but an all round view that includes the needs, fears and hardships that a person is facing. A physician from the orthodox school can also implement this holistic approach; it is mainly a question of time. A *second* – but not separate – approach takes into consideration the whole organism with its many interactions and distinguishes the global from the local perspective. If only one organ is examined and a medication for stabilising that organ is administered, then side effects ('undesired effects') often occur, which affect other parts of the organism. This is one consequence of a limited perspective, which is often accepted.

Some people may consider a *third* facet of holistic medicine to consist of including as many different medicine systems as possible, using their respective knowledge and applications. Of course, implementation of this ideal faces practical limitations. In any case, this represents an intensified expectation for complementary medicine to expand the '*both ... and*' principle. In fact, this is not true holism because it is quite possible to use several different therapies and still not cover all aspects of the patient's ill health. In addition, different therapies can interfere with or counteract each other so that in the end the patient might be receiving less benefit than with one therapy used alone. However, if therapies are capable of being used together (for example, nutrition therapy together with healing and aromatherapy) then they may combine to form a holistic system.

In addition, there is a particularly subtle *fourth* facet of holism, which appears to mean the exact opposite of what was just discussed. There are homoeopaths and practitioners of Traditional Chinese Medicine, for example, who claim that their therapy, used by itself, is holistic – that it covers everything and nothing more is required. You could dismiss this opinion as boastful and this might really be the case in some situations, but this claim does contain a certain amount of truth. For, if you believe that everything is interconnected, if the organism really is an interconnected whole system regulating itself, then it is possible to be successful with any one of a number of very different therapy systems that intervene at different locations of the network. Then the crux of the matter seems not to be whether you are trained in many methods but whether you are very skilled in one. As a result, some people might claim that every medicine system is holistic medicine. This is what orthodox Western medicine might claim for itself. Thus, the Austrian title 'Dr. med. univ.' (Doctor medicinae universae) already contains a claim to universality and the often-found dismissal or devaluation of every other method also implies the belief that one's own knowledge is sufficient. However, it is important to remember that ultimately the question of whether or not a therapy is holistic lies not in the therapist and his skills but in the therapy itself and its methods. Treating one part of the patient in a way that may result in harm or imbalance in other parts cannot be termed holistic.

However, a connection can be made between facets *three* and *four* despite their apparent irreconcilable differences. For, in practice it is not enough that *in principle* every illness or every patient can be treated with any medical method. There are patients who respond better to Ayurveda and those who respond better to homoeopathy. Others still are best treated with a suitable combination of various methods. Moreover, the frequently occurring side effects of orthodox Western medicine show how it, too, affects the whole organism – even if those effects are not desirable. A part of the organism is treated, but the whole organism is affected. Every medicine system should be aware of what (self-)regulative processes, for example, it can trigger. However, orthodox medicine in the Western world does enjoy a position of dominance and so is not forced always to be explaining and justifying its methods, as is the case for complementary medicine that is constantly engaged in emphasising the holistic aspect of its therapies.

I had a conversation on this topic with an Austrian physician who first studied orthodox Western medicine and, later, Traditional Chinese Medicine (TCM) (two complete curricula). When asked which side effects could be expected in TCM, she replied that there were no side effects if the therapy was used correctly (see also Porkert 1992, p.370). I then asked her whether she combined the knowledge gained from both fields of expertise or whether she focused on one of the two systems. Does she still think in orthodox fashion or according to the theories of TCM? She told me that although she utilises the orthodox system for clarification, she uses only TCM in her practice. According to her, the two thought systems are so different that one has to decide in favour of one or the other. It would seem that this applies to TCM but not to acupuncture, which is simply a technique used in TCM and represents only a small aspect of this method. Acupuncture, in a form based on scientific thinking, has already been integrated into our Western system. We will come back to this later.

There is one more thing to be considered concerning the frequently severe side effects of orthodox Western medicine and the claim that other systems are largely or entirely lacking in adverse effects. Some Western pharmaceuticals are based on natural plants or medicinal herbs as are, for example, the remedies used in TCM and Tibetan medicine. Nevertheless, there is a great difference. In the West, because of concerns about standardisation and reproducibility, only the primary active agent (or a few active ingredients) are isolated and administered as medication. This concept is contrary to that of the complementary approach that claims that the natural combination of herbs should preferably not be changed. The justification for this is often based on the assumption of a similarity of all living beings. This might seem interesting or ridiculous to us. However, Tibetan medicine remedies are produced by mixing dozens of ingredients and/or plants or parts of plants. Sceptics might like to consider how effective this form of treatment has been over the millennia. Another point is of especial interest to us: Tibetan doctors claim that often it is a very few of the ingredients that produce the desired effect, while the others are necessary simply to neutralise the side effects of the few strong active agents. If this is true, then they are way ahead of us in this respect. Investigating this claim would in any case be worthwhile.

By analogy, it is conceivable that combining certain therapy methods might be used to minimise side effects. Only focusing on the main active agent is often not enough. From every highly effective substance and every highly effective therapy we must expect side effects (albeit not necessarily adverse ones) due to the organism's interconnections. One example of a successful combination is the psychological or spiritual support of patients who are seriously ill or undergoing major operations. The 'side effect' of fear, which can also aggravate physical adverse effects via psychosomatic processes, is alleviated through this support. No matter whether methods are combined or the best method is chosen, knowledge of some medicine systems is necessary. Comparative literature can offer a first introduction into this issue, but at the same time it also brings up the question of assessment (by the authors as well as of the books themselves).

In the West, it is customary to use science as a guideline for assessment. Examples of this viewpoint are Federspiel (1996) and Bettschart et al. (1996). Both books are primarily meant as guidebooks for patients. The assessment of various alternative methods for the listed diseases is primarily made from a Western perspective. The methods themselves generally come off badly and are often judged ineffective, with the justification that there is no *scientific* evidence for their effectiveness. Two very different conclusions can be drawn from this: Either alternative medicine is practised entirely by charlatans or reference to scientific standards falls short (both arguments are popular). From the second viewpoint, some Western statistical tests, for example, do not do justice to many Far Eastern methods. Conversely, who knows what an Australian aborigine's assessment of orthodox Western medicine would be from his (outsider) viewpoint? Most of us do not care in the least about that, but that is another story.

Contrariwise, there are books describing complementary medicine systems from an insider's point of view with positive criticism, e.g., Baumgart (1995), Schmiedel & Augustin (1997), and Dillard & Ziporyn (1999). Their approach is not to instruct but to inform and support. The advice, which is repeated frequently in the last-mentioned book, is that in the final analysis one has to see the picture for oneself. This means that the authors concede more independence to the patients than is the common practice. Furthermore, there are books that are about midway between the above-mentioned two approaches. Examples are Jonas & Levin (1999), Micozzi (1999 & 2001), Reisser et al. (2001), Pelletier (2002), Jonas (2004) and Freeman (2004).

Within complementary and alternative medicine (CAM), many designations can be found:

- Holistic medicine (Diamond 2001)
- Energy and information medicine (Ludwig 1994 & 1999)
- Mind/body and spiritual medicine (Benor 2002, Schlitz et al. 2004)

Interestingly, several inputs to CAM come from holistic dental medicine (Kobau et al. 1996, Rossaint 2002 & 2005).

When the restriction to a single method, branch or focus of medicine is transcended, again several expressions can be found: Comparative, integrative (or integrated) and integral medicine.

As to comparative, integrated and integrative medicine, see Diamond (2000), Kratky (2003a-c), Lasker & Kratky (2005) and Coyle-Demetriou & Demetriou (2007).

As to integral medicine, see Schlitz et al. (2004) and Wilber (2000, 2001 & 2007). By the way, Wilber considers the integral approach in a general sense, also outside of medicine.

In the present book, the above-mentioned spectrum will be dealt with. In this context, however, we concentrate on comparative and integrative medicine.

Chapter 2

Understanding between Ages and Cultures

2.1. Language, Thought and World Views

Problems of comprehension start with language itself, which is an important means of communication but not the only one. Let us begin by examining words. They are characterised by their denotation, connotation(s) and the feelings associated with them, where the latter has a lot to do with evaluation and devaluation. The meaning of a sentence is given by the words and their combination, but the actual meaning of the words is given by the sentence. Thus, this comprises a circle; interpretation always contains an active, constructive element. Even understanding a sentence in one's own mother tongue is no simple process and, for this reason, does not always proceed satisfactorily. The imprecision of a natural language is also the reason for developing technical language in science and technology, where unambiguousness is achieved by limiting the area of applicability (an extreme example being computer languages). However, it is exactly this development which makes interdisciplinary work more difficult. An improvement in *intradisciplinary* communication is thus opposed by an aggravation of difficulties in the *interdisciplinary* field. No one can master all scientific languages. In the end, the vernacular is mostly used as a kind of 'Esperanto' for the various technical languages. Besides, the advantages of imprecision have recently been rediscovered by the sciences (the keyword here being fuzzy logic).

Everything is further complicated when translating from one natural tongue to another and possibly to languages which originated in different eras and cultures. Nevertheless there are also aids at hand: similar sounding words with comparable meaning in related languages, following the change in meaning of words during the course of history of one's own language, and apparently worldwide 'constants' in thinking, concepts and world views of peoples and cultures. For example, the word 'heal' is, in German, 'heilen'. The meanings around the word *'heilen'* include *'heil' (whole),* and *'heilig' (holy)*. To heal (making hale, healthy), then, has something to do with making whole (holism) and with making holy (a religious reference). The latter helps us to recognise the origin of all healing traditions. In ancient

cultures, these three activities often were not separated and were performed by priest physicians, shamans or medicine men. Since there are also culture-specific expressions and ideas,
it is necessary to attune ourselves to these. The aim is an understanding that is (almost) 'from
within' in order to avoid a (neo-)colonising process by means of our own language, thinking
and world view. This work is an attempt to reach this goal. The reader may assess whether
this attempt proves successful. The arguments will be presented in a language as natural as
possible in accordance with the above-mentioned considerations. However, the adopting of
individual terms that are indispensable to a special branch of science (or to a certain culture)
cannot be avoided. We shall put this issue to the test at once by means of an example from
linguistics, namely with the terms *syntactics, semantics*, and *pragmatics*, which generally
refer to sentences and texts.

Syntactics relates to formal correctness (including grammar) whereas semantics refers to
meaning (interpretation, coherence). Pragmatics (unlike the colloquial use of the term) concerns itself with the intent, purpose, and effect of a text. Let us imagine you are writing a
book. There are three aspects. Firstly, the formal aspect of grammar and spelling must be
fulfilled. Secondly, it has to make sense and to have meaning. You intend to express something. Though these two aspects have been supported, as long as no one is reading your book,
it has still not served its purpose so far, i.e. to gain numerous readers who in turn should be
inspired to rethink their attitude towards the issues that you have addressed. On the level of
words syntactics relates to correct spelling, semantics to the objective meaning (use) and
pragmatics to the associated feelings (subjectivity and valuation, which trigger feelings and
reactions). Discussions concerning linguistic and political correctness are part of pragmatics.
This book in particular faces an almost impossible task in using terms that prove to be comprehensible on the one hand (semantics), while on the other do not present any offence
(pragmatics).

Natural science, especially basic research, aspires not only to produce facts but also to
stay neutral in respect to both the facts and the consequences. The corresponding technical
languages attempt to neutralise any associated feelings, so semantics becomes the main
concern. During the application (e.g. medicine, technology) the pragmatic aspect steps into
the foreground. Pragmatics is also important in everyday life, and in advertising may be
dominant. Ever since the computer has entered the world of research and publishing, there
has been a risk of setting back semantic content in favour of syntactic as well as the
pragmatic aspect (expenditure of time due to an intolerance of formal errors, possibilities of
aesthetic presentations of formulae, tables and graphics). More on this subject can be found
in Kratky (1998b).

After these considerations regarding language, we will now address *world views*, bearing
in mind that thinking acts as a building bridge between these two issues. If we want to explore world views of different cultures, we should also ask "what exactly is our own world
view?" To start, let us confine ourselves to scientific theories while figuring out how they
have evolved, and how we can assess whether they are true or false. In doing so, we will need
a little background. First of all such theories are based on a few basic assumptions that not
only require prior understanding but are also hiding terms and assertions which cannot be
scrutinised any further. Furthermore, on the one hand there are (secondary) terms deriving
from definitions and, on the other, rules of derivation that specify how to get from the basic

assumptions to subsequent assertions or theorems, where the terms are linked together. Thus, a theory consists of a web of basic terms, assumptions, definitions, rules of derivation and other theorems.

Therefore, the basis of a theory cannot be challenged. The lack of basic definitions seems to be especially unsatisfying. For *'definition'* means the explanation of a term with the aid of well-known terms. After several steps (mentioned above) one approaches basic terms which can no longer be defined within the frame of science. Here, prior understanding is required, which generally derives from the non-scientific colloquial language. Even the exact science of mathematics must rely upon everyone 'knowing' what a number is. Accordingly, medical science is unable to define health and illness. Of course, these terms can be described – and many alleged definitions are in fact only descriptions, as in the above-mentioned case of the introduction of the terms *syntactics, semantics,* and *pragmatics*. If several theories are combined into one larger theory (i.e. a *paradigm)* or if reasoning is based on a specific world view, a number of basic terms and assertions will suddenly turn into derived terms and assertions. Here, the problem will only be shifted to the larger theory.

So let us return to our two questions: "How does a theory come about" and "How can we assess its correctness?" It would appear that the second question is easier to answer: by scrutinising the internal consistency on the one hand and, on the other, by conducting experiments that can thereby also be disproved in praxis. This method, however, might provide pitfalls, but that is a different argument. We would just like to point out that an experiment checks only a single statement, not the entire theory. Even trickier is the question of how a theory comes about (the problem of induction). Since there is no direct logical path, it will rather require inspiration and intuition. Observations and experiments can only suggest certain assertions. All in all, the whole structure ultimately resembles belief systems. Once a scientific theory has been developed, one is able to verify or falsify the assertions via experiments within the frame of logic. To venture beyond science or even beyond the Western point of view is only possible to a very limited degree.

We now need to address various ways of thinking: *causal, systemic,* and *symbolic* thinking. The first of these deals with *logical* progressions of cause and effect. This can be symbolised by the succession of arrows in Figure 2.1a (a simple representation of mono-causality). In addition, these arrows can also be interpreted as a *chronological* succession, which gives an even better account of the Western way of thinking. The transition to (scientific) modern times is especially characterised by the change from the questions *'why?',* *'whence?'* and *'what?'* to *'how?'*. Thus, Newton described the movement of planets in his law of gravity but neither addressed the question of the 'actual' cause of this movement nor that of gravitation itself. Nevertheless, in science as well as in medicine, we often talk about causal-analytical proceedings, and for this reason I've chosen the term 'causal thinking'. However, at the same time, one must always keep in mind the very limited understanding of the term 'cause'.

Now let us look at systematic thinking as represented in Figure 2.1b. What is new here is not the fact of it being a more complicated representation (that would be multicausality) but something else: The arrows do not travel just in one direction. There is at least *one* feedback loop, which further complicates the situation. In fact, this represents a more realistic assumption, since every discussion exhibits such interplays. Even the above-mentioned Newtonian law of gravity contains retroactions that may be neglected due to unequal masses within the solar system. Only by taking the entire range of interactions into account will the existing complexity of planetary movements be disclosed. Systemic thinking has only made its way into our consciousness in the last decades, but now can be found not only in chaos research and ecology, but also in psychotherapy (e.g. systemic family therapy) and in biofeedback. Chs. 3, 4 & 6 in particular will be dedicated to this way of thinking.

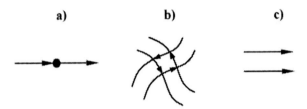

Figure 2.1. Representation of three ways of thinking: (a) causal, (b) systemic, (c) symbolic.

In Figure 2.1c, two parallel arrows represent symbolic thinking. In this case, we deal with significant connections without any causal interactive effects. You can visualise this by conceiving identical principles being mirrored on different levels. This will become clearer not only by reading further (Chs. 2.2 & 2.3), but also by considering Far Eastern methods of healing (Chs. 7 & 8). Symbolic thinking also comes into play in connection with placebo effects as well as rituals and other forms of ethnotherapy. Psychophysical parallelism, which relates to the question of how body and mind interact, gives a historical Western example. It states that body and mind always work in parallel without directly influencing each other: the body displays what is going on in the mind and vice versa. Although one could easily dismiss this way of thinking, it turns out that we are constantly working at this level in the fields of language, arts, and formulae, which serve as symbolic descriptions of processes of nature. The Newtonian law of gravity will again serve here as an example. Ideally, the results of mathematical calculations correspond to the movement of the planets, i.e. one thing can be translated into the other. However, neither does the law of gravity clearly follow from the dynamics of the solar system, nor do the planets – while solving differential equations – move according to the rules of Newton. The planets just move the way they move. The result is that, although one would tend to associate natural science at first glance only with causal thinking, it also exhibits parts of systemic and symbolic thinking.

2.2. Different Perspectives and Approaches to Reality

From the above-mentioned considerations we can conclude that we use all three ways of thinking, though not always with the same intensity or at the same time. Often we accomplish translation without even being aware of it. If we look at it literally, we see that translating from one language into another is difficult because we have to reconcile the meaning and the associated feelings of the original text with the translation. Furthermore, the way of looking at the world is not the same. This is comparable to the 'translation' between two different medicine systems. It is necessary to become attuned to both systems and to switch on demand from one perspective to the other. By means of the epistemological distancing technique of "strangification", it is possible to vary one's points of view. It is particularly helpful to look at our own ways of thinking through the eyes of someone else. Consequently, we start to challenge viewpoints that would otherwise remain unquestioned.

The occupation with 'otherness' is the professional task of ethnology (i.e. cultural anthropology). However, it is surprising how similar some 'foreign' views are to ours. This is evident, for example, in the Huna, the Hawaiian mentality and healing tradition. Contrary to many other cultures (including our own) life is not seen as a battle against external foes but as a game, a challenge, and an adventure (King 1998). For this reason, curiosity and trust dominate over defence and mistrust. Huna talks about four worlds or levels of reality. This means that we can approach one another in four complementary types of reality, which in the end always remain entirely or partly hidden from us. Depending on the situation, one way or the other might be especially obvious, but we always have the opportunity to choose our approach or perspective. Since the Huna approach is very useful for our comparison of medicine systems (and we shall use it frequently), we shall subsequently abbreviate the four possibilities as perspectives 1 to 4 (P1-P4), where the world view is reflected in the corresponding perspective.

Table 2.1a. Various perspectives (P1-P4) or approaches to reality

Perspective	Symbol	Occurrence	Designation	
P1	→●→●→	Classical natural sciences	Logical	/ Systematic
P2	◁▷	Chaos research, Social sciences	Dynamic	/ Systemic
P3	═	Humanities	Constructivist	/ Symbolic
P4	●	Spirituality	Holistic	/ Symbiotic

Table 2.1b. Perspectives P1-P4: characteristics and examples

P1	Everything is limited by time and space.	'Either – or', 'if – then'
P2	Everything is connected to everything else and moves in cycles.	'As well as'
P3	Everything is a symbol and stands for something else.	'On the one hand – on the other' 'TWO sides of a coin'
P4	Everything is one, forms a unity.	'Two sides of ONE coin'

P1	Objectivity, hierarchy, reproducibility, predictability
P2	Subjectivity, reflexivity, exchange, complexity
P3	Analogies, rituals, metaphors, hermeneutics, mirroring, placebo
P4	Identification, mystical experiences of unity, mass panic, ecstasy

Let us take a closer look at the possibilities with the aid of Table 2.1a&b. It contains statements made by King (2001) and Ulmer-Janes (1998, pp.17-50). The first three approaches relate to sayings like *"Everything will pass"* (P1), *"Everything turns, everything moves"* (P2) and *"There are two sides to every coin"* (P3). If you regard the further characterisations of P1-P3, you will recognise surprising parallels to Figure 2.1 and find that the thoughts of Ch.2.1 are a shortened but otherwise little-changed version of Kratky (1998b) – a work that I had completed before discovering Huna. In comparison to this work only the succession of b and c in Figure 2.1 are interchanged, so that it now corresponds to the Huna sequence. This close match of two systems which come from very different cultures is rather surprising and is easiest to understand in the sense of P3. Huna still has one more perspective to offer, P4, which has no place in science and can be characterised by the sentence: "Everything is one". In the final analysis, this approach is just as extreme as "Everything is separate from everything else", another way of formulating P1. A popular example for P4 would be the statement *"We won"* being used by someone who has seen the team that he supports win but has played no part in the victory. It expresses the experienced identification with the victor. This is what is meant in Huna.

The word 'everything' needs to be put into perspective (as is the case with the other approaches to reality) in the sense of 'everything which I count as part of it'. From this perspective the 'opposites' P1 and P4 can even merge. *"These are my compatriots and those are strangers."* Here, too, the separation into two groups – each experienced as uniform – is influenced by one's own experience but not forced. The comparison of P3 and P4 is also tantalising, namely under the aspect 'there are two sides to every coin', where P3 and P4 emphasise different words (Table 2.1b). Dialectic thinking is located in this area of overlap. *Thesis* and *antithesis*, which contradict each other, are followed by the dialectic step of *synthesis*, where according to Hegel the contradiction is '*aufgehoben*' (German 'aufheben' = eliminate; lift; preserve), and that in the three senses of the word: it is eliminated, preserved and lifted to a higher level (Pietschmann 2002, p.33f). In these three meanings, we find in sequence P1, P2 & 3 and P4. 'Preserved' refers to P2 or P3, depending on whether thesis and antithesis are seen as complementary (P2) or as reflecting one another (P3). Complete dialectics, therefore, encompasses everything. The referenced book by Pietschmann contains further considerations regarding contradictions.

Hofkirchner (2001) also works with four modes of thinking, which relate differently to parts and the whole. He states two *monistic* modes of thinking: *mechanistic*, which attributes everything to parts (this also includes interactions in his view), and *holistic*, which attributes everything to the whole. Then there is a *dualistic* thinking, where parts and whole stand side by side and cannot explain each other completely. These (to him) inadequate modes of thinking are not overcome until their *dialectic integration*, the fourth mode of thinking. Here, in a way, he meets with Pietschmann. The two monistic variants correspond to P1 (& P2) or an extreme of P4, the dualistic one has a connection with P3 – which, by the way, is also mirrored by the chosen symbolism of Table 2.1a. The dialectic integration corresponds to P4, which sees the whole but does not forget the parts (compare with *symbiosis*).

The meaning of the German word 'aufheben' as 'lifting to a higher level' and the concept of the dialectic integration have already implied that we are talking about meta-levels. Let us take a closer look at Table 2.1a&b with regard to this. First, we can see it as a list of four completely disconnected perspectives. This resembles P1 itself and can be seen as meta-perspective MP1. If we emphasise the overlap of perspectives, we come to MP2. Interpreting the list as sequences by analogy that are meant as a symbolic connection, then Table 2.1a&b leads us to MP3. If we are, however, of the opinion that this ostensible multiplicity really points to a fundamental unity, then this corresponds to MP4, which brings us back to synthesis as unity on a higher level, i.e. dialectic integration. As far as that goes, the latter is also to be placed at a higher level, a meta-level, according to Hofkirchner.

Further interesting considerations concerning perspectives and pluralism in medicine can be found in Matthiessen (2002), concerning thinking styles as a whole in Sternberg (1999). But now let us return to our perspectives P1-P4. We shall now utilise these to look at the historical development of world views and the healing methods associated with them. A rough division is displayed in Table 2.2.

Table 2.2. The historical development of world views and associated healing methods

Period	Time estimate	Healing methods
Archaic	For about 20000 years	Shamanism, religious/magical medicine (P4,3), cf. Achterberg (1989, p.25)
Ancient	About 2500 years ago	Roots of today's dominant medicine systems (P3,2) – hardly any change in Asian traditional healing systems since then
Modern	For about 200 years	In the West: scientific medicine (P1) and homoeopathy
Post-modern	For about 30 years	Renaissance of P2 in the West (chaos research, psycho-neuroimmunology) and multiplicity of paradigms

We can see at first glance that the process of change has accelerated. The older method has not been completely replaced but has only been superimposed by each new development. All approaches to reality are still represented today but with varying regional emphasis. Generally, a shift from P4 to P1 can be noted, at least until recently. The succession of perspectives and world views is closely connected to the often-mentioned transition of paradigms, which, however, originates from an old paradigm being overcome (Kuhn 1997). Especially in the last (postmodern) decades, however, a coexistence of several paradigms, a multiplicity of paradigms, has come into our awareness (Hütter et al. 1992, Pietschmann 1993). There are authors who favour the idea of a competition of cultures (Huntington 2002) or paradigms (Sokal & Bricmont 2001), which, in the final analysis, boils down to saving 'our' P1. Unfortunately, we cannot go into detail concerning this exciting discussion. For us, Huna is important for the very reason that its perspectives P1-P4 do not form a hierarchy but are considered equal. With its aid, various cultures and healing methods can be compared without running the risk of evaluating one approach as superior. Within Huna, a multiplicity of paradigms exists. This allows us to choose the approach to reality – in considering a particular healing method – which best corresponds to the method. Thus, P1-P4 are complementary in this system.

2.3. The Ancient Greeks

We shall now look at European Antiquity, in particular the Ancient Greeks. Not only can the roots of contemporary Western medicine be found there, but also we can come back to it for purposes of comparison with Asian healing methods. Table 2.3 lists the essential steps of development (rounded to quarter centuries). Some of this information comes from Schlote (2002). In early times, man strove to discover what exactly the world is based on. Thales postulated water as the primal substance. With this he attempted to separate 'physical' statements from the divine realm. Anaximenes considered air to be the central substance, as a symbol of breath, not only in the sense of the physical but also of the spiritual. For us Heraclitos is of special importance. He not only said that in his opinion fire is the most important element – this could be perpetuated with the other elements – but he also brought in the aspect of dynamics. The other elements (including earth, which still needs to be discussed) are rather static, while fire is dynamic and carries with it an aspect of transformation of the other elements. For this reason, Heraclitos remained something of an outsider in Greece. His saying, "Everything flows", is closer to the Chinese way of thinking (P2 being more important than P3) than the common Greek perspective (P3 dominating P2).

Table 2.3. Approximate dates of important developments in Ancient Greece (elements, medicine)

Thales	575 B.C.	Water	As primary substance
Anaximenes	525 B.C.	Air	Breath, soul
Heraclitos	500 B.C.	Fire	Dynamics
Empedocles	450 B.C.	+Earth	Fourfold scheme
Philolaos	425 B.C.	4 Elements	4 regular polyhedrons
Aristotle	325 B.C.	+Ether	+Dodecahedron
Asclepios Cult	until ca 600 B.C.	Healing	Magical/religious
Pythagoras	525 B.C.	Music	Numbers, harmony
Hippocrates	400 B.C.	Medicine	(Pre)scientific
Galen	175 A.D.	Medicine	Completion

Table 2.4. Sequences by analogy of the four Greek elements in Late Antiquity

Water	Air	Fire	Earth
Phlegm / mucus	Blood	Choler / bile	Black bile
Brain	Heart	Liver	Spleen
Phlegmatic	Sanguine	Choleric	Melancholic
Cold & damp	Warm & damp	Warm & dry	Cold & dry
Salty	Sweet	Bitter	Sour, pungent
White	Red	Yellow	Black
Winter	Spring	Summer	Autumn

The threefold system of water – air – fire was considered natural and held its ground for some time. Not until ca 450 B.C. did Empedocles postulate earth as a fourth element for logical reasons (P1). For, as can be seen from Table 2.3, the elements were also associated with physical characteristics such as temperature and dampness in terms of a bivalent logic (pairs 'cold/warm' and 'damp/dry'). With the threefold system, only three of the resulting four possibilities had been concretised (the elements water – air – fire with the bodily fluids mucus – blood – bile). The missing combination cold/dry was now assigned to *earth*. Subsequently, bile (formerly fire) was divided into a *yellow* (fire) and a *black* bile (earth). Later four temperaments were also assigned to the four elements. We shall come back to this later (see Table 2.3). At the same time, ca 450 B.C., autumn was added as a fourth season to the three already existing – winter, spring and summer (Asshauer 1993, p.20). Apparently at that time a general shift from a threefold to a fourfold system occurred.

Now let us return to Table 2.3. Philolaos found a correspondence between the four elements and the four regular polyhedrons – cube, tetrahedron, octahedron and icosahedron. Plato again adopted this, but a fifth regular polyhedron or 'platonic solid', the (pentagon) dodecahedron, had been discovered in the meantime. Accordingly, Plato postulated a fifth element, ether. Later on, the word 'quintessence' (or fifth essence) was derived from this (Bialas 1998, p.140).

Parallel to the steps mentioned here, we find a development in Ancient Greece towards mathematics and the natural sciences. Pythagoras made the interesting observation that the harmony of sound intervals is related to simple proportions of the length of the string and thus bridged formal and aesthetic characteristics. Pythagoras and his students investigated music as much as the mysticism of numbers and formal mathematics, which brings to mind the Pythagorean Theorem that is still taught today. At that time, philosophy, philosophy of nature and forerunners of the natural sciences were still one and the same thing. Aristotle is a good example here. However, since he stressed the importance of observation, he was also an important trailblazer for today's natural sciences.

The hypothesis of the fourfold causation of all processes is also due to Aristotle. He distinguished between causa materialis, formalis, efficiens and finalis. From today's point of view, these can be interpreted as material basis (matter, structure), general framework (boundary and initial conditions, parameters), cause/effect relationship, and purpose (goal), respectively. The last aspect is central to pragmatics, which has been discussed earlier. In classical science, however, cause/effect relationships play a central role, which points to the already mentioned limitation of meaning concerning the word 'cause'. This fits in with P1 and the characterisation 'if – then', cf. Table 2.1a&b.

And what about the development of medicine? Until ca 600 B.C. (and, in some temples, until the end of the millennium) medicine was a magical/religious affair practised by Asclepios sects. There are several versions of Asclepios, depending on their date of origin: in some, he was a man, a hero who once lived on the earth and practised as a physician; in others, he was a god or a serpent that served a god or was itself raised to the status of a god. Most often he is depicted as a god with a serpent (aesculap snake, Asclepios = aesculap). It was with the aid of Asclepios that the priests healed the sick. After a lengthy preparation phase (e.g. in caves), where the patients presumably experienced altered states of consciousness, the Asclepios priest would instruct them to sleep in the temple at a certain location.

They would then be healed by a dream. It might be that the god Asclepios appeared and performed a healing, or it might be that the patient had a dream which had to be interpreted and the interpretation would lead to a path of healing. Many clay tablets with reports of healings have been found near such temples. Sleeping in the temple apparently worked, whether it was Asclepios, the effect of a ritual, a placebo effect, imagination or psychological suggestion by the Asclepios priests. Today we would call this psychotherapeutic or perhaps a spiritual method of healing (P3,4).

About 500 B.C. much changed in this area. At some point, people were no longer satisfied with a religious medicine and physicians aspired to a 'scientific' medicine, although not necessarily in our sense. Hippocrates who, interestingly enough, practised in Kos in one of the most famous of the Asclepios temples, deserves special mention here. Not only did he introduce the scientific approach to medicine in the form of his theory of the circulation of humours (P2) but also the Hippocratic oath replaced the Asclepian oath. If we look at what 'healthy' and 'ill' mean in terms of the theory of the four humours or in terms of humoral pathology (humour = fluid), we see that they do not depend on whether a certain part of the body is ill or healthy but whether the flow of bodily fluids is harmonious. If this is not the case, if something is stagnating somewhere or there is a surplus or lack of one fluid or the other, then there is a risk of falling ill. Thus, three things come together in the Greek scenario: logic (P1), thinking in cycles (P2) and thinking in visual analogies (P3). You could say that the circulation of fluids and the tables of analogies are a theoretical construct, comparable to the theory of the circulation of qi in the meridians in Traditional Chinese Medicine. However, in the end it is a question of whether the constructs are useful and successful. We believe that we are much more 'objective' with modern science. Particularly in the field of modern theories of physics, however, we find constructs (P3) again and again, such as wave functions in quantum physics. They cannot be observed or directly measured. Nevertheless, if one presumes their existence, one can draw conclusions that can be tested with experiments. This situation is not that far removed from sleeping in the temple: Even if it always worked, it would be no proof of Asclepios' existence.

In Late Antiquity, as we have already mentioned, the theory of the four temperaments (phlegmatic, sanguine, choleric and melancholic) was developed (see Table 2.4). These types have been preserved in our thinking – and in some psychology books – to this day. Figure 2.2 shows how pairs of characteristics result in a four-way scheme (by Eysenck, referenced in Aerni 2000, p.598). The horizontal axis (Greek: *cold – warm*) is interpreted psychologically as INTROVERTED – EXTROVERTED or as calm state – aroused state, the vertical axis (*damp – dry*) as STABLE – UNSTABLE or as enthusiasm – apathy, respectively. Altogether, there are four types. One could speak of the INTROVERTED and EXTROVERTED, the STABLE and UNSTABLE types along the axes. In relation to these, the four temperaments can be found on an axis rotated 45° and this makes possible another correlation: The sanguine types, for example, tend to be more stable and extroverted. Such a yes/ no logic can be carried over to a higher dimension, but then the number of types will vary (e.g. in three dimensions: six types along the three axes, eight rotated 45°).

The fact that these four temperaments have survived until today shows how engrained these types are. This scheme, however, runs the risk – as much as the statics of the Greek elements with the exception of fire – of being rigid and artificial (stereotyped thinking), so there is a tendency to think "This man is a choleric, so I know exactly how he will behave." On the other hand, it is helpful to have an idea of what to expect. The medical relevance lies in the possibility of catering to the various types with different therapy methods, for example, knowing that a choleric will not respond to a certain medication, even if it would be indicated by his current condition. Such considerations are common in homoeopathy or Ayurveda but rare in orthodox Western medicine.

If we return to Table 2.4 we can see that sequences by analogy (P3) are helpful but neither unambiguous nor logical (P1). This is also true for the sequence by analogy in Table 2.4, despite the efforts of Empedocles to be logical. Thus, fire can be understood in terms of warm (hot) and dry, but air can be dry as well as damp. Table 2.4 also associates air with the heart and with spring. This seems pretty arbitrary and can only be fathomed from the Greeks' way of thinking. Why is fire associated with bitter taste? This, by the way, agrees with the Chinese association, which argues that meat turns bitter with roasting. Other assignments such as water – mucus – brain on the other hand appear intuitively plausible. Nevertheless, the general question remains: By what means does a sequence by analogy come about? If such sequences were completely arbitrary, then there would have to be hundreds of these sequences by analogy. Nonetheless, the Greeks, in essence, only handed down the above-mentioned sequence – and some of it coincides with Indian and Chinese assignments.

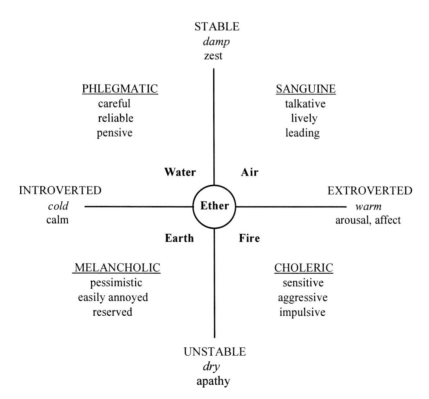

Figure 2.2. The four temperaments with psychological interpretation. The Greek assignments of *cold* /*warm* and *damp* /*dry* and the elements are also indicated. To complete the picture, the fifth element, ether, is drawn at the origin.

From today's Western viewpoint, humoral pathology seems obsolete. This might be true of its antique version. Some facts, however, should give us cause for consideration. Thus, in Ayurveda and Tibetan medicine (Ch. 8) we find three regulatory principles or 'fluids': wind, bile and mucus. They correspond to the Greek fluids blood, (yellow) bile and mucus (elements: air, fire and water) and thus largely to the three Greek elements. In Ayurveda, incidentally, there are five elements – in other words, it works with a different number of fluids and elements. The Indian elements are water, air, fire, earth and ether, corresponding exactly to a late European version, where ether was added as a fifth element. Furthermore, there is a direct historical line from Greek medicine via Islamic medicine (Arabs: Avicenna; Persian medicine) to Unani medicine, which is officially recognised in India, Pakistan and Indonesia. It is, so to speak, the current Asian version of the Greek theory of the four humours. Its name, incidentally, calls attention to its origin ('Unani' or 'Yunani' means Ionian). It is also – apart from Ayurveda, orthodox Western medicine ('allopathy') and homoeopathy – the fourth fully recognised healing method in India; see Nadkarni (2000), where primarily herbal medicines are described, including their use in therapy systems that we have already mentioned. India, therefore, currently offers the ideal setting for studying the functioning of the mode of thinking found in complementary healing methods. Furthermore, humoral pathology is enjoying a comeback in Europe in a new guise; see below.

2.4. Recent Developments in Europe

Greek medicine as depicted here was summarised and refined ca 175 A.D. by Galen (Table 2.2). Afterwards comparatively little changed for many centuries. Paracelsus (1st half of the 16th century) went back to a threefold system (tria prima or tria principia: sulphur, sal, mercury), which – a little later – changed European culinary habits (Laudan 2000). In the 16th century a paradigm shift to P1 occurred in natural science (Galileo, around and after 1600), which did not have any influence on medicine for a long time. However, during the last 150 to 200 years much has changed. Around 1800, dissatisfaction with medicine had grown to the degree that it inspired two developments: homoeopathy and orthodox Western medicine. Thus, both have existed for the same amount of time. Today, orthodox Western medicine appears to be dominant. Our own time and our own culture are, of course, the most important to us, but as a result we forget that what is medically standard for us has only been in existence for a relatively short time, and was first limited to Central Europe.

Orthodox Western medicine became established by stages during the 19th century. First, there was *anatomy*. Autopsy was an important aid to facilitating an analytical and objective medicine. The principles governing disease became more important than the patient's individual symptoms (Porter 2000, Ch. 5). Then *physiology* emerged, which saw function as being more important than structure. Around 1850, Helmholtz, du Bois-Reymond, Brücke and Ludwig met and established an anti-vitalistic programme, in which physiology was to be based on physics ('psychophysics', see Baatz 1989 and other contributions in Clair et. al. 1989). Then, in the second half of the 19th century, Virchow developed *cellular pathology* ('illness is located in the cell') and Koch, among others, sought and found an external foe as the cause of illness ('illness is caused by pathogens'), see Risch (1998, p.15).

Thus, in the 19th century, the cyclic thinking (P2) of humoral pathology gave way in university medicine to the local thinking (P1) of solidism (organ pathology, then cellular pathology, cf. Ch.1.1). Surgery – as the primary domain of this way of thinking – made enormous progress in the 20th century, especially due to the two world wars. Whenever a part of the body was injured or destroyed, it was operated on, repaired or replaced, constantly advancing into smaller and smaller regions. However, in genetic engineering, an exaggeration of solidism, which is increasingly gaining importance, we witness the paradox of the tiny locale of a gene under some circumstances influencing larger areas or even circulations in the body and, with that, bringing holism back into the game.

Interestingly, for some time now, developments in medicine and psychotherapy have been showing the interconnectedness of the organism and have brought cyclic thinking back into focus. The keywords here are psychoneuroimmunology (and the older term, psychosomatics) and systemic family therapy. Psychoneuroimmunology in particular (Kropiunigg & Stacher 1997) is extremely non-local, since it deals with correlations between the nervous, immune and endocrine systems. The circulatory systems (particularly the cardiovascular and lymphatic) are playing an important role again. Pure cellular thinking is no longer enough; the extra-cellular matrix (Heine 1997), which concentrates on what happens between and thus outside the cells, and which is especially important for good health, comes into focus more and more.

In psychotherapy, the focus used to be 'local' as well, concentrating on one person, the patient. In systemic methods, this is no longer the case (Brandl-Nebehay 1998, Simon & Rech-Simon 2002). A single 'defective' family member is not just repaired or treated, the family's communication network is also considered. The goal is to achieve an unhindered flow of communication in the family. The (alleged) patient is merely seen as a symptom carrier. If he recovers, another member of the family can take over the role of patient. Thus, the fact that one individual always has to be the patient depends primarily on the dynamics of the system, not on one certain individual. An example may be found in the world of business: After a particularly unpleasant or mean colleague is sacked, the atmosphere in the office will not improve for long, because this negative role has to be taken on by someone else – someone who had not come to anyone's attention in this way before. The idea that one person is not by himself healthy or ill, mean or loving, but that this also depends on the surroundings and the prevailing circumstances, can in itself ease the burden of individual responsibility for problems.

Orientation in cyclic thinking, and thus in P2, can also be found in the natural sciences, namely in chaos and systems research. This research has only become possible in the last few decades with the appearance of adequately powerful computers. This is a paradox insofar as the computer is a typical product of P1. In the next two chapters, we will address this topic in depth.

Chapter 3

Systemic View I: Chaos and Fractals

3.1. When does Chaos Occur?

Our Western way of thinking is determined by logic, see Figure 2.1a. Possible interpretations of the arrows are: cause – effect, stimulus – reaction, input – output, diagnosis – therapy. The succession moves in *one* direction only. The suggestive expression 'linear' is sometimes used but is not advantageous because this term has a different meaning in mathematics from that in the natural sciences (see below). The less well-known expression 'lineal' used in psychotherapy (Böse & Schiepek 1989, p.105f) fits much better. Therefore, if something is going in just one direction, we shall call it a lineal process. If there is a closed loop, cf. Figure 2.1b, depending on the circumstances, one refers to a feedback loop, self-reference, reflexivity, recursivity, cycle or circularity. We can imagine the parts ('spheres') as members of the family and the links (arrows) as channels of communication. Feedback interrupts the hierarchy and enables discussion of 'who started the fight'. In terms of logic, paradoxes and circular reasoning come about, which classical logic attempts to avoid. Thus, we are talking about the fundamentally different perspectives, P1 and P2 (Table 2.1). Therefore, we can identify P1 with lineality and P2 with feedback (or the occurrence of cycles).

A generalised approach always takes the existence of cycles into consideration. If circularity is only weakly developed, we can still neglect it if the particular case warrants it. Our Western thinking, however, proceeds in reverse: As long as we can get away with it, we repress the existence of closed loops to the extreme case of assuming *monocausality*. This results in massive ecological and also, subsequently, economic problems. Indeed, it is much simpler and cleaner to argue lineally (P1), but this way of thinking encompasses neither the entire environment nor all aspects of complex, e.g. living, systems. For the last few decades physics, too, (where the keywords are chaos and systems research) has been engaged in investigating complex phenomena, which exhibit completely new characteristics which are difficult to explain with Western medical thinking (for example, problems with reproducibility and predictability, and with side effects). This could be confronted, however, by including circularity (P2), which again corresponds to complementary medicine systems.

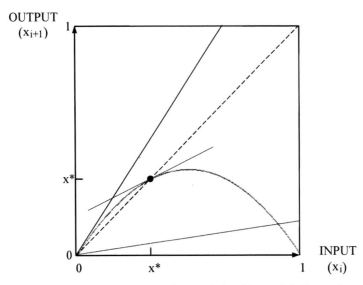

Figure 3.1. Linear and non-linear relationship, straight line and curve, respectively. For details, see the text.

We can quote a simple example to illustrate this problem. When I raise a child, I am not aware of the existence of a feedback loop. Nevertheless, the child slowly changes me as well, depending on how he or she reacts to my wishes and orders. We all consider ourselves the centre and livef under the impression that we manipulate our surroundings. We prefer to overlook the fact that we, too, are manipulated by our surroundings. However, these feedback loops bring about surprises, loss of control and similar situations. Chaos research illuminates the question of how it comes about that we do not have control over everything.

We shall now look into how it can be that individuals, groups, technical devices and so on can behave in an unexpected manner and why there is a great deal we cannot understand and control. Just thinking about the example of a human being, we can easily understand this. In comparison to a single person, a group of people, consisting of many individuals, is more likely to exhibit uncontrollable behaviour (mass hysteria, lynching, panic, etc.). But even the individual organism is quite complicated. It consists of many individual parts (such as cells). The question is how far down can you go, what so to speak is the simplest system that can exhibit surprising behaviour. From physics we know that systems which seem to be very simple can show surprisingly complex behaviour. We already know one necessary condition – circularity or non-lineality. A second is non-linearity, which we shall discuss now (see also Kratky 1989). The system does not even have to be complicated – in other words, it does not require a great number of parts or variables.

Referring back to Figure 2.1b, we can see that, there, we are not looking at the entire network of the system but are picking out an arbitrary cause/effect (input/output) relationship (see Figure 2.1a as the interpretation of a detailed section from Figure 2.1b). In the simplest case, we have a so-called linear relationship, as in the four straight lines in Figure 3.1. Three of those go through the origin. These correspond to a proportional relationship (doubling the cause produces double the effect') . Linearity and in particular proportionality are so engrained in our Western way of thinking that, in general, we are not aware of it. Nevertheless, non-linear situations with deviations from the straight line are more realistic. Curves, in particular, (as in Figure 3.1) occur more frequently, e.g., in the relationship of tax with the Chancellor of the Exchequer's revenue, in the cost of a ticket with the efficiency of the transport system, in the relationship of nervousness to performance, etc. If the cause is small (the curve being close to the origin), the cause/effect relationship will almost be a linear one. Higher values, however, will result in greater deviations from linearity, until finally the direction is reversed. Thus, the Chancellor of the Exchequer would not have any revenue with a tax rate of 100%. Nobody would continue to work, if nothing was left after deductions.

Complex behaviour requires non-lineality as well as non-linearity. More precisely, the system's network must contain at least one feedback loop, and at least one of the relationships in the system must be non-linear. These relationships are generally not depicted graphically but in the form of systems of equations. The question of linearity, however, is more fundamental. Non-lineal but linear systems of equations can not only be made lineal via transformation of variables, but can also be put into separate equations (which greatly simplifies calculations). In other words, this enables a return from P2 to P1.

Why is linearity, which is so rare in real situations, engrained in us? Why are there so many linear relationships in the study of mathematics and the sciences? Not because they are so realistic, but because they are the ones that can be handled mathematically with great ease. This corresponds to a narrowing of our attention. We do not see the world in its surprising diversity but only focus on that part which we can master, the part we can deal with mathematically – and we believe that this is all there is. Linear equations can be calculated with paper and pencil and it is for this reason they always have been, and still are, so popular. However, the computer has brought changes. With its help, non-linear systems of equations can also be solved and this is the reason why chaos research is only about 30 years old – sufficiently high-performance computers have only been around for that long.

In reality, non-lineality and non-linearity are the norm – for example, in an interconnected, feedback system. In technology, complexity is often simplified by assuming lineality, (e.g. information processing only in one direction, input/output relationship). A video camera, for instance, might record an object that can simultaneously be seen on a monitor with the correct cable set-up. If the recording device were perfect (linear, among other things), the monitor would show an exact image of the recorded object. Small faults do not attract attention. However, turning the camera towards this monitor closes the loop (video feedback). Small errors now build up with this method of application, which was not intended by the manufacturer (for example deviations in colour could allow this to be used for a particularly exact form of quality control!). An image originally appearing on the monitor quickly dissolves; a self-organised pattern arises. This pattern can remain the same, but it can also rotate, pulsate or change in any number of ways – all of this without changing the position of the camera (which might be set on a tripod). There is no external cause for the succession of images. Crutchfield (1984, 1987) was a pioneer in this field. It is fascinating to see the arising patterns – some even look like biological forms.

But first the question arises of how this can come about from the original image. It could possibly be generated by reflections of furniture in the monitor. What happens, however, when the room is completely dark and even the light of the monitor is turned off so that no external influences can affect the feedback process? A dark monitor will remain dark, but it is possible to set an initial image by flicking a lighter, for example, in the line of sight between monitor and camera. In a perfect technical system the image of the flame would be 'frozen' on the monitor – in other words, the externally produced image would be fixated internally. However, since the system is not perfect, patterns arise, which can be explained by the internal conditions of the system. The flame merely represents a necessary trigger.

The question of the relationship between internal processes and external influences is also important in medicine. Just think about the role of therapists – are they *only* a trigger for healing processes which, on the whole, then proceed autonomously, or is their role more extensive? It is obvious that there are a number of feedback loops within the human being. Thus, occurrence of complex behaviour depends on (non-) linearity. Distinguishing between linearity and non-linearity is also important in considering the question of interactions of therapies, e.g. drugs A and B. Let us suppose that the effects of A and B have been scrutinised in clinical studies, but A and B have not been tested together – it is not feasible to study all combinations. What do we do if a certain patient requires both drugs A and B? As long as no adverse effects are known, the general assumption is that A and B do not affect each other. Then the effects E of the drugs A and B can be added in order to get the total effect E (A+B), see (3.1a). It can be shown mathematically that this only applies if all partial processes in the organism (including the interaction of A and B) are linear. Of course, this prerequisite is not met. Nevertheless, it is surprising how often this assumption can be applied with good results.

As a linear equation: $E(A\&B) = E(A) + E(B),$ (3.1a)

As a non-linear equation: $E(A\&B) = E(A) + E(B) + RE(A,B).$ (3.1b)

More precisely, an interaction term ('reciprocal effect' RE) should be included, (3.1b), even if it complicates the calculations. The existence of this correcting term can be recognised in the description accompanying the medication. There, we find a list of interactions and contraindications. For the latter A is the therapy and B another circumstance. For example, if a certain drug A has an adverse effect on pregnancy B, then it is contraindicated for pregnant women. Not much is generally known in this respect. Usually one assumes that this interaction term is zero. Then, once a harmful effect occurs, we have a scandal on our hands and a great deal research is begun in this particular field. As a result the drug description might be changed to "Drug A must not be taken by pregnant women."

3.2. The Logistic Map

Now we come to the logistic map, the simplest system exhibiting complex behaviour. Let us go back and take a closer look at Figure 3.1 and, first of all, focus on the two steep straight lines (linear case). The solid line is steeper (slope 1.5) than the dashed one (slope 1.0). The latter is at an angle of exactly 45° to the two axes and is known as a diagonal. It will serve us as a reference line. Now we will interpret the horizontal axis as input and the vertical as output. If we choose an input value x_o, then the output according to the solid line is $1.5\,x_o$. If this were to represent a bank account, this would mean that at the end of the year it would contain 1.5 times the amount which was present at the beginning of the year (in general, r times as much). This means a hypothetical interest rate of 50%. The diagonal on the other hand represents an account balance that does not change over time (no interest, $r=1$). If $r=0$ then there will be no money left after one year. What happens to the balance if you let 'the money work for you' and you invest it at a fixed interest rate over several years? The output (final balance) of the 1st year equals the input (starting balance) of the 2nd year. The same is true in general for the transition from year i to year (i+1). In mathematical terms:

$$x_{i+1} = r \, x_i \quad (r \geq 0 \text{ fixed, but arbitrary}); \text{ thus } (x_{i+1}/x_i) = r \equiv e^{(\ln r)} = e^\lambda. \qquad (3.2)$$

The identity $r \equiv e^{(\ln r)}$ comes from the fact that the exponential function, e, and the natural logarithm, *ln*, are inverse functions. Linearity corresponds to a constant slope r, which can also be expressed by the so-called Lyapunov exponent $\lambda = \ln r$. As long as $r>1$ ($\lambda>0$) the account balance will increase every year. If $r=1$ ($\lambda=0$) it remains the same and if $r<1$ ($\lambda<0$) it steadily decreases. The first case corresponds to the solid straight line in Figure 3.1 ($r=1.5$), the second to the dashed line ($r=1.0$) and the third to the flat dotted line ($r=0.15$). If you consider this process over a period of several years, this recursive behaviour of output to input represents a circular, i.e. non-linear, system. It is also called an iterated map, because the same scheme is applied repeatedly. Since the individual steps are linear, the solution can be given explicitly:

$$x_i = r^i x_0 = e^{\lambda i} x_0, \quad \lambda = \ln r ; \qquad (3.3a)$$
$$\delta x = r^i \delta x_0 = e^{\lambda i} \delta x_0. \qquad (3.3b)$$

It is a little confusing that a linear relationship if applied again and again with $r>1$ ($\lambda>0$) would lead to an exponential growth. However, we know this process from calculating compound interest. The same is true for the earth's population, when $r>1$ (r: constant); $r<1$ would result in an exponential extinction of the human race. Eq.(3.3b) shows that with $\lambda>0$ an *uncertainty* factor δx of the value x also builds up exponentially during the course of time whenever the initial value is not known exactly. This is the real reason why Lyapunov exponents are defined. We will come back to this later.

For the following considerations, let us assume that the variable x represents the number of animals of a certain species per square metre (population density) in a zoned area, where x_i represents the ith generation. We will assume for the sake of simplicity that the generations are strictly separated – for example, the entire generation dies off in the winter, in the spring the next generation is hatched and x_i is always measured at a certain day in the autumn. The parameter r represents the fertility of this species but also the available food source in the summer. With $r>1$ we will have exponential growth, which cannot continue ad infinitum. The food source, for example, would eventually be depleted, which leads to a decrease in fertility due to stress etc. The simplest mathematical deviation from the straight line that can take into account such corrections is the parabola, the curve in Figure 3.1:

$$x_{i+1} = r \, x_i - r \, (x_i)^2 = r \, x_i \, (1-x_i), \quad 0 \leq r \leq 4. \qquad (3.4)$$

From the x-value of a given step, the value for the next step (year, generation) can be calculated. Eq.(3.4) is called a logistic equation or map. The non-linearity is announced by the square term, and the slope of the curve (change in x_{i+1} with respect to the change in x_i, see Figure 3.1) is no longer constant even with r fixed but depends on x_i. The parabola goes through zero at $x_i=0$ and $x_i=1$. Now the chosen units come into play. x_i can be interpreted as the population density relative to the maximal density ($0 \leq x_i \leq 1$). In order for this also to apply to x_{i+1} and thus to make the equation consistent, r must fulfil the condition $0 \leq r \leq 4$. For very small x_i the factor $(1-x_i)$ in (3.4) can be neglected and the linear relationship (3.2) results, which is a very good approximation. One also talks about the process of linearisation. Figure 3.1 depicts this situation clearly. The corresponding line represents the tangent to the *parabola* through the origin. The greater the value of r, the steeper the parabola and its tangent line and the higher the maximum value of the parabola ($r/4$ at the place $x_i=\frac{1}{2}$, which does not exceed the value 1).

If there is no initial population, i.e. $x_o=0$, it will remain so (trivial equilibrium or fixed point $x^\#=0$). By the way, the maximum population density $x=1$, will lead to the species' extinction in the next generation, $x_{i+1}=0$, and will then remain at 0. But what happens when the initial value is somewhere between 0 and 1? If we look at Figure 3.1 (parabola with $r=1.5$), we find an area of x_i (smaller values), where the curve is above the diagonal. This means the population density will increase in the next generation. At the point of intersection with the diagonal there is no change in population (equilibrium or fixed point x*), and for larger values the population density decreases in the next generation. Although it is clear what happens from one step to the next, the situation as a whole is confusing. There is also no general solution such as (3.3a), but the use of a computer is necessary to calculate the succession numerically. Nevertheless, it turns out that long-term behaviour is easily understood. As you can see from Figure 3.2b (where $r=1.6$), the succession of values (trajectory) approaches the constant value x* after a transitional phase. $x^\#$ and x* can generally be easily determined as points of intersection of line and parabola:

Fixed point $x^\#=0$,   stable for $0 \leq r < 1$,   (3.5a)
Fixed point $x^*=1-(1/r)$,   stable for $1 \leq r < 3$.   (3.5b)

For $r < 1$, $x^\#=0$ is stable, attracting (or an attractor). This term is locally defined, which means it attracts all points near it (every small x_o) and the population becomes extinct. Conversely, $x^\#=0$ is unstable, repelling (or a repellor) for $r=1.5$ and 1.6. It repels every x_o, no matter how small, initially into an almost exponential growth. Near $x^\#$ the parabola (3.4) can be approximated by the line (3.2). The latter corresponds to the solid line through the origin in Figure 3.1 (case $r=1.5$). However, as soon as the population has become large enough, the local approximation is no longer valid. What happens then can be estimated by observing the fixed point, x*. For $r=1.5$ the fixed point is an attractor according to (3.5b), it attracts all points near it and the population density levels off at x*. 'Near' indicates a local characteristic. In the case of a logistic equation, however, it is true that every r has exactly one global attractor. For $r<1$, the population will die off in the long run in every case, since it cannot reproduce. Thus, $x^\#=0$ is the global attractor (see Figure 3.2a, $r=0.8$). For $r=1$, x* replaces $x^\#$ as global attractor, which according to (3.5b) increases with increasing values of r (see Figure 3.2b&c, r=1.6 & r=2.4). For $1 \leq r < 3$, all initial values $0 < x_o < 1$ lead to x* in the end. This is interesting, because then the (long-term) effect does not depend on the (initial) cause x_o at all. If you want to talk about a 'cause', you must link it to the parameter r, which determines the long-term effect, x*. If a logistic equation can be applied to an observed system and r is known, a clear long-term prediction can be made for the value of x without knowing its current value!

It really gets interesting when r=3. From this value on, x* is unstable – there no longer exists a stable fixed point. Figure 3.2d shows the case for r=3.25. The long-term behaviour is a periodic movement (cycle or oscillation). More precisely, this is a twofold period: the population density goes back and forth between the values x_A and x_B. This twofold period is globally stable and therefore is called a global periodic attractor. Almost all initial values converge to it (the exceptions being $x_o = x^\# = 0$, $x_o = x^*$ and those which converge to one or the other fixed points after a few steps). The initial value plays a role only inasmuch as either the even or odd generations converge to x_A (reverse for x_B), but that is unimportant in principle. On the other hand, what is remarkable is the long-term dynamics in the form of an oscillation, although the equation is always the same and the parameter r remains constant. At first glance, observing such fluctuations could lead to the assumption that huntsmen decimate the population every other year. Instead of external influences, however, there are internal laws, in the form of logistic equations, which are responsible for these fluctuations. They result by themselves, so to speak. Instead of a clear transparent causal correspondence, a complex behaviour emerges, which is also characterised by the term self-organisation. Fluctuations in populations can be observed in nature over and over – but in times gone by, we did not know how they came about.

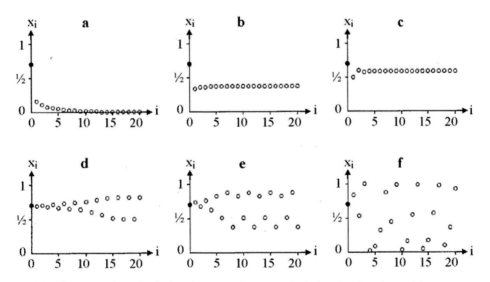

Figure 3.2. The succession of x during the generation i (small circles) for six values of the parameter r, the initial value x_o is always 0.7 (black dots on the vertical axis). Based on Briggs & Peat (1990, p.83). **a)** r=0.8, **b)** r=1.6, **c)** r=2.4, **d)** r=3.25, **e)** r=3.52, **f)** r=4.0.

This rather simple case of a logistic equation has even more surprises in store. In continuing calculations for higher and higher values of r, a succession of periodic doubling occurs: the twofold period becomes an attractor of first a fourfold period (see Figure 3.2e, r=3.52), then an eightfold period and so on in increasingly rapid successions until r=3.56999 exhibits non-periodic or chaotic fluctuations. We shall talk about chaos in more detail in Chs. 3.3 & 4.2. Now let us scan through the range of r. If you keep increasing r after the first appearance of a chaotic attractor, periodic windows will emerge from time to time (for example, threefold periods), where chaos becomes unstable. Chaos is most pronounced when you reach the final value of r=4. This case can be seen in Figure 3.2f. This situation can be demonstrated by an imaginary medical example – the effect on the blood pressure of an antihypertensive drug. If we increase the dosage slowly over a few weeks, the blood pressure continues to fall. After reaching a critical dose, the blood pressure goes up abruptly and keeps changing in an unpredictable manner with a constant increase in dosage. Not a very pleasant situation.

If you want to know more about the questions that we have covered so far, have a look at Leven et al. (1994) and Worg (1993). Both of these link formulae with graphics, with the formulae predominating in the first book and the graphics in the second. We also want to examine chaos in more detail. For certain parameter ranges of r the logistic equation results in chaotic solutions, which are non-periodical, or, in other words, form an infinite period. For chaos, however, another aspect is even more important – the aspect of the impossibility of predicting the development of the variable x in the long run by knowing the current value approximately but not exactly. Our intuition tells us that the predictability should be limited by random disturbances for which, however, there is no term in our model. It is strictly deterministic and for this reason is called deterministic chaos. Hence, there is no randomness and the aspect of disorder contrary to self-organisation is not valid (Kratky 1992). We shall come back to this. To adapt a quotation from Shakespeare, one could say "Though this be chaos, yet there is method in 't."

Let us stay with the logistic equation. While, for a (global) fixed-point attractor and a periodic attractor, the initial value x_o plays practically no role in the long-term behaviour, in the chaotic case only exact knowledge of x_o can help making long-term predictions. How it is possible that the same equation behaves is such a diverging manner for different values of the parameter r? The following consideration on doubling periods gives a partial answer – as long as $1<r<3$, the fixed-point attractor $x^*>0$ (formally a single period) is reached in the long run. This does not depend on x_o, except that x_o must not equal 0 or 1. In the case of the twofold period, whether the sequence reached the value x_A in even or odd steps i, in the long run depended on the initial value. We shall take a closer look at this now. Let us continue to double the periods and designate x_A to be the highest value of the corresponding period. Then we get 4, 8, 16 ... nested regions of x_o, which determine in which of the 4, 8, 16 ... successive generations x_A will appear (all other values then result automatically). If one aspires to such precision, one has to know x_o more exactly with every doubling of the period. The limiting case of a period with infinite length requires an infinitely exact knowledge of the initial condition in order to make statements about the future and not just say: "So, now we have chaos."

Chaos can be characterised by the statement 'small causes, large effects'. This has to do with the fact that two very close x-values will be separated by a great distance due to exponential growth (with a positive Lyapunov exponent). Uncertainties and inexact calculations also grow exponentially (Schamanek & Kratky 1994, Kratky 1995a). Surprisingly enough, especially for r=4 (greatest chaos, maximal $\lambda=ln2$), the logistic equation can be solved explicitly, which gives a better understanding of the circumstances of how chaos develops in the first place. There will be more on this in Ch. 3.4, together with further comments on the logistic equation.

3.3. Fractals – and their Relevance in Medicine

Now we shall look at graphically iterated processes, a geometric variant of the iterated map, which will lead us to so-called *fractals*. An example of this is Koch's curve (Figure 3.3). We start (step i=0) with a line of length 1, take out a third in the middle and replace it with two lines of equal length (in this case 1/3). The result (step i=1) is a continuous curve consisting of four line segments of a total length 4/3. In each further step the same scheme is applied – every line segment of the previous step is replaced with two new line segments. Figure 3.3 shows the steps 0 to 3. The image becomes either coarser or finer with each step and, at the limit, approaches the (complete) Koch's curve with its length going to infinity. This is very unusual for curves. Let us take a closer look. For the ith iteration the length of a segment, ε_i, the number of segments, N_i, as well as the total length, L_i, is given by:

Koch's curve: $\varepsilon_i = (1/3)^i,\ N_i = 4^i,\ L_i = (4/3)^i,$ (3.6a)

In general: $N_i = (1/\varepsilon_i)^D,\ L_i = \varepsilon_i N_i = (1/\varepsilon_i)^{D-1}.$ (3.6b)

D denotes the dimension. Through comparison, we get for Koch's curve:

Dimension (Koch): $D = ln4 / ln3 = 1.262.$ (3.6c)

The important thing here is this: The usual dimension D of a curve is 1. That it has a well-defined length corresponds to the fact that L_i is not dependent on step i, which means D−1=0 in (3.6b). If D>1 then the length tends to infinity and that the more quickly the larger D is. In this case we have a generalised or fractal (broken) dimension. 1<D<2 can be interpreted to mean that Koch's curve is between a normal curve (D=1) and an area (D=2). In general, we speak of fractals whenever their generalised dimension is not a whole number. Another characteristic of Koch's curve, which also applies to fractals in general, is its *self-similarity*. For example, the last third of the curve in the 3rd step looks like the entire curve of the 2nd step. If you approach a segment of the complete Koch's curve or, rather, zoom into it, you cannot estimate the distance. You keep seeing smaller and smaller segments with more and more detail, but the overall impression remains the same. This stepwise self-similar construction, then, corresponds to a self-similar impression in analysis, studying shorter and shorter line segments, a finer and finer decomposition of Koch's curve. In any case, no matter how small a part of the curve you study, it reflects the entire curve.

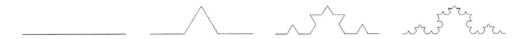

Figure 3.3. The first steps (i = 0 to 3) for constructing Koch's curve.

Koch's curve appears to be a special case. Indeed this is the case due to its rigid construction, which actually leads to its 'self-equivalence'. During the course of the last three decades, the study of irregular, self-similar fractals has become more and more important. It has also been discovered that living and inanimate nature exhibits many forms that can be described well with fractals. In this process, of course, not an infinite number but typically 3 to 5 iterations are observed. Just think about trees with their trunks branching out into thick and then thinner and thinner branches. Often structures with (almost) fractal surfaces can be found whose surface area (through branching and coarsening) can become quite large. This is how the cardiovascular system is able to supply the entire body with blood – despite a relatively small volume – by repeated tree-like branching, the surface area is increased to such an extent that a sufficient exchange of substances is possible. A similar situation is found in the lungs, where there is a surface area of ca 100 m^2. The diverging values for surface areas found in literature point to the fact that they are less valid than the fractal dimension D. Thus, the surface of kidney arteries results in a D of 2.2 to 2.3 (Sernetz 2000). That the transport-limiting internal boundary layers of human beings and of many animals have almost the same fractal structure can be seen in the fact that the basic metabolic rate G, in terms of the body length L, increases with D=2.22 ($G=L^{2.22}$). Unfortunately, we cannot go into more detail here.

It is certainly plausible that fractal structures that develop in the embryo come about as a result of genes repeatedly applying the same steps of construction (iterated processes). On the other hand, drainage systems or networks of rivers, which only obey physical laws, when seen from the air look exactly like the living circulatory and bronchial systems. Correspondingly, the border between land and water is very long. Incidentally, research on fractals had been in progress for decades only by a few pioneers (such as van Koch, who gave his name to Koch's curve). It was Mandelbrot, who coined the term fractals and who made this field popular and systematically investigated it, especially using computer graphics, which had started to improve a great deal around 1980 (Mandelbrot 1987).

It is clear that fractals occurring in *inanimate* nature do not arise by deliberate steps of construction but as a 'by-product' of complex physical processes. Here, too, the connection between cause and effect is blurred. Thus, clouds emerge because of meteorological processes, mountains and river systems owing to geophysical processes. However, even simple mathematical iteration rules can bring about a variety of patterns whose connection to the rules – contrary to Koch's curve – cannot be fathomed. One example of this is the Mandelbrot set ('little apple man'), which we will not discuss in detail here but just point to the aesthetic pictures in Peitgen & Richter (2000). This raises the question: Is the converse true, i.e. can arbitrarily complex forms in general be constructed from a few simple equations? If you are interested in this fascinating field, we refer you to a study of iterated systems of functions (Barnsley & Hurd 1993). Fractals and chaos research were finally integrated into an extended medicine by Toifl (1995) and Hanzl (2002).

Now let us address the frequently heard objection that fractal geometry is unsuitable, since strictly speaking there are no fractals in nature in the mathematical sense. Indeed, most often the process stops after 3-5 steps. Nevertheless, this argument applies just as well to classical geometry, which works with points, straight lines or spheres. For example, a 'point' drawn on the board is not really a point; otherwise you would not be able to see it ($D=0$). In the final analysis, the tools we use in approaching reality are always only constructs. New tools bring these flaws more into focus than old ones, less known tools more than the well-known ones, others' tools more than one's own. This, by the way, is also true for the sometimes tense relationship between orthodox and complementary medicine.

Conversely, new discoveries allow new terms to be developed with which one can approach previously unnoticed phenomena. So nowadays many fractal patterns are being discovered in natural objects. Fractals come in handy for modelling processes (Kratky 1994). One example of self-similarity in the human being is the sensory and motor homunculus, where an image of the entire human being can be found in a part of the cortex of the brain (the connection is given here via the nervous system). The somatotopies (reflex zones), which have been known in acupuncture for a long time, also fall into this category; see Gleditsch (1988b) and Gleditsch & Ogal (2002). There, the body's surface is represented in its entirety in a small part of the body. Many acupuncture points are found along the course of the twelve major meridians. The idea of qi ('energy') flowing in the meridians resembles the Greek theory of the four humours (P2). Therapy consists in stimulating these points (see Ch. 7). However, in various locations on the body we find everything again in a smaller version, for example in the ear (Gleditsch 1988b, Ch. 2.2) or in the hand (Yoo 1994). In fact, one could speak of fractal acupuncture. Which physiological processes are responsible for this is not clear. One can utilise the idea of analogies, P3, and approach ear acupuncture with a mindset of treating the whole body. Fractal acupuncture points have the advantage of being more easily accessible and can also be used for diagnostic purposes. Points that need treating tend to be particularly tender. We will return to this problem in Ch. 7. What now follows is a mathematical advancement. Those people who are not especially interested in this may skip it.

3.4.* More on the Logistic Map

For the logistic map, time is assumed to be discrete, i.e. discontinuous. The expansion of the linear relation (3.2) to the parabola (3.4) is apparently not the most general case, since both terms on the right side have the same coefficient r. The more general case would include two coefficients, r and s; in addition, we now call the variable y instead of x for formal reasons:

$$y_{i+1} = r\,y_i - s\,y_i^2 = r\,y_i\,[\,1-(s/r)\,y_i\,].\qquad\qquad(3.7a)$$

This parabola has two zeros: at $y_{i+1}=0$ and $y_{i+1}=(r/s)$. That this case, however, is not more general than the one previously considered, can be seen by the transformation of variables $y=(r/s)x$. Substitution results in:

$$y = (r/s)x: (r/s)x_{i+1} = r(r/s)x_i - s(r/s)^2 x_i^2 = (r/s)[rx_i - rx_i^2], \qquad (3.7b)$$

$$\text{thus } x_{i+1} = rx_i - rx_i^2. \qquad (3.7c)$$

This leads us back to (3.4). x and y are equivalent; they relate only to different units (like different currencies). $y=(r/s)$ and $x=1$ correspond to the maximum values, respectively. Now, the logistic equation can also be expressed as a differential equation, which describes the change from step to step:

$$\Delta x_i = (r-1)x_i - r(x_i)^2, \qquad\qquad \text{with } \Delta x_i = x_{i+1} - x_i, \qquad (3.8a)$$

$$\Delta x_i / \Delta i = [x_{i+1} - x_i] / 1 = (r-1)x_i - r(x_i)^2, \qquad \text{with } \Delta i = (i+1)-i=1. \qquad (3.8b)$$

(3.8b) is just a more complicated way of writing (3.8a). However, it allows us to make comparisons to a representation, which relates to the time passed per step, $\Delta t = \Delta t_i$.

$$\Delta x_i / \Delta t_i = [x_{i+1} - x_i] / \Delta t = [(r-1)x_i - r(x_i)^2] / \Delta t, \text{ where } \Delta t_i = \Delta t = \text{const}. \qquad (3.8c)$$

Making the transition from a difference equation, in which time is treated as discrete, to a differential equation, in which time is continuous, such as the ones used in Ch. 4, corresponds to considering smaller and smaller steps of time, which at the limit approach zero (formally: $\Delta t \rightarrow dt$).

Now let us look at the stability of the fixed point, x^*. The logistic map (3.4) represents a parabola, whose slope (mathematically: derivative or differential quotient at point x_i) is therefore not constant but depends on x_i.

$$x_{i+1} = rx_i(1-x_i) = rx_i - r(x_i)^2, \quad \text{slope: } (dx_{i+1}/dx_i) = r(1-2x_i), \qquad (3.9a)$$

$$\text{Fixed point } x^* = 1 - (1/r), \qquad \text{slope: } R = 2-r. \qquad (3.9b)$$

Eq. (3.9b), for which (3.5b) was used, gives the actual slope at fixed point x^*, which we will call R. Now we can answer the question of when the fixed point x^* of the logistic map is stable or unstable Formally, the behaviour near x^* can be understood as a *linearisation* of the parabola around x^* (see tangent at x^* – dashed line through x^* in Figure 3.1). By (3.9b) it has slope $R=2-r$. Thus, near x^* we have:

$$x_{i+1} = x^* + R(x_i - x^*), \quad R = 2-r, \qquad (3.10a)$$

$$|(x_{i+1}-x^*)/(x_i-x^*)| = |R| = e^{(ln|R|)} = e^{\Lambda}. \qquad (3.10b)$$

Therefore, the distance to x^* decreases step by step when $|R|<1$, i.e. the Lyapunov exponent $\Lambda < 0$. This is the case for $R=2-1.5=0.5$, where x^* is an attractor. The general boundaries for stability given in (3.5a&b) now make sense. Geometrically we can see that when the tangent through a fixed point has a greater slope (is steeper) than the diagonal, the fixed point is unstable. If its slope, however, is less steep, the fixed point is stable and thus a fixed-point attractor. Now we can see at first glance in Figure 3.1 why $x^{\#}=0$ is unstable and x^* is stable. The tangent line to the parabola at zero is steeper and the one at x^* flatter than the diagonal. The more negative the Lyapunov exponent is, the faster the corresponding trajectory approaches the fixed point; the more positive it is, the faster the trajectory diverges from the associated fixed point. In the limiting case of the diagonal, the values do not change at all.

Now to the explicit solution to the logistic map for $r=4$ (largest chaos), which is addressed in Ch. 3.3. First, eq. (3.11a) is made linear (3.11) by means of a substitution:

Logistic equation: $x_{i+1} = 4\,x_i(1-x_i)$,   (3.11a)

Substitution $x = \sin^2\xi$: $\xi_{i+1} = 2\,\xi_i$,   (3.11b)

General solution: $\xi_i = 2^i\,\xi_0 = e^{(ln2)i}\,\xi_0$,   thus $x_i = \sin^2(2^i\,\xi_0)$.   (3.11c)

The linear relation in the variable ξ leads to exponential growth with $\lambda = ln2 = 0.6931...$, cf. (3.2), (3.3b). The explicit solution for x_i is given by back substitution, cf. (3.11). So where does this uncertainty come from? Let us stay with the ξ-representation and assume that although we do not know the initial value exactly, there is only a small degree of uncertainty, $\delta\xi_0$. This uncertainty builds up exponentially, namely with the Lyapunov exponent $\lambda = ln2$:

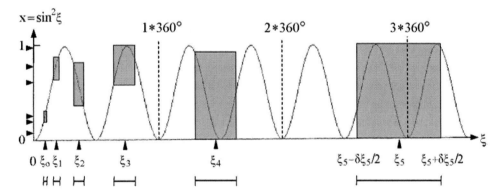

Figure 3.4. General solution to the logistic equation with $r=4$. The impact of an initial uncertainty in ξ_0 or x_0 on the next steps is displayed. The assumed initial uncertainty, $(\delta\xi_0, \delta x_0)$, results in a complete loss of information regarding x after just 5 steps: $\delta x_5 = 1$ because $\delta\xi_5 > 180°$.

$\delta\xi_{i+1} = 2\,\delta\xi_i$, $\delta\xi_i = 2^i\,\delta\xi_0 = e^{(ln2)i}\,\delta\xi_0$,   (3.12a)

$(\delta\xi_{i+1}/\xi_{i+1}) = (\delta\xi_i/\xi_i) = (\delta\xi_0/\xi_0)$.   (3.12b)

Since the value itself also grows exponentially, the *relative* uncertainty remains the same. For this reason, uncertainty does not play a central role with the usual exponential growth; see (3a&b). However, if we substitute back into the original equation, we get a different picture (see Figure 3.4). While the ξ-values and their uncertainty are doubled from one step to the next, the x-values and their uncertainty are bounded by the $\sin^2$ function, i.e. they lie between 0 and 1. The uncertainty eventually reaches the entire set of values. As can be seen from Figure 3.4, the uncertainty traverses an entire $\sin^2$ period after just a few steps, and thus the original knowledge regarding ξ is completely lost. Only knowing the initial value exactly (and performing the computation exactly) removes all problems with predicting future values. However, precision would require an infinitely exact knowledge, which is unrealistic. An initial uncertainty, no matter how small, results in the impossibility of long-term predictions (see the grey rectangles). One could argue that we chose a relative large uncertainty $\delta\xi_o$ in Figure 3.4 for graphical reasons. This is true. The smaller the initial uncertainty, the longer the period of predictability. Due to the exponential growth, the gain, however, is negligible. When certainty of ξ_o is doubled, the predictability is only extended by 1 step, e.g. from 17 to 18 steps.

Thus, the bottom line is this: We have just seen how a completely deterministic relationship, which can even be solved explicitly, can result in chaos.

Chapter 4

Systemic View II:
Self-Organisation and Chaos Control

4.1. Processes of Self-Organisation

Graphic representation of complex processes in general, and fractals in particular, necessitate sophisticated computer software, which only became available fairly recently. The use of a computer is necessary for calculating formulae as well as for the graphic representation of the results. Although it can neither recognise nor interpret these phenomena, the computer is indispensable as a tool for making new discoveries. Dealing with computer graphics, incidentally, has also led us to take a closer look at the human visual system (optical illusions, ambiguous images). It turns out that seeing is not a passive but an active, constructive and self-organising process. It is accompanied by subconscious assumptions, such as the direction, from which the light emanates (constructivist aspect, perspective P3). In this process, a complete and consistent image is produced from limited information, with a three-dimensional image from a two-dimensional picture. Strictly speaking, this is an optical illusion. We do not perceive it as such, because it leads to a 'correct' impression.

The above considerations also apply to this book (and every other). An information bottleneck between sender and receiver occurs because of many factors (cf. *The Tree of Talking*: Norretranders 1997, Ch. 5). In the process of writing a book, a great deal must be left out. In addition, the receiver reduces the amount of information by way of selection and pre-processing and replaces it with his own knowledge (Vester 2002, p.22f). You, dear reader, are trying with the aid of your prior knowledge and world view (as well as assumptions about my prior knowledge and world view) to make this text into a coherent whole and are trying to reconstruct my original thoughts as closely as possible, which, of course, can never completely succeed (P3). If we then ask what statements the individual chapters contain, we must expect a variety of answers.

We are surrounded by processes and modes of behaviour, which demonstrate certain recurring patterns but, nonetheless, always harbour surprises in the concrete case. Examples include human behaviour, the progression of falling ill and convalescence, and the weather.

Comparatively small influences such as solar flares millions of miles away can change the weather on earth in wide areas. So why else is forecasting the weather so difficult? Does randomness play a role here? The phenomenon of weather as a whole is indeed rather confusing. Nevertheless, for this very reason, it is interesting that studying simple weather phenomena can lead to profound insights. Lorenz (1963) investigated such a phenomenon and as a result became the father of chaos research. That is to say he found chaotic (he called them non-periodic) solutions to deterministic equations. These equations do not depend on chance. We will discuss this system of equations, which, incidentally, is continuous in time, in more detail later. Lorenz's research allows us to conclude that weather can be unpredictable in the long run, even if chance plays no role at all. Similar phenomena keep repeating (high and low pressure, thunderstorms, etc.). Nevertheless, in the medium or long run, it cannot be predicted where and when such phenomena will recur and with what intensity. Predictions are limited to a few days, because the uncertainties – depending on the values of the parameters – can build up exponentially. It is no wonder, then, that meteorology is a crucial root of chaos research.

The bottom line of Lorenz's research is often formulated as the *butterfly effect*. One of the many versions runs as follows: If a butterfly beats its wings in the Vienna Woods, perhaps in a different manner from the usual, it can produce a change which, after a few days, can cause (or prevent) a hurricane in the Caribbean. The butterfly is quite unaware of what it can provoke, but there are also many other butterflies which can cancel out the effects of the first. Deterministic chaos, then, has a great deal to do with instability. As long as everything is stable, everything has its 'order'. Whenever instabilities arise, very small disturbances or changes can have very large effects. This, of course, does not only apply to butterflies. This paradoxical view of being able to produce a very small effect and, at the same time, a very large one without even being aware of a connection between cause and effect, applies to each and every one of us. By just putting one foot wrong, we might have got into great mischief somewhere in the world without knowing it. Even so, we do not need to worry about that, because there is someone, somewhere, who can cancel out our action again, also with very small influences and without his being aware of it. This is the strange world view to which chaos research and systems approach has brought us. It corresponds to perspective P2, "everything is connected with everything else." (cf. Ch. 2.1) The question then is: Is it easier or harder to control chaotic processes because of that? We shall come back to this in Ch. 4.3.

As we have already mentioned, chaos does not deal with randomness – not for dogmatic reasons but on a provisional basis: one tries to get along without it. Chaotic processes become unpredictable so quickly that they practically cannot be distinguished from randomness. Thus, with deterministic equations we are able to follow processes that seem to be random. Quantum mechanics takes the reverse approach: randomness is central here. For this reason, it has to explain why there is, in addition, so much order in our macroscopic surroundings. Chaos research compared to quantum mechanics is narrower in one sense and broader in another – it is not related to indeterminacy. In other words, all values can be determined with arbitrary precision. On the other hand, this does not help at all, since an arbitrarily small imprecision can destroy predictability. Thus, within the scope of chaos research – as opposed to quantum physics – Laplace's demon is still alive, though toothless. As long as he knows the universe exactly in all its details, he can predict the future exactly (*weak* causality). We used to conclude from this that if we knew the present fairly well but not exactly, we would be able to predict the future fairly well, though not exactly (*strong* causality). However, this is just what is not true for chaotic processes. Incidentally, quantum theory also utilises P2, even postulating non-local connections. Thus, both theories leave the classical/scientific perspective (P1) behind, which is connected to many questions of comprehension.

4.2. Difficulty in Forecasting the Weather

Equations and/or systems of equations which are *discrete* in time (discontinuous, step by step) or *continuous*, can be used for modelling processes. One example of the first type is the logistic equation, which was addressed in Ch.3, see (3.4). An example of the second type (differential equations) is the Lorenz equations (4.1a-c), which we shall now discuss in detail. Differential equations relate to a state at a time t (e.g. of the variables x, y and z) and specify its instantaneous velocity of change with respect to time (symbolised by dx/dt, dy/dt and dz/dt). If the correspondence between the two representations spurred your interest, we refer you to Ch.3.4, especially (3.8). It needs to be pointed out that the computer transforms continuous systems of equations into discrete systems and solves them as such. This is not without problems however, as the chaotic case in particular demonstrates (see below).

Let us move on now to the Lorenz equations, which also show the connection between chaos and fractals, among other things. This system of equations models the meteorological phenomenon of air coils (cloud streets). Whenever a layer of air has a higher temperature (T_+) at its lower edge than at its higher edge (T_-), a collective circular motion in form of air coils can develop once a critical temperature difference, $\Delta T = T_+ - T_-$, has been reached, which can result in air tubes many kilometres in length. One coil is located next to another; neighbouring coils always turn in opposite directions so that they experience as little friction as possible. (This type of movement can be demonstrated if a container of fluid is heated from the bottom, resulting in fluid coils that can be observed.) Lorenz studied the behaviour of one such coil with the aid of the equations which were named after him and which represent a milestone (unacknowledged for many years) on the path to chaos theory. They are three coupled differential equations, which represent a stark simplification of the real situation but, nonetheless, can make relevant statements. From the current state (values of the variables at time t), the velocity of the change of the variables, e.g. dx/dt, can be calculated:

$$dx / dt = -\sigma x + \sigma y, \tag{4.1a}$$
$$dy / dt = -\underline{xz} + rx - y, \tag{4.1b}$$
$$dz / dt = \underline{xy} - bz. \tag{4.1c}$$

x, y and z are linked *variables*, where x represents the coil's velocity of rotation, e.g. x>0: clockwise, x<0: counter-clockwise, x=0: no rotation (and no coil). The variables y and z make statements about the distribution of temperature within the coil in the horizontal and vertical direction, respectively (see Kratky 1992). The terms on the left side are so-called *differential quotients*. On the right side, we have two non-linear terms – the underlined products $\underline{xz}$ and $\underline{xy}$. The three parameters σ, b, and r represent characteristics of the air. Usually $\sigma = 10$ and $b = (8/3)$, which we will assume from now on. The *control parameter* r is proportional to the temperature difference ΔT between the upper and lower edge and scaled in such a manner that its critical value is $r = 1$ (for higher values of r, coil formation x deviates from zero). r is chosen arbitrarily and remains constant throughout the calculations, or is varied so slowly that the system has enough time to adapt to the change. In order to study the behaviour of the variables over time independent of the selected r, this system of equations must be solved numerically with the aid of a computer. On the other hand, the following fixed-point solutions can be calculated analytically. They are stable in the corresponding ranges for r – in other words, they represent *fixed-point attractors*:

$$0 \le r < 1: \quad \mathbf{x}^{\#}: \ x^{\#} = y^{\#} = z^{\#} = 0 \qquad \text{(only thermal conductance)}, \qquad (4.2a)$$

$$1 \le r < 24.7: \ \mathbf{x}^{*}_{\pm}: \ x^{*}_{\pm} = y^{*}_{\pm} = \pm[(8/3)\,z^{*}_{\pm}]^{1/2}, \ z^{*}_{\pm} = r - 1 \qquad \text{(convection)}, \qquad (4.2b)$$

the power ½ meaning the square root. For $r < 1$, (4.2a), every disturbance in air layer is damped until the air, from a macroscopic standpoint, comes to rest again. This is the trivial fixed point $\mathbf{x}^{\#} = \mathbf{0}$ (vector notation, $\mathbf{x}$ contains all three coordinates x, y and z). This fixed point is, incidentally, also stable for $r < 0$, representing the case of the temperature being lower at the lower edge than at the upper edge ($\Delta T < 0$). Now, the 'natural place' for warmer air is up – just think about high rooms in winter, where the temperature at ceiling level is warm or even hot, while the temperature at floor level is cool. This distribution of temperature is then further supported or stabilised by $\Delta T < 0$ ($r < 0$). Only the opposite case, $r > 0$, affords the possibility of instability, where two opposite tendencies are in competition with each other. In the following, we return to this case, especially to the critical value $r = 1$.

At $r = 1$, the system tips over and the trivial fixed point $\mathbf{x}^{\#}$, (4.2a) becomes unstable. From then on, the coil starts to move, (4.2b), namely with the two mutually symmetrical solutions $\mathbf{x}^{*}_{\pm}$ (clockwise or counter-clockwise movement). One also speaks of a *bifurcation* (forking) and a *break in symmetry* connected with it. Seen from the symmetry of the real system or the Lorenz equations, no rotational direction is specified. As r increases, $r > 1$, so does the rotational velocity. The initial value [x(t=0), y(t=0), z(t=0)] determines to which of the two fixed-point attractors the trajectory will tend. Thus, each of the two fixed points has its own basin of attraction. The movement in this abstract three-dimensional space (state or phase space of the variables x, y, z) must be distinguished from the directly visible movement of the coil in regular space. Every point (x, y, z) corresponds to a certain rotational velocity and temperature distribution of the coil in regular space. Movement towards a fixed point corresponds to the development of a coil rotating with constant velocity.

Now let us look at the transition from thermal conductance (4.2a) to convection (4.2b) near $r = 1$. First the system is at the fixed point $\mathbf{x}^{\#}$. This fixed point becomes unstable as r grows beyond $r = 1$. To which one of the fixed points $\mathbf{x}^{*}_{\pm}$ will the system go (clockwise or counter-clockwise rotation)? Alternatively, will it stay at the now unstable fixed point? You could say 'it is down to chance'. A more precise argument would be to point out that the Lorenz equations represent a simplification of the real situation. Simplification does play a role just when one is considering a critical point. Thus, a disregarded bumblebee flying counter-clockwise can cause this huge air formation to follow its lead. These things can happen at or very near such a point of instability, where tiny causes can have huge effects (in chaos, which links stability with instability, this occurs again in a complex fashion, see below). If r now keeps increasing slowly, the coil will turn faster and faster but will no longer change its rotational direction by itself (stability). To achieve this one would have to have a great influence on the system, e.g. with huge rotors.

From $r=24.7$ on these coils, too, become unstable, cf. (4.2b). Due to non-linearity chaos comes back, starting with $r=24.7$. Thus, for $24.1 < r < 24.7$ there are three attractors (two fixed points; chaos) with their respective basins of attraction. All this from these rather simple equations! In contradistinction to the discontinuous case, where one single equation suffices (an example was given in Ch.3.2: the logistic equation), three coupled differential equations are necessary for chaos to appear, which is the case for the Lorenz equations. What is especially remarkable is the co-existence of several attractors. This is not the case for the logistic equation, but it can also occur in the video feedback situation, which has already been mentioned. Depending on the initial conditions, different patterns emerge with the camera remaining in a fixed position. This is also interesting as a metaphor for medicine. One could interpret the various attractors as different healthy or unhealthy modes of behaviour. Then it would not be necessary to change an ill person (his 'system of equations') in order for him to get well. We only have to get him to move towards the 'right' attractor by means of a suitable stimulus, which would also allow treatment by a nonspecific therapy, maybe several times, until the right 'basin of attraction' is reached.

Another model for therapeutic intervention represents changing a parameter that determines human behaviour. Let us again consult the Lorenz equations. The control parameter r can be seen as a knob, wheel or a joystick, with which one can change the system and thus its dynamics, and work out different modes of behaviour. The system of equations itself remains the same. The only thing changed is the intersection of the system and the external world, which is represented by control parameters (generally more than one). In the case of air coils, r is determined by the sun's radiation. Of course, in practice, the air coils themselves affect the temperature difference ΔT and thus r, since convection causes the heat to rise more rapidly. This feedback effect is neglected in the Lorenz equations. We would need an additional differential equation for r, which would turn r from a parameter into a variable. This additional equation, however, would contain a new parameter, which takes into account solar radiation, etc. In any case, solar radiation as the single external influence determines the system's behaviour, more precisely the range of behaviour. Changing the equations themselves would correspond to a massive external intervention (e.g. a large-scale propeller use to change air movement), resembling some practices in orthodox Western medicine. However, there is another rather elegant way of influencing the system, which we shall address in this chapter – and that is chaos control.

Remaining with the Lorenz equations for now, it is interesting to see how simple scanning $0 \leq r < \infty$ leads to a complex succession of modes of behaviour (cf. Bergé et al. 1986, pp.308-312; Kratky 1992). It results in a succession, and sometimes coexistence, of non-chaotic and chaotic attractors. The relationship between r and this behaviour is difficult to fathom and does not correspond to a direct cause/ effect correlation. It rather resembles self-organisation initiated or triggered by external influences. Thus, even chaos, which arises for certain values of r, is a phenomenon of self-organisation and not contrary to it. Finally, we should point out that chaos does not come about for small values of the parameter (r<24.1) and for very large values (r>214.4). This can be interpreted to mean that *resonance*, which leads small causes to a build up to large effects, only comes about with medium external influences. The system is able to counter-balance small influences, so to speak, but it cannot keep up with larger influences. This resembles common resonance phenomena in physics.

Let us take a closer look at the dynamics for r=28. At this oft-regarded value, there is only one chaotic or strange attractor, the Lorenz attractor. Except for the three now unstable fixed points of (4.2a&b), every initial value leads to this global attractor. It depends on the representation, however, whether you recognise it or not. If we look at Figure 4.1, we see that it shows a typical timeline for r=28, where the variable x(t) is observed. There is a going back and forth, which is different each time but similar. A closer look reveals that these are pendulum-like movements around x_+^* and x_-^*, which correspond to the x-values of the unstable fixed points $\mathbf{x}_+^*$ and $\mathbf{x}_-^*$. One of the fixed points repels the trajectory until it nears the other and is repelled again by it. In real space, this looks like a coil turning clockwise, which wobbles more and more and then topples into a coil turning counter-clockwise. You could set up a game of fortune and bet on how many rotations the coil goes through before it topples back again. No randomness is built into the equations; it is a case of chaos. In any case, everything looks rather unmanageable, also with regard to predictability. For this reason, the weather forecast is unsuccessful even in this restricted area, although r is fixed and random-ness does not come into play. Similar processes keep on in a similar manner, albeit only in the short run.

The dynamics can also be represented in a very different way, namely as a trajectory in three-dimensional phase or state space, Figure 4.2. This graph represents an extended piece of the trajectory after the transient phase – in other words, the long-term behaviour. The geometric shape of the attractor, which draws in all trajectories, is clearly recognisable. It looks like two records turning in opposite directions, whose centres are the two fixed points $\mathbf{x}_+^*$ of (4.2b). Every point (x,y,z) corresponds to a certain rotational velocity and temperature distribution of the coil in regular space. The dynamics is represented by the small arrows. The attractor appears to be plane-like (D=2), but closer analysis by zooming in on the attractor reveals that every assumed piece of curve splits into closely neighbouring finer pieces of curve. Finally, a fractal results since chaotic attractors in general are fractals. The Lorenz attractor, incidentally, has with D=2.06 (Bergé et al. 1986, p.126) a negligibly higher dimen-sion than a plane.

Because of D<3 the attractor has a volume of V=0 in three-dimensional phase space. A point chosen arbitrarily within a cube of phase space including the attractor would land on the attractor with probability zero. This means that from this standpoint we know *a great deal* about the behaviour of the system by knowing the attractor. The representations of Figures 4.1 & 4.2 disclose two complementary standpoints on the dynamics of the Lorenz equations. Different systems of equations exhibit different chaotic attractors, which can be aesthetically very pleasing. We see nothing of 'randomness' and 'disorder', which are often associated with chaos, in this perspective; it is more like a clever and sophisticated order. Graphics representing complex processes have even won prizes in artistic events and art shows. It is something that speaks to us, probably because we see something of ourselves in it, because all the processes inside us presumably also have a chaotic element. For this reason, the irregularity of a babbling brook is much more pleasant than, for example, the regular ticking of a clock.

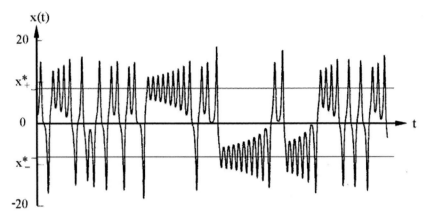

Figure 4.1. Dynamics of Lorenz equations (r=28). Chaotic time sequence of x(t). Figures 4.1 & 4.2 are based on Bergé et al. (1986, p.124f).

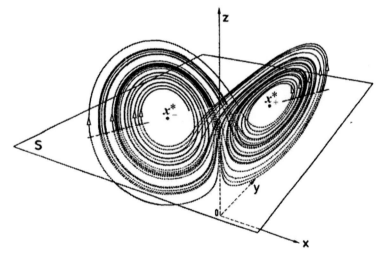

Figure 4.2. Lorenz attractor in three-dimensional phase space, (x, y, z), with r=28. Trajectory over a lengthy period of time, the direction of movement is indicated by arrows. The intersecting plane S is characterised by z=r−1=27. It contains the two fixed points, cf. (4.2b). They are represented in vector notation as x_+^* and x_-^*.

The computer plays an ambivalent role in finding chaotic solutions to systems of equations. On the one hand, it is necessary for making calculations but on the other, different computers turn out different representations in the long run (as in the case of Figure 4.1) because every computer works a little differently from every other computer (e.g. the number of decimal places or rounding rules). Especially in chaotic solutions, the smallest differences will eventually lead to large discrepancies (where there is no certainty of whether the coil is 'actually' turning clockwise right now). In the representation shown in Figure 4.2, however, everything is again consistent: the same attractor results with great precision. However, it was precisely the effect of differences in representation due to rounding shown in Figure 4.1, which led Lorenz to the discovery of chaos.

There is another reason, which we have already mentioned, why the computer does not calculate exactly. It turns differential equations into discrete equations with respect to time. Additionally, due to the finite decimal representation, the values themselves become discrete – in other words, there is only a finite number of values available. Starting at an arbitrary point in time the computer, for example, in solving the Lorenz equations (4.1a-c), inevitably comes to the same combination of x, y, z after a very long time. Since the equations and the manner of computation are the same, the trajectory also continues in the same fashion – that is to say, it is a matter of periodic movement. The computer that we draw on for calculating chaotic movement is, strictly speaking, not able to yield chaos at all! In practice, however, these 'artificial' periods are of such a length that they do not stand out. In the representation of Figure 4.2, this looks like a periodic attractor, which is very similar to the Lorenz attractor, but the trajectory closes in on itself after many revolutions, which is not the case with a chaotic attractor.

Now let us come back to the discussion from Ch. 2.3 of how to interpret, from a modern standpoint, the four causes described by Aristotle. A few statements to this effect can be made which also allow inclusion of the various perspectives P1-P4 with the aid of the Lorenz equations. To start with, equations express – as is customary in the sciences – the causa effi- ciens (P1, Table 2.1a&b). However, due to the coupled (feedback) equations, a connected- ness of all parts is also expressed. The expression connected to P2, 'everything is connected to everything else and moves in cycles', fits in very well here. This connection is represented by the air molecules and their interactions. Mutually completely independent particles could not form matter, as we know it. In this respect, P2 relates to causa materialis. On the other hand, what generates the form of the cloud streets (causa formalis)? It is the fact that the tem- perature of the lower layer is higher than that of the upper layer. This can be found in the pa- rameter r, which provides the framework for the formation of structure. One could also consider it part of the boundary conditions. There is a connection to P3 in the sense that although r belongs to the system of equations, it actually (also) represents the effect of the surroundings on the system.

The question remains as to whether there is also a goal (causa *finalis*). While the causa efficiens drives or *pushes* a development from a given starting point to a future further and further away, the causa finalis *pulls* a state to a desired future. The Lorenz equations enable both possibilities, which are reflected in Figures.4.1 & 4.2. Applying the equations (causa efficiens) results in the system being drawn into the Lorenz attractor (causa finalis). Names and terms such as 'attractor' can be somewhat treacherous, since they suggest movement towards a final goal. Indeed, Newton was held in low esteem by his continental European colleagues for using the term 'attraction' for gravity.

Even the Lorenz equations themselves offer two interpretations, if one considers them not as a causal relationship but as a description of a succession of events. How do the variables change depending on their momentary values? Calculating from a starting point into the future is only *one* possibility, even if it is the more common. However, we can just as well use them to compute the past. The collapsing of equations and their application or interpretation and questions of reversibility of time are very interesting topics, which are examined by Coveney & Highfield (1994).

It should also be mentioned that the term 'collective phenomena' within the frame of self-organisation hints at P4. A single air coil does not just behave as if it was monolithic, but in chaos it also changes rotational direction together with the other coils as if moved by a ghostly hand. In the end, this can all be led back to basic physical equations. However, perspectives do not concern themselves with true or false but with fitting or not fitting.

Incidentally, a few years ago the end of the butterfly effect was announced somewhat prematurely (Robert 2001). Far more complicated weather models than Lorenz used were computed, which did not, on the whole, result in chaos. However, the author could not be pinned down on the question of the long-term predictability of weather. Another critique can be found in Wehr (2002). A great deal could be said about this but we shall limit our comments to the following. Even if we assume that the weather is never (or rarely) chaotic in a strict mathematical sense, this cannot do much to the butterfly effect. It is primarily a symbol, a metaphor for the possibilities that have been disclosed by chaos research. Just as it has often been 'proven' that Columbus was not the first to set foot in America (of course not, since the native Indians were already there), nevertheless he is still considered the discoverer of America – as a (also questionable) symbol for the strength of Western civilisation, which could discover and conquer new continents.

From one perspective, perhaps, the weather is not quite as chaotic as has been assumed. On the other hand, however, it seems more and more that the solar system – which has often been considered to be like clockwork and capable of being predicted arbitrarily far into the future – also has chaotic elements (Lecar et al. 2001). These chaotic processes, however, play out in a time frame that should not unduly concern us. After all, we have the moon, which stabilises the earth's axis, to thank for life on earth (Laskar et al. 1993).

4.3. Chaos Control and Stochastic Resonance

Let us now focus our attention on chaos control, which we have already mentioned briefly. For this, we shall look at the stability of chaotic attractors. For discrete representations it was the Lyapunov exponent λ that indicated (in)stability: For $\lambda > 0$, we observed exponential growth, for $\lambda < 0$ exponential *damping* of errors, disturbances or inaccuracies during the course of time; see (3.3b) & (3.12a). For *differential* equations, Lyapunov exponents can be defined in an analogous manner. In a system of three coupled equations, e.g. (4.1a-c), there are three such exponents characterising (in)stability. For chaotic trajectories the largest exponent λ_+ is greater than zero:

$$\lambda_+ > 0, \quad \lambda_o = 0, \quad \lambda_- < 0. \tag{4.3}$$

It is this positive exponent that causes two neighbouring initial values to be dispersed. It expresses the unstable component of chaos. More information on this and other exponents can be found in Ch. 4.4. The connection between Lyapunov exponents and fractal dimensions of chaotic attractors is also explained there. For periodic attractors, incidentally, the largest exponent is zero, and for fixed-point attractors less than zero.

Now, the question arises by what means unstable fixed points or periodic trajectories – possibly at the expense of a chaotic attractor – can be stabilised. We talk about controlling complex systems, in the latter case of chaos control. We shall examine this now for continuous systems of equations such as the Lorenz equations (4.4a-c), (cf. also Kratky 1995b, 1996a&b). Our goal is to stabilise periodic trajectories, since these are hidden in chaotic attractors. If we look at Figure 4.2, we see that the Lorenz attractor closely resembles a closed eight, likewise a loop which leads back into itself after *two* eights etc. Closed trajectories correspond to periodic orbits. It is our goal now to stabilise these and analyse the hidden behaviour of the system at hand. Pyragas (1992), one of the pioneers of chaos control, augmented, for example, the second Lorenz equation (4.1b) by the additional term, F(t), the other two equations remained the same:

$$dy/dt = -xz + rx - y + F(t), \quad \text{with} \tag{4.4a}$$
$$F(t) = L[y_i(t) - y(t)] \quad \text{or} \tag{4.4b}$$
$$F(t) = K[y(t-\tau_i) - y(t)]. \tag{4.4c}$$

The two versions stated are called *external force control* (4.4b) and *delayed feedback control* (4.4c). K and L are constants and $y_i(t)$ is the y-component of the ith periodic orbit, which remains hidden at first. In the first version, it must be given externally in order to produce it in the system. The second version is more elegant. In (4.4c) the difference between the value before an orbit and the present value is used. No knowledge about $y_i(t)$ is necessary. τ_i can be deduced from the chaotic behaviour: it is a good approximation of the time elapsed, in which the chaotic trajectory almost returns to itself (τ_1: the mentioned eight, $\tau_2 \approx 2\tau_1$: a double eight, etc.). The stabilising K-region must be found empirically. K must not be too small but also not too large. It is like walking a tightrope. The counter-balance must not be too much or too little. Whenever the control is successful, F(t) rapidly becomes negligibly small, and the periodic orbit can be held stable with very little effort. We should also mention here that, in the meantime, several new developments regarding 'delayed feedback control' have taken place, see Pyragas (2006). An overview of the possibilities of chaos control can be found in Schuster (1999).

What is remarkable is that chaos control works at all and with comparatively little effort. Chaos makes medium- to long-term predictions impossible. A mere bystander to these processes does not stand a chance. Particularly due to their sensitivity to small disturbances, these systems can be controlled very well as long as the intervention is suitable. With 'delayed feedback control', the system is led back into itself and stabilises by itself. All that is needed is finding suitable τ's and the range of K. This assumption suggests that regulative or control processes in the organism behave in a similar fashion: quickly, intelligently and with little effort. In this case, it may even be advantageous for the underlying processes to be chaotic. Whenever physiological processes have been studied in the last 30 years under the aspect of chaos research, it comes as a surprise to find chaos cropping up again and again (West 1990, Goldbeter 1997). This was surprising inasmuch as chaos had always been associated not only with flexibility but also with unpredictability. Under the aspect of controllability, this subject takes on a different meaning.

Many processes are chaotic or nearly chaotic in an organism. Therefore, we must be able to control instabilities. We are like tightrope walkers, so to speak, who keep themselves on the tightrope with little effort. As a matter of fact, the effort *must* be minimal or we would fall. Life, then, is very uncertain and dangerous, but it enables us to control many processes with little expenditure of energy. As soon as it was clear that chaos is essential, the electrocardiogram (ECG), the electroencephalogram (EEG), hormone fluctuations and so on were investigated. This led to the discovery of almost universal fluctuations of a more or less irregular nature. It was also discovered that in some cases it was not the mean value of a variable, not even the range of fluctuations but the type of fluctuation process that was important for diagnostic purposes. The mean values (for example, of hormone levels) and even the range of fluctuation can be normal, but an excessive periodic movement can nevertheless be a sign of illness.

We can take as an example osteoporosis, which mainly affects women after the menopause. As far as can be analysed mathematically, the blood levels of parathyroid hormone, as well as the calcium which it regulates, fluctuate in a chaotic fashion (Kriz 1997, Ch. 5.1). Osteoporosis can be correlated to a situation when the parathyroid hormone is no longer fluctuating chaotically enough – calcium is then leeched from the bones or can no longer be embedded in sufficient amounts (in Ch. 11, we will look at this example again from the aspect of chronomedicine). Thus, for an accurate diagnosis, one would have to determine a time sequence. Frequent measuring is, of course, difficult when it comes to hormones. On the other hand, it can be done easily with electroencephalograms and electrocardiograms. There is one more development we should mention. In principle, it is possible to reconstruct the dynamics of the entire system from a single time sequence – in the case of an electro-encephalogram, for example, from a single encephalogram derivative. In case of the air, coil knowing the rotational velocity of the coil, $x(t)$, suffices for reconstructing the three-dimensional Lorenz attractor. In the same manner, it is possible to reconstruct a higher dimensional attractor from the one-dimensional electrocardiogram (Morfill & Scheingraber 1991, Ch. II.4).

The idea is to extrapolate the behaviour of the entire system from knowing a small part of it. For example, if something goes wrong within a family and communication goes awry, then it suffices to observe a *single* family member in a natural family setting. Without knowing what the others are doing, one could get a good idea about the idiosyncrasies of a family system. The observed component must, however, not be separated from the system. If, for example, a child is observed apart from its family situation, it will not exhibit its usual modes of behaviour. However, if one leaves the part embedded in the whole, then it should be possible to reconstruct the entire situation by means of this small part. This is a programme implemented again and again in the research of complex systems. This example also has an impact on medicine. For example, a doctor may look only at the liver and its function within the whole body. With this knowledge, he can then gauge in principle how the other functions of the organism are performing. If seen in this light, orthodox Western medicine, which only examines one part, in principle can become holistic medicine.

In conclusion, we shall look at one more interesting aspect of complex systems – stochastic resonance (Hänggi 2001). This deals with how disturbances (fluctuations, noise) influence signal perception. It seems evident that such an influence can only be negative. For this reason, an attempt is made in technology, for example, to suppress noise as much as possible. The phenomenon of stochastic resonance, however, deals with the fact that the noise itself improves signal perception in certain cases. This means it is advantageous to increase noise whenever it is too low! A comprehensive, partly also mathematical description can be found in Moss (1994). But let us look at the example of an egg carton, modelled after Hänggi (2001), where a ball is lying in one of the depressions. If we do not hold this egg carton exactly level but rock it slowly a little to one side then the other, the ball will remain in the same depression and only move about a bit at the bottom of this depression. If the egg carton is jiggled in addition, the ball might pop into a neighbouring depression.

The expression 'resonance' refers to the fact that there is an optimal jiggling intensity, in which the duration of oscillation to and fro of the egg carton is transferred to the time span that elapses between two transitions (popping into a neighbouring depression). If the jiggling subsides, there are no transitions, with rigorous jiggling the ball jumps around a lot, but this has nothing to do with the gentle rocking motion. Thus, weak oscillations can be strengthened in a certain sense by optimal noise. In the biological field, the surprisingly capable sense organs are good candidates for stochastic resonance, such as the human ear, which can perceive lower noises than it 'should be able to'. For us, the positive aspect of noise will play a role in maintaining health (Ch. 13.3). Thus, chaos control as well as stochastic resonance are utilised by the organism in order to sustain its functioning.

The question is, of course, where does the noise come from? The expression 'stochastics' refers to random processes, which brings us back to the question of chance and randomness, cf. Freund & Pöschel (2001). The field of tension of randomness and chaos is treated in detail by Ruelle (1993). He speaks of deterministic noise, a seeming randomness produced by chaotic processes. Indeed, there is a mathematically polished theory on treating random processes, but a concrete case is impossible to prove to be 'true' randomness. At the most, one can assert that the series of events at hand pass the corresponding tests. At the end of his contribution, Moss (1994) addresses the question as to whether there is also something like chaotic resonance. This question has since been answered positively (see Reibold et al. 1999). Thus, randomness is not needed for this effect either.

4.4.* More on Predicting Complex Systems

First, we shall take a closer look at the stability of chaotic attractors in three-dimensional phase space, for reasons of simplicity, because they connect stability to instability. Let us imagine an arbitrary point, $P(0)$, on the attractor at a certain time, $t=0$. Let this point be the centre of a very small, imagined sphere (cloud of points in the form of a sphere) with radius $\rho(0)$. Due to the dynamics, the centre P as well as any other point of the sphere will move and, after a short time, will form an ellipsoid (with centre P). This ellipsoid then keeps moving not only in phase space but also turns with respect to the fixed axes of the variables x, y and z. The ellipsoid is characterised by three so-called *eigenvectors* (radii ρ_+, ρ_o, ρ_-), which make statements about stability and instability. In the direction of the trajectory (groove of the record, see Figure 4.2), the length (ρ_o) does not change in essence. Across the trajectory, however, within the attractor (across the groove but *on* the record) an expansion (ρ_+) in the form of exponential growth (instability) can be observed. The transverse direction perpendicular to the attractor (on the record) results in a contraction (ρ_-, exponential shrinking, i.e. stability). This can be described formally by three Lyapunov exponents, λ_+ (expansion), λ_o (along the trajectory) and λ_- (compression):

$$\rho_+(t) = \rho(0)\, e^{\lambda_+ t}, \ \rho_o(t) = \rho(0)\, e^{\lambda_o t}, \ \rho_-(t) = \rho(0)\, e^{\lambda_- t}; \tag{4.5a}$$

$$\text{with } \lambda_+ > 0, \ \lambda_o = 0, \ \lambda_- < 0; \ \lambda_+ + \lambda_o + \lambda_- < 0. \tag{4.5b}$$

The Lyapunov exponents are to be seen as analogous to (3.2) and (3.3b), where we considered them for the one-dimensional discontinuous case. All in all, compression (stability) outweighs expansion (instability) and the total volume of the ellipsoid gets smaller and smaller (dissipative or irreversible system). Thus, the expression *attractor* is justified. Points lying outside the attractor are drawn into it, but inside the attractor two neighbouring points will repel each other exponentially due to $\lambda_+ > 0$ – as long as they do not lie exactly along the trajectory, which is arbitrarily improbable. Thus, small inaccuracies build up ('small cause – large effect').

Figure 4.1 shows a picture of the dynamics. Including also y and z will result in all Lyapunov exponents λ_+, λ_o and λ_- – Figure 4.2 (without arrows) shows the attractor with the fractal dimension D; a static, 'frozen' picture. Only movement along the trajectory (the direction marked by the arrows) combines statistics and dynamics. For three variables (for example, the Lorenz equations) the connection between the 'static' dimension D and the dynamic Lyapunov dimension D_L is given by:

$$\text{General case:} \quad D \cong D_L = 2 + [\lambda_+ / |\lambda_-|]; \ \text{due to (4.5b): } 2 < D < 3; \tag{4.6a}$$

$$\text{Lorenz, r=28:} \quad D = 2.06, \ \lambda_+ + \lambda_o + \lambda_- = -41/3, \ \text{thus: } \lambda_+ \cong 0.9, \ \lambda_- \cong -14.5; \tag{4.6b}$$

see Leven et al. (1994, p.111) concerning the formula for D_L. Because $\lambda_+ > 0$ (chaos), D is greater than 2, because $\lambda_+ < |\lambda_-|$ (stability outweighs instability) D is less than 3. Thus, the chaotic attractor is also fractal. In general we can say that for a fixed-point attractor (D=0) all Lyapunov exponents are negative. For a periodic attractor (a closed finite curve, D=1) one of the Lyapunov exponents, the one along the curve, is zero; all others are negative. For more information see Leven et al. (1994, p.73). For a periodic attractor (D>2, generally fractal) there is at least one positive exponent and the sum of all exponents is negative; cf. (4.6b). The negative sum applies, of course, especially to fixed-point attractors and periodic attractors.

Chapter 5

Homoeopathy and Related Methods

5.1. Arndt-Schulz Law and Simile Principle

In this chapter we shall introduce the principles of homoeopathy and relate them to the other chapters. Figure 5.1a shows a particular type of dose/ effect relationship, which is called hormesis (Calabrese 2008) or dose dependent *reverse effect* (Linde 1991). We can take as an example a medication that, if taken in small but steadily increasing doses, will lower the blood pressure with increasing effect. If the dosage is raised still more, however, the effect decreases, drops to zero and, after this, further increases in dosage actually cause the blood pressure to *rise*. Such a possibility is usually not considered. It does not fit in with our linear world view of proportional relationships between dosage and effect (the straight line in Figure 5.1a). The presumed linearity, however, extrapolated from well-researched high doses to low doses, overlooks the region of low doses, where the medication has an opposite effect. Hormesis is not an exotic case but occurs frequently (Oberbaum & Cambar 1994). There are individuals who find that drinking a weak cup of coffee will help them to sleep but strong coffee will keep them awake. One cannot claim that coffee acts just in one direction. There are also individually different (type-specific) effects or dose/ effect relationships. This opens up new possibilities.

The so-called Arndt-Schulz Law fits in with hormesis, and one version states the following: Therapies (interventions, medications, treatments) are stimulating (strengthening, promoting) in small doses, no longer have a promoting effect in medium doses, are weakening in higher doses and in large doses even suppress the organism. Acupuncture is subject to this law as well, which should actually be called a rule. Acupuncture points can be tonified (stimulated) or sedated (calmed) as necessary. Gentle needle stimuli have a stimulating effect, vigorous stimuli a damping effect. If one is not careful in the second case and stimulates too vigorously, it can lead to a collapse. Stimuli that are too strong suppress biological activity. (The basic terms outlined here such as hormesis and Arndt-Schulz Law are summarised in Table 5.1 to enable an overview).

Examining the time/ effect relationship is also interesting (Figure 5.1b). A therapeutic intervention can have a positive effect in the short run but have adverse effects in the long run (or vice versa). Thus, whether an effect goes in one direction or the other also depends on which point in time one refers to. In homoeopathy, such a temporary reverse effect is known as initial aggravation, which is followed by improvement of the condition after hours or days. Some homoeopaths believe that an optimal treatment avoids this initial worsening. Others welcome it because it is a strong indication that the correct remedy has been prescribed. The successes of orthodox Western Medicine, which often lie in treating acute conditions, can be seen as producing an initial improvement. However, if the treatment does not incorporate other strategies in the long run, taking the same medication over a long period of time can lead to a long-term worsening of the condition. Indeed, orthodox Western medicine does experience difficulties in treating chronic diseases. One could say it is because of the frequently occurring temporary reverse effects that it runs into trouble and causes long-term problems. It is not necessarily always so, but the possibility of dose- and time-dependent reverse effects should be taken into consideration.

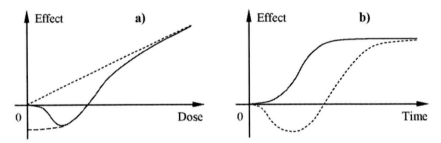

Figure 5.1. a) Varying dose/effect relationships. Effect is determined at a certain time after therapeutic intervention. Solid curve (non-linear): dose-dependent reverse effect (hormesis); dashed line through the origin: the usual linear dose/effect relation. Dashed curve: non-disappearing effect with potentisation instead of sheer diluting. **b)** Time/effect relationship at a certain dose depending on the time elapsed after therapeutic intervention. Solid curve: usual progression. Dashed curve: reverse effect after some time.

We are talking about highly non-linear effects such as we discussed in previous chapters. The difference between short-term and long-term thinking can be found in the West in the difference between (presumably) economic and ecological thinking. Let us take as an example the building of a new road for easing traffic. In the short-term, it is bound to have the desired effect. In the medium-term, however, drivers are alerted to the possibility of avoiding the traffic jams and this draws more traffic to the new road. In the long run the situation (more people driving more cars) can paradoxically get even worse than if no new road had been built at all. In the therapeutic situation, this is certainly a difficult position: a therapist cannot refuse to help a person with an acute problem just because the long-term consequences are unclear.

Now to the origin of modern homoeopathy. It all began with cinchona bark, an already well-known remedy for malaria in Hahnemann's time (ca 1800). Hahnemann discovered in an experiment on himself that ingesting a rather high dose induced symptoms corresponding to a weakened form of malaria. Here we find the idea of an opposite effect again. However, now we are not concerned about a difference in dosage or time but the fact that the effect on a healthy person is the opposite of that on an ill person (as long as the patient has an illness corresponding to this remedy). This was formulated by Hahnemann as the *simile principle* (from Latin: similis, -e = similar), cf. Table 5.1c: *"A remedy which induces a certain pathology – the remedy picture – in a healthy person is capable of curing an illness corresponding to this pathology."* The use of the terms *symptoms* and *illness* are important since they are the focus of some debate between orthodox and complementary medicine. Orthodox Western Medicine is often accused of only treating the symptoms and not the cause of illness. However, homoeopathic remedies are prescribed based almost entirely on the symptom picture! Another point of contention is whether the focus is on the ill person or the disease. We shall return to this later.

Table 5.1. Overview over important terms concerning homoeopathy

a) *Hormesis: Dose-Dependent Reverse Effect* (Calabrese 2008)

In many cases, the action of a low concentration of an otherwise poisonous substance has a stimulating effect. Conversely, in low doses it is possible for an otherwise promoting substance to have an inhibiting effect.

b) *Arndt-Schulz Law* (various versions, cf. Oberbaum & Cambar 1994)

Weak stimuli increase, strong stimuli decrease, and very strong stimuli suppress biological activity.

c) *Simile Principle* (cf. Dellmour 1992, pp.7f & 17; Endler 1998, p.22f).

* A remedy that induces certain symptoms – the remedy picture – in a healthy person is capable of curing an illness that exhibits these symptoms.
* Simile: highest possible agreement between known remedy picture and current symptoms.
* Drug proving in healthy individuals: utilises simile principle for finding homoeopathic remedies for the ill.

d) *Generalised Simile Principle* (cf. Kratky 1993)

We are looking at a remedy with a certain symptom picture. The actual effect of such a remedy on an ill person (time behaviour, strength and direction of effect) depends on the following circumstances:

* Details of the manufacturing process, prescription and ingestion (e.g. time) of the remedy as well as the general constitution and the special condition of the patient,
* Degree of agreement between the patient's symptoms and the symptom picture of the remedy.

Further generalisations are possible with regard to every kind of treatment or therapy....

Hahnemann, incidentally, merely *rediscovered* the simile principle, the core of homoeopathy. The basic idea of this principle was already known to Paracelsus and even Hippocrates and can also be found in Homer's Iliad and the Old Testament. During the Trojan War (see Locker 1999), King Telephos of Lycia was wounded by Achilles in a battle with the Greeks and, since the wound would not heal, he consulted the oracle, which told him: *"That which struck you will heal you."* He then asked the Greeks for splinters from Achilles' spear which, scattered into his wound, healed it. This story is interesting inasmuch as it is not about the symptom level, which is paramount in homoeopathy, but about a causal connection between the trigger of an illness and the remedy. This is close to *isopathy*, which can be seen as a special case of homoeopathy, but is often not regarded as part of proper homoeopathy (*isos* Greek = equal; *homoios* Greek = similar). An example from isopathy is that of an allergic person who is given the allergen prepared homoeopathically as remedy. Naturally, there are always only *similarities* – the splinters are not the whole spear and the homoeopathic preparation does not correspond exactly to the original allergen.

The following narrative from the Old Testament (numbers 21:6-9) is also quite instructive. On the Israelites' journey through the desert many people died from snakebites. God ordered Moses to erect a bronze snake on a pole. The people who had been bitten were told to look at this serpent and they would recover. Here homoeopathy is linked with a symbolic principle or principle of analogy. This approach can also be found in magical forms of healing (e.g. Asclepios cult, shamanic rituals) and corresponds to perspective P3. The snake as an ambivalent animal (standing for evil and sin but also for healing powers – another homoeopathic idea?) appears again and again in symbolic representations, for example as an aesculap snake winding around a pole (the staff of Asclepios still used today as a symbol by pharmacists). We need also to mention here the caduceus, or staff entwined by twin snakes, of Hermes (Greek) or Mercury (Latin), the messenger of the gods. According to Benedikt (1986, p.246), it is a symbol of the integration of positive and negative forces. This also corresponds to the ambivalent role of Hermes or Mercury. Today the caduceus as the staff of Mercury is a symbol of the Anthroposophists.

Hahnemann stated the simile principle more precisely and transformed it into a manageable technique (dynamisation or potentisation). That is to say, he developed a practical method of application from the theoretical concept. We shall come back to this topic in Ch.5.3. First of all, though, we shall address the difference between orthodox Western medicine (allopathy, *allos* Greek = different) and homoeopathy. This difference is often characterised in the following manner:

SIMILIA SIMILIBUS CURENTUR
(may like be cured by like)
Simile Principle (same sense, homoeopathy);   (5.1a)

CONTRARIA CONTRARIIS CURENTUR
(may opposite be cured by opposite)
Contrarian Principle (opposite sense, allopathy or, more precisely,
contrarian therapy as a frequent variant of allopathy)   (5.1b)

Curentur ('may be cured') instead of *curantur* ('will be cured') also points to the fact that healing success is not guaranteed in either system. Homoeopathy focuses on the *organism* and its *regulation*. Use of – from the perspective of orthodox Western medicine –

harmful substances can be seen as stimulative or regulative therapy. After the homoeopathic initial aggravation, a reaction expected by orthodox Western medicine, the organism's over-compensating counter regulation achieves the therapeutic effect. *Stress* put on the organism by homoeopathy contrasts with *de-stressing* the organism by orthodox Western medicine. The latter does not focus on the organism but on the *illness* and its *trigger*. Both are seen as foes, for example intruding bacteria or viruses, which are often combated directly by by-passing the immune system. Indirectly this supports the immune system. However, at times the foe is combated by impairing the immune system, which leads to another type of stress. Orthodox Western medicine is a war medicine in two senses. First of all it enjoyed a great boom due to the two world wars (see Ch. 2.4), and secondly its vocabulary contains many warlike or militant expressions, such as the following *anti*-expressions: antibiotics, antibodies against antigens, antiarrhythmic drugs (which could just as well be called rhythmic drugs, since they stabilise heart rhythm). This corresponds to the contrarian principle of allopathy as opposed to the simile principle of homoeopathy, to which we shall now return.

5.2. Generalised Simile Principle and Remedy Proving

After our considerations regarding hormesis and the Arndt-Schulz Law, an obvious next step is to *generalise* the simile principle. We shall now move on from concentrating on the effect on healthy and ill people to a wider context. A remedy's effectiveness (behaviour over time, strength and direction) can depend not only on the dose but also on the time of day it is ingested (an idea from Traditional Chinese Medicine and also chronobiology). The exact formulation can be found in Table 5.1d. Different but very similar therapies can have oppo-site effects (according to chaos research, small causes can have large effects; subtle differ-ences are crucial). At one time the simile principle and, at another, the contrarian principle will come into play. For this reason the work in which I first introduced the generalised simile principle (or the resonance principle) is called "*The generalised simile principle as a joint framework of allopathy and homoeopathy.*" (Kratky 1993). The trials conducted by Endler regarding stimulation or *inhibition* of the metamorphosis of tadpoles by use of poten-tised thyroxin constitute one example which demonstrates how the direction of results is sensitive to the various conditions of an experiment. A Table of Overview can be found in Endler (1998, p.62).

We are faced, however, with a *fundamental* problem resulting from hormesis. What is considered similar and what opposite or contrary depends on one's individual viewpoint. Let us take the simplified example again of a substance that in small doses *lowers* a healthy individual's blood pressure and in high doses *raises* it. This substance (for example, one that has been homoeopathically prepared) is given to a patient suffering from, among other things, high blood pressure; in the concrete case it may have a blood pressure *lowering* effect. Does this correspond to the simile or contrarian principle? First of all the terminology itself must be questioned. If a substance has a blood pressure lowering effect in a healthy person, allo-pathy assumes that it will work in the same fashion in a patient with *high* blood pressure (could be seen as 'similar') and homoeopathy will assume the opposite ('contrarian'). Thus, one has to know what is meant in order to classify 'correctly' the terms similar and contrarian.

Having looked at these principles using blood pressure as the variable, we shall now take a concrete example in connection with the variable ('axis') temperature. If someone has burnt his hand, for example, then it is obvious that the therapy has something to do with heat and cold. Should the patient now receive (homoeopathically) more heat or (allopathically) cold water or a cold compress? You could think of this in terms of axes (here with the temperature axis), which we shall come across in dealing with Far Eastern modes of healing (Chs. 7-8). But now let us take an actual example to do with burns. Glassblowers in a Swiss glassworks react to burns on their hands with a method that prevents blisters from forming, if the burn is not too severe: They immediately put the burnt hand as close to an open fire as they can tolerate and then change the distance over time corresponding to the change in their sensation of pain. After about 20-30 minutes, this self-treatment is completed. Experience shows that this is more effective than cold water and works with the feedback loop *distance to the fire – individual pain sensation.*

Here this thinking in axes is very concretely implemented; a burn is treated with heat but it must be the right dosage. If the burnt hand is placed in the fire, it will get not better but worse. Another example is that of cold compresses (Kobau 1993, p.292f). There are cold compresses for cold and cold compresses for heat. If you make a cold compress and let it take effect for about 30 minutes, it cools. If you leave it on for 40-70 minutes, it warms. After another 50 minutes, you will even start to sweat. Here, too, the time effect needs to be observed. One cannot just say that in order to cool the body one needs a cold compress, but one must also take the time element into consideration in order not to achieve the opposite effect.

There are other examples of such ambivalences:

- After a heart attack, the doctor may order either rest (de-stressing) or a mild exercise (stress).
- The homoeopathic remedy belladonna (deadly nightshade) can provoke either dilation or constriction of the pupil, the former more often than the latter. The pupil size, so to speak, is the axis on which belladonna has an effect. In a healthy person, however, who ingests belladonna for proving this remedy (see below), whether the pupils will dilate or constrict depends on the individual.
- In the summer, cold drinks (allopathic) are preferred, but physicians recommend hot teas (homoeopathic)! Especially when it is very hot, you should drink hot beverages.
- Coffee with its contradictory effects has already been mentioned.
- Various diets with their partly contradictory recommendations must also be seen in this light.

Another interesting aspect relates to *vaccinations.* Passive and active immunisations correspond to a *de-stressing* (battle against the intruder, *contrarian principle*) and a *stressing* (preventive stimulus therapy, *simile principle*) of the organism, respectively. One would think that the latter meets with the approval of homoeopaths. Interestingly though, homoeopaths criticise this practice of vaccinations. This is a special kind of resonance effect, which merits further investigation.

Now let us turn to the question of how (new) homoeopathic remedies are developed. Here the simile principle shows the way (Table 5.1c) by means of 'proving' in healthy subjects. In this process, a healthy individual ingests a chosen substance over several days. Symptoms, signs and modalities which arise (general term: *symptoms*) are then recorded in great detail. Hahnemann did this for many years (in self-experiments and experiments on his large family and his colleagues, which, at times, resulted in injury). However, drug proving provides the means for discovering individual *remedy pictures*. The homoeopathic remedy can then be used to treat for patients exhibiting comparable symptoms. Of course, sometimes the illness may not yet exist – as in the case of Aids. Some homoeopathic studies in the treatment of Aids are promising hope, for example Rastogie et al. (1993). In this study, various homoeopathic remedies were administered depending on the individual symptomatology of Aids patients. Unlike orthodox Western medicine, which immediately puts lots of money into researching the newly emerged foe, homoeopathy consults the existing textbooks – humans change very slowly compared to viruses.

Regarding the terminology of homoeopathy, *symptoms,* in a narrow sense, refer to the usual symptoms of an illness, *signs* to other noticeable reactions (such as the patient's dreams). Furthermore, *modalities* refer to indications such as whether the discomfort gets better or worse at a particular time of day, whether it is helpful to lie on your right or left side, whether movement or rest eases the discomfort. Many rather fine distinctions have been recorded and can be found in the textbooks. Two kinds of representations, which complement each other, need be distinguished. The 'Materia Medica' starts with the homoeopathic remedy and describes a complete remedy picture. The 'Repertory' on the other hand lists symptoms, signs and modalities along with the range of homoeopathic remedies – in order of importance – to be considered in these cases. By the way, such cross-referencing is not uncommon: The medical student learns the symptoms related to various diseases and, in his medical practice, the doctor must diagnose the illness from the patient's complaints.

Finding remedy pictures and determining their application in homoeopathy is an empirical endeavour. During consultation, the homoeopath attempts to find the best match between the patient's symptoms and a remedy picture (P3). The closer the agreement, the higher is the probability of having found the / a simile. However, It can never agree in every respect, but the question is what is important. The more unusual and distinctive the symptoms, signs and modalities, the easier it is to find the correct homoeopathic remedy. The question of potency comes later. The problem often is not finding *a* simile but choosing from a number of similia, and deciding which one is the best match (*the* simile or simillimum).

The question now is to what extent a patient is treated as an *individual*. Complementary medicine in general and homoeopathy in particular make this claim. In principle, there are about 3500 homoeopathic remedies. In practice, however, only about 200 of these are well-tested and in actual use and about 80 of those are polychrests, which are prescribed predominantly. This seems to limit individual treatment to a great degree. Thus, if homoeopathy is to be successful, most patients must exhibit a symptomatology corresponding to the common remedy pictures. Furthermore, complementary medicine's claim of a strictly individual approach must be questioned in general. If every case were different, then one could never learn a method of treatment. No case that one has learned or studied in books is consistent with the case at hand. It is true that every patient is different, but if one wants to draw a conclusion from one case to another based on one's training, the case at hand must resemble cases one has studied. There must be some classification or typology and there might even be hundreds of different 'types'. One exception to the above mentioned limitation is given by feedback therapies (Ch.6). In spite of general rules, this approach affords individual therapy – as we have already seen in the case of the treatment of burns by glassblowers.

An interesting question refers to the *concrete* discovery of new homoeopathic remedies. In principle 'anything' could be tested via drug proving and then used in practice to find out if it proves beneficial as a homoeopathic remedy. Especially at the start, many poisonous substances were used. Snake venoms were tested one after the other because strong poisons produce numerous and dramatic symptoms. However, everyday foods and ingredients (such as parsley, onions, sugar, salt) were also tested. This shows in an unusual way how important it is what we eat: eating similar foods for several days may be an involuntary 'drug proving'! The doctrine of signatures, which Hahnemann himself dismissed, was also used to find homoeopathic remedies. This is how the Anthroposophists had the idea of using mistletoe in cancer therapy: Mistletoe proliferates on a tree much as a cancer tumour in the organism. This was seen as an indication that mistletoe could be effective in the treatment of cancer. This conjecture, naturally, had then to be tested. Thus, there are many ways of discovering something: by guesswork, through intuition or through principles. A theoretical concept can be found in Kratky (1994, 1998a, 2004) as well as in Kratky & Milavec (1994). From these articles, it can be concluded that the dynamical structure of homoeopathic remedies must be in accord with the structure of water.

To round things off, there is one more point, which, in fact, will lead us back to remedy proving. Complementary therapy is primarily a regulative medicine and the different approaches of orthodox and complementary reflect the difference between *organisation imposed externally* and *self-organisation* (Kratky 1990). In the former case, (massive) intervention is external but in the latter the organism's regulation, which was impeded or blocked in some way, is reactivated. Of course, this is in a way paradoxical since it is supplying *help for self-help.* It does not work all by itself; otherwise, the patient would not have sought treatment. If you take regulative medicine as regulation toward a medium value seriously, then the direction of stimulus does not matter as long as the correct kind of stimulus (the right axis) is found. If we take acupuncture as an example, we can see that, if the correct acupuncture (stimulus) points are treated, whether they are tonified or sedated is not that important – except in the short-term. If, for example, a certain point is sedated instead of tonified by mistake, then the organism must counter it by overreacting in the opposite direction but is only enabled to do so by the correct 'wake-up signal' (correct acupuncture point). A far more elegant solution is the *neutral* needle stimulus, which is achieved with a medium stimulus strength (corresponding to passing through the origin in Figure 5.1a). At the beginning of the training, often only this technique is taught for simplicity. The organism reacts accordingly in a correct manner (as if it had been tonified or sedated). A neutral stimulus, therefore, is not *no stimulus*, but a harmonising one.

Two opposing tendencies have resulted in this way. On the one hand, there is a sensitive dependence on delicate differences (generalised simile principle, divergence) and, on the other, a great insensitivity or robustness (regulation toward a medium value, convergence). Both are sides of the same coin, which says that cause and effect in complex systems are not linked as closely as in the systems usually investigated by the sciences. This requires much experience. In order to avoid complications, classical homoeopathy limits itself to remedies which have undergone provings and which are not combined or mixed with each other (*single* remedies). Of course, homoeopathic pharmacies also supply combination remedies, containing two or more remedies, which are sold for the treatments of conditions such as hay fever or the common cold. Classical homoeopaths reject the use of complex remedies, arguing that this is a shotgun method, which cannot replace a sound anamnesis. Another argument results from Ch. 3: non-linear systems contain an interaction term, see (3.1). The effect of a combination of two homoeopathic remedies can only be known if a *specific* drug proving has been made for this combination – knowing the effect of the two ingredients is not enough. However, it is interesting to note that single remedies, particularly those derived from plant material, may contain several individual substances but will have undergone proving as such.

5.3. Production of Remedies and Potentisation

Now we shall look at how homoeopathic remedies are produced. According to the simile principle, whatever is harmful to a healthy individual may be beneficial to the ill person. As we have already mentioned, Hahnemann made use of poisonous substances in his experiments. The problem with this was that the healing effect in the patient was always superimposed by the effect of the poison. For this reason, Hahnemann experimented with stepwise higher dilutions – in liquid states with water or water/ alcohol mixtures and in solid states with lactose as solvent, or rather, carrier substance. In the limiting case of an arbitrarily high dilution (disappearing dose), the effect vanished (see the solid curve in Figure 5.1a). This led Hahnemann to alter the dilution process in further experiments. He chose the result of a previous dilution as the starting point for the next dilution. Furthermore, he discovered that a certain type of shaking (in the liquid state) or grinding with a pestle and mortar (in the solid state) prevented the loss of the healing effect (see the dashed line after dose 0 in Figure 5.1a). In order to distinguish this process from mere diluting, Hahnemann coined the term *dynamisation*; today we call it *potentisation*.

Thus, adding energy in a suitable manner changes the result. This, incidentally, also underlies a much older process – spagyric production. When this procedure is used to produce aurum, for example, gold dust is placed in water, heated and evaporated (during which process a small amount of the gold is taken along) and then cooled. The (now diluted) condensate is heated again in further cycles. Altogether, this succession of steps combines dilution with supplying energy. The aurum used for healing purposes is a result of many cycles, where the final condensate contains practically no gold at all. There is an analogous procedure in Ayurveda, where metals are heated to 1600°C and then combined with buttermilk and oil, this succession being repeated up to 1000 times (Netzhammer 2000). This idea of repeating the same process over and over again (in the above examples, shaking or heating combined with diluting) resembles the iterated processes we discussed in connection with chaos research in Ch.3, which then led to the representation of fractals (Figure 3.4). This repetition corresponds to P2 (feedback, cycles).

In order to perform a homoeopathic potentisation, using a soluble substance, it is first of all dissolved in alcohol to form the mother tincture. In *D-potencies* (from Latin: *decem* = 10) every step dilutes by a factor of ten: 1 part previous potency and 9 parts solvent. (In English, D potencies are known as X potencies.) Usually water/ alcohol mixtures are used (43% ethanol) although water can be used alone. Starting with the mother tincture (D0, 0X), the potencies D1, D2, D3 (1X, 2X, 3X) etc. are produced in sequence through diluting and shaking. (Incidentally, the mother tincture may already be D1 or 1X corresponding to a 10% solution.) The potency D3 is obtained after three dilution steps by a factor of 10 each. This means a concentration of $10^3 = 1000$ times less than D0. Hahnemann discovered that numerous potentisations could be made without losing effectiveness. On the contrary, the effects seem to become more and more specific. Starting around D24 (24X) no molecule of the original substance is left – it consists only of solvent (see below). These high potencies appear to work more deeply on the mental/ emotional levels. On the other hand, lower potencies work more on the physical levels and are shorter acting.

The effectiveness of high potencies is one of the main contentions in homoeopathy's battle for recognition. Hahnemann himself preferred using high potencies, since their effect is more to the point. This is also the reason why experienced homoeopaths prefer prescribing high potencies, while conversely, with lower potencies an error in choice of remedy is not as precarious. Therefore, if the best simile is not chosen but the second or third best, this does not matter as much with a D6 (6X) as it does with a D15 (15X) or even a D30 (30X) potency because the effects will wear off more rapidly. These dilutions can be taken directly in liquid form or, more often, in form of saccharose pills (globules) which are coated with the remedy.

Homoeopathic remedies can also be prepared from substances that are not soluble in water by mixing them with lactose (trituration). However, this procedure is very time-consuming since, for every step of potentisation, the mixture has to be ground for about one hour. Once trituration D4 (4X) has been reached, the substance can be dissolved and the potentisation continued in liquid form. The first liquid potency thus produced is D5/ 5X (Dellmour 1992, p.47) or D6/ 6X (Dorcsi et al. 1991, p.73). In any case, it is interesting that the suitable solvents water, alcohol and sugar all have hydrogen bonds in common. Such bridges connect various molecules but are not as strong as ordinary chemical bonds. There are, for example, no tightly interlinked large clusters of water molecules, but molecules in close proximity bind together for a short time and then separate again. Corresponding physical models work with these hydrogen bonds (Kratky 1994).

In addition to the D-potencies there are also *C-potencies* (from Latin: *centum* = 100). Each step uses a dilution by a factor of 100. This is a faster way to reach smaller concentrations. For example, we consider C6 (or 6C in English). From a chemical point of view, this corresponds to D12 (12X) since they both have the same concentration of active agent. However, because of the different rules of potentisation, medium and higher D- and C-potencies cannot be compared offhand, although lower potencies can (see below). Hahnemann worked only with C-potencies for many years. Today in Germany, mainly D-potencies are used, whereas in France and England C-potencies are preferred. In addition, there are also LM- or Q-potencies (LM or Q stand for 50000, pseudo-Latin notation). The starting point of a LM 0 is the C3 (3C) potency of trituration. Each step dilutes by a factor of 50000 and this is done by alternating use of water/ alcohol and globules in a complicated way. The resulting potencies are known as LM I, LM II, etc. Hahnemann developed this method towards the end of his life and from then on only used LM-potencies, because they are more effective and gentle, and are less likely to result in initial aggravation even in higher potencies. However, aggravation can occur later in the process. There are fine differences between LM- and Q-potencies, but we shall not go into this.

As far as effectiveness of potencies is concerned, D5/ D6 (5X, 6X) might represent a 'magical' boundary. Up to then it is probably of minimal importance whether the remedy is potentised or merely diluted, a C2 (2C) corresponds to a D4 (4X), etc. It seems that enough of the starting substance is present for the chemical effect still to be important. In addition, in many cases solutions of colour or flavour additives in water can still be detected up to – but not beyond – a dilution of 10^{-5} and 10^{-6}, respectively – in other words, the water still appears coloured or tastes of the flavouring (Moser & Schwarz 1994, p.63). After that, the chemical substances somehow disappear in the structure of water. This is also approximately the border between lower and medium potencies. Up to D5 (5X) the potencies are considered low; beyond this point they are considered to be medium and this, in my opinion, is where true homoeopathy begins. Engler (1989) is of the opinion that remedies under D6 (6X) are characterised by their substantive effect and beyond that by their electromagnetic effect. We have already come across another indication of this boundary: For water-insoluble starting substances the higher potencies – from D5 or D6 (5X, 6X) on – are also available in liquid form. Dellmour (1994) points out that, later in his life, Hahnemann recommended using C3 (3C) triturations, corresponding to a concentration of 10^{-6}, as a starting point for further potencies instead of the mother tincture.

Let us now consider the high potencies – scientifically the most controversial aspect of homoeopathy. According to Loschmidt's or Avogadro's number, $6.02*10^{23}$, the probability of *not a single* molecule of the original effective agent still remaining in the homoeopathic potency grows with every successive potentisation step beyond a dilution of 10^{-24} (corresponding to D24/ 24X, C12/ 12C or LM IV). Often in this connection the question is raised of how such a high potency can be effective at all if there is NOTHING left in it. On the other hand, homoeopaths keep on potentising. Potencies of D1000 and C1000 (1M) can also be found. Thus, homoeopaths proceed on the assumption that potentisation is an effective procedure, although beyond about D24 (24X) only the solvent remains. The idea is that it does not depend on the chemistry of the active substance but on the information, which can be transferred to the dynamic structure of the solvent (Taddei-Ferretti & Marotta 1998). The chemical substance, then, only serves as a means to an end, which is reaching the right condition of water (cf. Kratky 1994).

Thinking in terms of information is supported by the fact that homoeopathic remedies can also be manufactured electronically (see the next chapter and Endler 1998, Ch.2.4). In this case, there is always only the pure solvent, which is imprinted with various electromagnetic fields. Thus, the laborious method of going from substance to pure solvent can be shortened by electronic means. This method is establishing itself more and more (for example, in the USA) if for no other reason than because of the prohibition of more and more 'normal' homoeopathic remedies due to the protected species of plants and animals necessary for their production. In Austria low potencies of homoeopathic remedies up to D5 (5X) containing pyrrolizidine alkaloids are prohibited, corresponding to the idea that homoeopathic remedies can be poisonous if they are in low potencies. On the other hand, there is talk about making high potencies generally available; 'there is nothing in them anyway' (the motto apparently being: "*If it doesn't do any good, then it can't do any harm either.*"). From a homoeopathic perspective, however, this makes little sense. High potencies have a more profound effect and can be regarded as stronger than lower and medium potencies. From this point of view, the use of high potencies in particular requires a thorough anamnesis.

Now the question arises as to how important determining the right potency is in relation to finding the right simile. A clear answer cannot be obtained from homoeopaths. Many believe that finding the right remedy is crucial and the potency secondary: if the organism receives the right information, then the exact potency and manner of production is unimportant. Anyway, some believe that acute cases need to be treated with lower potencies and chronic cases with higher potencies.

Imprinting water with a frequency to make a homoeopathic remedy and determining the frequencies of a homoeopathic remedy are complementary to one another. Ludwig (1999, Ch. 10.1) performed such analyses by means of physical devices. In this process, he found frequencies that initially were hidden in noise to such a degree that the analysis of a single remedy took him six weeks. On the other hand, apparently the organism is able to read this information in matter of seconds or minutes once the remedy is ingested. Thus, in spite of steady improvements in physical devices, they are still less sensitive than the human body. Smith used his own sensitivity to measure thyroxin in all D-potencies from D4/ 4X to D30/ 30X (Smith & Endler 1994). In contrast to D4/ 4X, D5/ 5X exhibited one single frequency (0.07 Hz = oscillations per second). Starting with D6 (6X) two new frequencies higher than the previous ones were added – such as 7.8 and 9.1 MHZ in D30 (30X). One could say that for thyroxin (and presumably for all homoeopathic remedies) a certain series of frequencies is characteristic. The lower the potency, however, the fewer frequencies that are actually activated (the lower ones). It is interesting to note that Smith did not find this characteristic behaviour for thyroxin until D5/ 5X or D6/ 6X – the 'magical boundary' that we have already mentioned.

5.4. Human Constitution and Hering's Law

Now we shall return to the simile principle, which concerns itself with congruence between remedy picture and current symptomatology. Hahnemann did not refer to this principle exclusively, since it did not always suffice to bring about healing. He recognised that not only the current symptomatology but also the underlying *constitution* or type of patient was important in the choice of the correct remedy (Gawlik 1990, p.10f). In later life, he also introduced the concept of miasms, which brought another theoretical aspect to the otherwise primarily empirical homoeopathy and which is still controversial today among homoeopaths. It recognised three fundamental illness types: p*sora*, s*ycosis* and s*yphilis*. This concept is difficult to interpret and the choice of terms is unfortunate – syphilis, for example, did not just refer to the disease itself but included aspects beyond this. Consequently, Hahnemann searched for remedies characterising these three types. He spoke, for example of anti-psoric remedies, an expression fitting in better with allopathy than homoeopathy. You can argue, of course, that this is merely a linguistic problem. According to Hahnemann, psora diseases are the most common. They also usually arise at the onset of illness. The outbreak of psora (and thus the outbreak of the illness itself), incidentally, was associated with the idea of original sin. These somewhat strange considerations will appear more plausible in the light of Far Eastern healing modalities (Chs. 7-8). Further chronobiological considerations can be found in Chs. 11-12.

Table 5.2. The three diatheses of homoeopathy – comparison with miasms, the Indian doshas and Krämer's Bach Flower typology

Nomenclature	Lymphatic	Lithemic	Destructive
Dorcsi	Fearful	Loud	Rigid
Ortega	Deficiency	Overabundance	Degeneration
Miasms	Psora	Sycosis	Syphilis
Ayurveda	Vata	Pitta	Kapha
Bach Flowers	Communication	Compensation	Decompensation

The controversial miasms were later interpreted as being constitutional – that is, they were converted from *types of illness* to *types of ill people* and were re-named *diatheses*. One can look at them as types of people (temperaments, cf. Ch.2.3) with their typical physical and psychological characteristics, their predispositions toward certain diseases, and a predominance of a certain regulatory principle. Diseases that come and go comparatively quickly may be checked against a personality that changes only slowly. Table 5.2 shows the nomenclature of the three diatheses with some typical characteristics and the corresponding miasms. The diatheses are called lymphatic, lithemic and destructive. Unfortunately, the third term has wider connotations. Ortega characterises these expressions with deficiency, overabundance and degeneration. One could also say that they represented too little, too much and different. Further characterisations can be found in Kratky (1997a).

Healthy:	a stressful stimulus is quickly followed by a reaction, which then subsides again.	(5.2a)
Lymphatic:	the reaction arises (too) late – or overcompensates.	(5.2b)
Lithemic:	dying away of the reaction is delayed	(5.2c)
Destructive:	unresponsiveness, disconnection from stimulus.	(5.2d)

In (5.2a-d) typical reactions to a stimulus are listed, cf. Pichler (1996): With the lymphatic diathesis, the reaction usually arises too late. With the lithemic diathesis, on the other hand, the same is true for the *abatement* of the reaction, which thus is too strong and over-compensating. With the destructive diathesis, we find unresponsiveness to a stimulus. This diathesis seems to be the final phase in an illness progression. Conversely, a healthy 'destructive' person could be called easy-going, someone who is not rattled easily. This goes to show how tricky this choice of words is. The best way to describe these types is to use the Indian terms vata, pitta and kapha, cf. Table 5.2. The Ayurvedic regulatory principles or doshas, which we shall discuss in detail in Ch. 8, correspond largely to the diatheses, but these foreign expressions do not evoke false associations. In any case, vata imbalances are the most common and diseases usually start with them. A parallel to psora already suggests itself. Another is hidden in (5.2b). According to Pichler the lymphatic diathesis also offers an often unappreciated second possibility, which corresponds to *too much* and not to *too little*. As we shall see, the vata type shows a similar ambivalence.

Now to the Bach Flower Remedies listed in Table 5.2. Krämer (1991, 1994) divides them into 'inner' and 'outer' flowers, of which the first group is by far the larger one. This group comprises three sections, which according to Krämer's description, can easily be assigned to the diatheses (Kratky 1996d, 1997a). He makes distinctions between communication, compensation and decompensation flowers. However, according to his own logic, communication should rather be called communication *disturbance*, *deficiency* or *loss*. An illness begins with a disturbance in communication. If this cannot be corrected, the afflicted organism attempts to master this situation by the expenditure of a great deal of energy (compensation or over-compensation). If this is of no use or the person becomes exhausted, he will go over to decompensation, where he no longer reacts to any great degree (Krämer 1991, pp.18-20). For the corresponding miasms, this means that the illness begins in psora and progresses via sycosis to syphilis.

As the patient progresses through different sages of the illness, different flower remedies must be administered, unless one is already working with several. If the patient is in the decompensation stage, he will need a corresponding decompensation flower essence. This will lead him to the compensation stage, from where a suitable flower essence will take him to the communication deficiency stage, and from there the right flower remedy can then lead to recovery. Thus, Krämer describes the path of illness progression as opposite to the path of convalescence. Homoeopaths think in a similar vein. In this connection Hering's Law is often cited, see Table 5.3.

A few comments on Table 5.3:

- *From the outside in*: conditions often begin with skin problems and then go steadily deeper (e.g. bronchitis, asthma) and can become chronic. To be consistent, in Ayurveda *skin* is primarily assigned to vata as well as *communication* (see Krämer's communication flower essences).
- *Reverse order of symptoms during convalescence* compared to falling ill: This means if the patient develops a rash during the course of treatment, the homoeopath is happy (as opposed to other doctors). He can be assured that his goal is almost met.
- *From bottom to top*: For example, homoeopaths have noticed that, as a cure progresses, symptoms such as pain can sometimes move down the patient, say from

back to legs to feet before finally disappearing completely. We will return to the relationship bottom – top in Chs. 7-8. At this time let me just mention that in Ayurveda the principles vata, pitta and kapha are primarily assigned to the upper, middle and lower regions of the body, respectively. The succession of falling ill from vata via pitta to kapha, then, corresponds to Hering's Law!

- *From less important to important organs*: It is plausible that for reasons of self-protection in the course of falling ill, first less important organs become afflicted. With growing severity and duration, more and more important organs become involved.

Table 5.3. Hering's Law
(cf. Dellmour 1992, p.36; Endler 1998, p.124f)

Symptom progression in serious illnesses (healing occurs in reverse order):
* from the outside in * from bottom to top * from less important to important organs

Homoeopathy is, of course, such a comprehensive field that one chapter of a book can only offer a brief glimpse. As we have already mentioned, we shall keep finding references to this subject in other chapters. Ch. 12, in particular, will be dedicated to questions concerning homoeopathy, and we shall treat the dynamics of miasms in more detail. We will close the present section with two references that deal with basic questions and research in homoeopathy: Endler & J. Schulte (Eds., 1994), Schulte & P.C. Endler (Eds., 1998).

Chapter 6

Feedback Diagnoses
and Feedback Therapies

6.1. Electro-Acupuncture as an Example
of Feedback Therapy

In Chs. 3.1, 4.2 & 4.3 we have already mentioned the importance of feedback loops. We shall now focus on this topic. Let us start with Figure 6.1a – a situation, where feedback has not yet occurred. The upper and lower halves of this figure both depict a simple relationship, and the arrows can have different meanings:

Arrows: Input – Output,   Cause – Effect,
          Stimulus – Response, Question – Answer.   (6.1)

The square box might represent, for example, a black box, a computer, a medical device or a living being, particular a human. Our thinking can often be represented by this simple type of relationship. A simple example is that of doctor/patient (upper/lower box). The patient comes to the doctor. From what he can see of the patient, the doctor is already getting information and drawing conclusions (flow of information in Figure 6.1a, top). In addition, he asks specific questions, which the patient answers (flow of information in Figure 6.1a, bottom). Finally, he makes a diagnosis and writes a prescription for medication. This again affects the patient and leads to a reaction which both doctor and patient hope will be that of the patient getting well again (again according to Figure 6.1a, bottom). If, however, you ponder this situation for a while, you will come to the conclusion that this process is actually circular and looks like Figure 6.1b. Doctor and patient move in a circuit of interaction and feedback. Feedback is already occurring during the process of consultation and examination for the purposes of diagnosis. The flow of information described in Figure 6.1a top and bottom cannot be separated. Analogous considerations hold for therapy. If the patient calls or is asked to come in for a check-up, the circuit of therapy and feedback – or a subsequent change in therapy – closes.

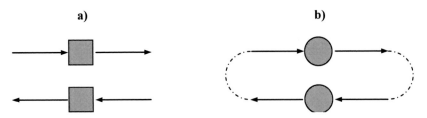

Figure 6.1. a) Simple cause/effect relations, **b)** Feedback loop.

Thus, usually diagnosis as well as therapy progression occurs in feedback mode. Seeing it this way corresponds to a change from perspective P1 (separation, hierarchy) to P2 (connection, cycles). At the same time, the viewpoint of patient's role and doctor's role changes as well, which is indicated by the other symbols (discs instead of squares in Figure 6.1b). The semicircles on the outside are dashed to indicate that they are often forgotten. In some cases this is not important, in others very much so (see below). Even taking into account *one* semicircle but not the *other* corresponds to the logic of P1; the feedback loop does not close. Thus, in simple cases diagnosis can be assigned to the *left* and therapy to the *right* 'semi-loop'. From the perspective P2, on the other hand, the whole loop is traversed – often more than once. The diagnosis, therefore, turns into a *feedback diagnosis*, and therapy into *feedback therapy* (two terms that I have suggested). In some forms of diagnosis and therapy, this terminology seems more appropriate than in others. In the end, it is not about right or wrong terminology but about the *perspectives* (P1 or P2). We are free to choose them to some extent and, which can be helpful, to a greater or lesser extent, depending on the case.

If P1 serves you well, then objectivity in general is not a problem. For example, a radiologist takes an x-ray of a patient and studies it. One can say that there is a circuit since the doctor turns on the machine in order to take the x-ray, the patient's body reacts to this step and the doctor looks at the result. This can be resolved, however, by a chronological succession. We will demonstrate how problems can arise even here with the example of electro-acupuncture by Voll (EAV; Voll 1976), from which related procedures have been developed: bio-electrical functional diagnostics and the VEGA test (see Matthiessen et al. 1994), as well as biological test medicine (Schramm 1992). In EAV, electrical resistance, or rather its reciprocal, electrical conductance, is measured at certain meridians – which is how it relates to acupuncture. We shall come back to this topic in Ch. 7 but, for now, we just want to mention that the meridians run through different sections of the body and come to the surface where the acupuncture points are located. In EAV, a current is run through the body by setting a small voltage across two electrodes. The cylindrical reference electrode has a large surface area and the subject always holds it with the same hand. The specific electrode is in the shape of a pointed stylus, which the physician presses into the acupuncture points.

Voll's system of meridians and acupuncture points, incidentally, does not agree completely with the Chinese system, but this need not concern us here. The measured values are often indicated by a needle (range 0 to 100): A value of 50 is normal, while higher values (i.e. higher conductance) indicate inflammatory processes around the meridians and lower values correspond to chronic degenerative processes. Another important marker is a drop in the measured value. If the stylus is pressed into the acupuncture point for a few seconds, the value can drop, for example, from 70 to 40. This is interpreted as a poor capability of the organism to regulate (rapid exhaustion). Since the patient is brought into an electrical circuit, and his reaction to the set voltage is measured, this is an example of circularity. Nevertheless, P1 could be saved (as in the x-ray example) by assigning the effect of the stylus to the right lower arrow in Figure 6.1a, the lower box to the patient (connected to the device) and the left lower arrow to the needle of the device.

Why then is EAV regarded with a certain amount of scepticism by orthodox Western medicine? For two reasons: medicine testing and the sensitivity of measured values to pressure. Let us take medicine testing first. If, as a result of looking at the measured values, the physician has a certain diagnosis or several therapy suggestions in mind, he can test corresponding orthodox drugs, or homoeopathic or other remedies. To do this, remedies are placed in succession on a metal plate contained in the circuit. When the right remedy is placed there, the needle shows a return to normal or a reverse in drop. How this works is unclear. As far as the pressure sensitivity of the values is concerned, the results are strongly influenced by the pressure applied to the stylus. Too weak or strong pressure affects a wide range of measured values (artefacts) and the question is raised as to what extent the doctor or the patient has contributed to the indicated value. The training for EAV is correspondingly lengthy and requires a certain talent. Not everyone can learn it. The lengthy training is justified because one has to practice a lot in order to place pressure – independent of all other influences – in the same way consistently. If this is true, then objectivity and reproducibility are assured. If this is not the case, then doctor and patient are inextricably caught in a feedback loop during the EAV test.

van Wijk & Wiegant (1994) investigated this important question with experiments, in which the applied pressure of the stylus was also measured (cf. also van Wijk 1998). The completely unexpected result is that electro-acupuncture by Voll is *not objective* but nevertheless *consistent* and *reproducible*! More precisely, EAV physicians found – independently of each other – consistent differences in readings or indicator drops in patients. However, this was primarily based on different stylus pressures for different patients; otherwise, the measured results would not have been significant. But how can it be that artefacts lead to the right diagnosis and choice of medication? There are two possible explanations: one relatively harmless in the sense of P2 and one unusual in the sense of P3 (Ch.6.3). However, for our purposes, P2 should provide an adequate explanation. It goes like this: We look at it in terms of a feedback loop between doctor and patient. Through the change in pressure, a weak effect on the side of the patient builds up to an externally visible effect – which a sensitive therapist subconsciously or semi-consciously senses. Here we go again, small cause – large effect, where the causes are so small as to be immeasurable (van Wijk & Wiegant 1994). The body as a complex system is therefore not always completely replaceable by a measuring device. Whoever finds this disagreeable can always wait for the discovery of more sensitive measuring devices. This raises another interesting question: Can a therapist knowing about these results continue to practise EAV without reservation or will he now be self-conscious about using the correct pressure? This feedback loop would be fatal, because it would mean that studying the work of van Wijk & Wiegant (1994) would result in their main discovery (the consistency of EAV) being lost.

The same questions can be raised concerning muscle testing, which is at the centre of kinesiology. Here the strength, or rather the resistance, of a muscle is tested (cf. Hey-artz 1996). The patient holds out his arm horizontally, for example, and attempts to keep it there against the downward pressure applied by the therapist. As in EAV, medicines are tested and amount of pressure applied can vary. Substances placed on the tongue or in a breast pocket either strengthen or weaken the arm. In addition, the patient's strength has to be seen as relative to that of the therapist's applied pressure. Here, too, one can assume that the therapist produces the result by applying more or less pressure but projects this to the patient and perceives him as stronger or weaker.

In the meantime, improvements have been developed in EAV meridian diagnosis as well as in muscle testing, which have the aim of objectifying and making both practices more approachable to Western thinking. The diagnosis and therapy control system Prognos, for example, which was developed in Russia, can be seen as an improvement on EAV. The set voltage is lower, the stylus placement area larger, and the amount of pressure is monitored automatically and held constant. In addition, anyone can learn to use this method with just a short training period. We shall go into this further in Ch.7.4. In addition, a muscle test has been developed which reduces or excludes the artefact on the part of the therapist. This is the myostatic test based on the O-ring test by Omura (Lack 1996). In this method, the subject puts the tips of his thumb and forefinger together to form a ring and the therapist attempts to open the ring by pulling the fingers apart. It is a mixed strength/ reaction test, which has been studied in detail by Heyartz (1996). It was possible to objectify this test by measuring the amount of tension applied. In order to exclude placebo effects, some of the patients were given counter-factual information ("*opening the ring is a good sign*"), without the results being influenced significantly. Thus Prognos, as well as the myostatic test, can in principle lead back to P1.

These results also suggest that EAV and the usual muscle tests have an objective founda-tion, which, however, is not strong enough to be measured by a device. Thus, sensitive individuals are needed to render feedback loops detectable (P2). Of course, there are phenom-ena in muscle testing and myostatic testing which may present problems to our way of think-ing. These include the test results being changed by insignificant influences such as having active agents placed on one's tongue or in one's breast pocket, taking off one's jewellery, cleaning one's glasses, or even by thoughts and moods in general and placebos in particular. In addition, there is the phenomenon of a surrogate test person (Lack 1996). For example, this means that it is possible for a mother to act as surrogate for her small child who is the patient. The mother places one hand on the child while her other arm is used for testing. The patient's strong and weak responses are then automatically transferred to the surrogate.

This sounds very strange but it works. Tibetan pulse diagnosis, which we shall discuss in Chs.7.5 & 8.1, offers an analogous phenomenon of *surrogate* or *substitutional pulses* (Qusar et al. 1997, p.26f). Traditionally, in Tibet and the surrounding regions, the patient travels to see the healer. However, if the patient is seriously ill or the region inaccessible, this may not be possible. However, the illness of a child left at home, for example, can be diagnosed using the mother's pulse. All this – as well as the medicine testing in EAV – points to a method of information transference of which we know next to nothing. Protocols of experiments can easily be conceived here which could explain the circumstances under which this transference no longer occurs. For example, the myostatic test using surrogates apparently requires a connection between the surrogate and the actual patient. What type of connection is needed (strength, type and location of bodily contact, by telephone or even just mental)? Must the connection be mutual or not? Answering these questions would pave the way for a more focused implementation of these phenomena.

6.2. Taking Symbolism into Account: Biofeedback

Another aspect of feedback loops is given by biofeedback. Unfortunately, it is utilised in medicine far too rarely. This probably has to do with the fact that it does not agree with the classical healing scheme but emphasises the aspect of self-experience and self-therapy. Among other things, it concerns the control of bodily functions, which are subject to the autonomic nervous system and therefore are usually beyond the reach of conscious will. Sensors are used to detect, for example, electrical conductance, skin temperature or blood circulation in a finger but also the heartbeat (electrocardiogram) or tension in various muscles. The measured values are shown on a computer monitor. The temperature might be coded by colours, from violet (cold) to red (hot) with green as medium temperature. Since skin temperature does not remain completely constant, this is also true for the colours on the monitor. The task is to feel into these colours and attempt to change the temperature in the finger. With the proper aptitude, it usually takes a few days to learn this technique. How it works remains a mystery. In any case, it is possible to raise or lower the temperature in a finger locally by 1°C relative to the normal temperature and that, after some practice, without the biofeedback device. Indian yogis can also do this. However, they need months or years to learn it. Apparently, the feedback device augments an individual's abilities enormously. Possible applications include relaxation training or learning the correct muscle contractions to treat incontinence.

Biofeedback shows aspects of self-therapy and encompasses diagnosis and therapy. The patient learns to interpret the signs on the monitor (the colours as signs of temperature, tension, etc.) and to influence them actively. That signs and symptoms are changed simply by observation and measuring is a well-known fact. Influencing a quantity to be measured simply by measuring it is something that also comes up in physics. In a personal communication, Gerhard Bujak gave me the following medical example: For the purposes of practice, several students performed Chinese pulse diagnosis on one and the same test subject. This resulted in a substantial change of pulse characteristics in a matter of 15 to 30 minutes. From my own experience, I know that whenever my pulse is too fast before I fall asleep, it normalises as soon as I can hear or feel it through 'pillow feedback'. The idea that the diagnosis is already the first step in therapy, or is even therapy in itself, comes up again and again. Even so in psychoanalysis, which finds its conception based on the idea that merely bringing a childhood trauma into consciousness helps the patient to process it. A more recent example is that of a bioresonance device which had been designed simply to measure abnormalities in the body's electromagnetic fields but was found to partly normalise these just by measuring them (Noemi Kempe, personal communication).

Closing a feedback loop can have astounding consequences in other ways as well. We met such an example in the physical-technical field in Ch.3 in form of a video feedback, where aesthetic and at times apparent biological structures emanated 'out of nothing' simply by training the video camera on the monitor in a suitable manner, which in turn mirrored what occurred in the camera's view (Crutchfield 1984). It would be just as novel to influence the behaviour through focused feedback. It is possible, for example, to change the relationship of singular and plural in a conversation partner through slight nodding of the head or frowning (whenever singular or, resp., plural is used by the conversation partner independent of the content) without him knowing what's going on (Giselher Guttmann, personal communication). This can be interpreted as feedback (praise and punishment) minimally influencing all modes of behaviour which were activated immediately before feedback. Through frequent repetition, the desired behaviour is reinforced. Such considerations are not only important in upbringing but also offer an enormous potential in medicine, which should be utilised for focused development in feedback diagnoses and feedback therapies.

This building up of processes supported by feedback leads to dynamic and sometimes even chaotic behaviour (cf. Chs.3-4). Since there is a multitude of feedback loops in the human organism, the complex dynamics of living processes is not astounding. This field of chronobiology and chronomedicine is discussed in more detail in Ch.11.2. It also expresses itself in the altered dynamics in the case of illness. The term "dynamic diseases" is also used (Glass & Mackey 1988, Ch.9). Bringing in well-defined external feedback loops, to which the organism nonetheless reacts in an individual manner, enables individual therapy, despite general rules (cf. Ch.5.2). We have already mentioned one example of this – biofeedback. Its individual aspect is apparent in the fact that not all patients can work with it equally well. According to Achterberg (1989, pp.136-140), it primarily depends on trust and willingness to participate but also on aptitude for imagination and altered states of consciousness.

Due to the crucial role of feedback, biofeedback is an expression of P2. In addition, the symbolic representation of temperature with colours, in particular, points to a relationship to P3 (*"everything is a symbol and stands for something else"*, Table 2.1) – hence the title of Ch.6.2. The translation of the monitor's colour information by the organism also remains a mystery. Presumably, everything works so well because we, too, function on a symbolic level. Whenever we see or hear something, it is coded into our nervous systems. The colour or tone is constructed by the brain. We are already working with coding, symbols and analogies. Thus, the fact that a colour on the monitor represents a temperature fits in well and can be processed by us.

This brings us to the possibility, which has already been mentioned, of regarding the forms of diagnosis (EAV, kinesiology, pulse diagnosis) discussed in Ch.6.1 in the light of P3, which expresses itself in symbolism, analogies and mutual mirroring of various planes. Clues to this are: a) surrogate testing or surrogate pulse, where *one* person instead of *another* is examined, b) EAV measuring, where the *doctor* (co-)creates the needle deflection but projects this to the *patient* and/or the *device*. In the sense of P3, the patient's condition is possibly mirrored in the surrogate or therapist, who then only has to listen inwardly. To do this, however, he must be able to turn off his own scepticism, which tells him that something like this is not really possible and which therefore blocks his own abilities. The remedy is: external actions and projecting onto the external world. In archaic and ethnic forms of therapy, the healer calls on external powers or goes on a spiritual journey but this may be simply a way of activating his or her abilities. Rituals and symbols would then be used not only to impress and distract the patient but also to influence one's own consciousness. Today's fetish is technology. It is a very useful tool, allowing one to hide one's own sensitivity behind a pointing needle and to project one's skill onto a technical device in order to circumvent any blocks that the use of this skill might provoke. Achterberg (1989) even talks about the possibility of listening in the body without a biofeedback device (p.273), which presumably has something to do with the unconscious mind purposefully arranging for the body to heal itself (p.264). In the usual form of biofeedback, the patient also goes on an inner journey and enters a realm where information about healing is accessible (p.138).

Altered states of consciousness ('trance') often arise in ethnotherapy. Among other things, they could serve to overcome the scepticism of rationality or of normal waking consciousness. Van Wijk (1998) also speaks – in the case of electro-acupuncture by Voll – of a change or shift in the doctor's consciousness, which allows him to perceive tiny changes in the patient. The transpersonal perspective offers another way of looking at such phenomena (Zundel & Loomans 1994, Brückner 1999). Achterberg (1989) also comments on this. According to p.10, imagination can affect one's own organism (communication with one's own organs, preverbal visualisation of healing) or another's (transpersonal visualisation of healing). On p.73, Achterberg addresses the important role of the healer's ability to visualise. If this is sufficiently large, then rituals and symbols are only necessary for the patient. Discoveries that are more recent point to the fact that transpersonal and spiritual ideas are not necessary for explaining the phenomena of healing but they are easy to work with (p.156 & 214). On p.261, the author makes a connection between *symbols* and *symptoms*, whose combined meaning is a concrete, comprehensible object standing for an incomprehensible idea (a circumscription of P3!).

Table 6.1. Medical concepts (Dossey 1995, pp.65-72) and healing imagery (Achterberg 1989, p.10); compare with perspectives P1-P4.

Dossey:	*Era I* (from 1850 on)	*Era II* (from 1950 on)	*Era III* (in progress)
Characteristics	Local	Local	Global
Synonyms	Substance medicine	Mind-body medicine	Transpersonal medicine
Description	Causal, deterministic	Impact of consciousness	Beyond space and time
Examples	Surgery, medicinal plants	Biofeedback, hypnosis	Prayer, therapeutic touch
Achterberg	–	Preverbal (inner aspect)	Transpersonal (outer aspect)
Table 2.1a–b	P1 & 2	P2 & 3	P3 & 4

Dossey (1995, Ch. 2) also discusses the role of consciousness in various forms of medicine. His is also a chronological arrangement, which in a certain way is a reversal of a longer-term development (cf. the considerations of this work, Ch. 2.2). However, he assesses the times of transition as earlier. Table 6.1 gives a brief account of Dossey's statements and makes a connection to Achterberg and the approaches to reality of P1-P4. There are some overlaps: with the aid of P2, a bridge can be drawn from era I to era II, with P3 from era II to era III.

Finally, let us also elaborate on Weil (1995), who draws interesting conclusions concerning *spontaneous healing*, which fit in well with the above. On p.146, he talks about the problem of our autonomic nervous system not being directly subject to our will, which blocks healing reactions. This impediment can be circumvented, according to Weil, by projecting our belief in healing onto something external. The strongest correlation between psyche and healing consists in accepting the illness, which brings about internal relaxation as opposed to the constant stress of resisting, which is often connected with surrender to a higher power.

On p.280, Weil offers a similar idea from a different perspective. In daydreams, the visual cortex is relieved from processing visual information and can connect psyche and mind via the control mechanisms of the autonomic nervous system and thus trigger spontaneous healing. This statement brings to mind that, when the subject's eyes are closed, an electroencephalogram of the visual cortex will show an α- instead of a β-rhythm, which indicates relaxation. Moreover, in a trance one's gaze is pointed inward and the usual focus on what is visible externally largely loses its significance. On p.342, a paragraph on religious healing is presented (cf. Table 6.1, era III). It points out that the patient's belief in the effectiveness of the prayer being said for him is important (and could then be explained within the frame of era II), but that prayers can also be effective even if the patient does not know that they are being said (here we need era III).

6.3. Bioresonance and Autologous Therapies

Let us now concentrate on the *therapeutic aspect* of what has been discussed in Chs. 6.1 & 6.2. This information transference, which we have mentioned several times, can also be used to manufacture remedies electronically, in particular those used in homoeopathy (cf. Ch. 5.3). There are two versions, one direct and one indirect:

a) The homoeopathic remedy is placed into an input beaker in the device and the information is transmitted – via a high-power amplifier – to the pure solvent (in the output beaker), which thus becomes an electronically produced homoeopathic remedy.

b) The information is first stored on a CD. Whenever a corresponding homoeopathic remedy is to be produced, it can then be read electronically off the CD.

More on this subject can be found in Endler (1998, Ch.2.4 & p.64). According to Endler, there was no significant difference, in the cases he investigated, between the homoeopathic remedies manufactured in the usual way and those made by the above methods.

What has been said so far in Chs. 6.1 & 6.2, together with the following considerations can also be looked at from a different angle. In Ch. 6.1, we looked at the organism's reaction to an externally set electrical voltage or information (external or exogenous aspect in the foreground). Then, in Ch.6.2, we discussed biofeedback, where diagnoses and therapy, as well as internal (endogenous) and external (exogenous) reference, are inseparably intertwined. And now we shall explore methods in which information is taken from the organism and fed back to it in altered form. The internal starting point and the therapeutic aspect are central in this case. For example, bioresonance therapy is based on the MORA device by Morell and Rasche, but since they first made theirs, there have been many different versions made by a number of manufacturers. In principle, electrodes with large surfaces are placed on the hands and feet, which then read the weak body signals and feed them back in altered form, triggering a therapeutic effect.

How this alteration of signals occurs and what form they take often remains a mystery. There is talk of frequencies with pathogenic components, which have to be eliminated. After scrutiny, one finds a gap between physical science and technical/electronic application. In this case, there seems to be a particularly blatant disparity between the respective approaches of scientist and electronic 'tinkerer'. When I asked two competent scientists in this field how these bioresonance devices really worked, both said that, although they were very interested in the subject, the official information was unsatisfactory. Thus they would need to build such devices themselves (or had already built one) in order to establish some clarity on its function and to use it for further research.

Two borderline cases of conversion to which the device can be tuned and which always come up with regard to this topic, are in-phase feedback and inverting. In the former case, the signal is amplified (stimulus, homoeopathic approach) and in the latter, it is cancelled out (de-stressing, allopathic approach). This is especially interesting for us, as we have examined the ambivalence of these two approaches several times already. Interestingly, Ludwig (1999, pp.86-88) writes that originally the signal was inverted, but now it turns out that it makes no difference whether it is inverted or amplified! We have encountered a similar situation (cf. Ch.5.2) in acupuncture when considering whether tonifying (stimulating) or sedating (calming) has an *opposite* or *similar* effect. According to Ludwig, it depends on the change, which serves as an alerting stimulus and thus apparently triggers a regulation. He gives the example of a ticking clock, which one no longer hears once one is used to it, so that one can fall asleep next to it without difficulty. Noticeable changes, such as the clock ringing or stopping ticking (which corresponds to cancelling) will cause one to wake up. In much the same way, constant pathogenic signals in the organism are interpreted as signals of a normal, healthy state and so are no longer counter-regulated.

Since bioresonance devices, first and foremost, serve as therapy, they are used in combination with other methods, which have been mentioned in Ch.6.1, for the purposes of diagnosis or progress control. There are also several versions of bioresonance therapy, such as dual biosignal modulation (Lack 1997). In order to find a common term for this far-ranging field, Ludwig speaks of *system information therapy* or *informative medicine* (Ludwig 1994, 1999). Endler & Schulte (1996) and Endler & Stacher (1997) also investigated the relationship between homoeopathy and bioresonance therapy. In Kratky (1995b, 1996a&b, 1998c), first-principle considerations concerning feedback therapies were made, which can be found under the keyword *chaos control* in Ch.4.3. We refer the reader who is interested in questions regarding regulation and bioelectrical phenomena to Bergsmann (1994).

It is not only electromagnetic signals that can be taken from the organism and fed back to it in altered form, but also substances. In this case we shall refer to them as *autologous therapies or procedures, cf.* Gedeon (2000). There are, for example, autologous blood and autologous urine therapies (Schmiedel & Augustin 1997). It seems absurd to reintroduce a substance (especially a product of excretion) into the body from which it was taken. According to Ludwig, however, it could also be a signal, which alerts the organism to a change. Just the mere external introduction (and the negligible but unavoidable chemical alteration) results in a new situation which is only *similar* to the pre-existing one. This similarity brings to mind homoeopathy, especially when the substance has also been changed in some way (for example, when blood is exposed to a magnetic field before re-injection). Otherwise, a comparison to *isopathy* suggests itself (cf. Ch.5.1). In any case, something must have changed for an alertness signal to take effect. Incidentally, the argument concerning the alertness signal implies that an ideal isopathy (identical instead of similar) would not work. Then a homoeopathically prepared arsenic potency, which is administered in isopathy in a case of arsenic poisoning, is only similar to the toxic trigger (being different in terms of concentration and production). It appears, then, that the simile principle works *because of* its similarity (simile, simillimum) and not *despite* a lack of agreement (exactum). However, the similarity must be sufficient in order to have an effect in the form of resonance.

Whether or not something is effective in this way might also have to do with the site at which a substance is introduced into the body. To this effect, Sukul (1998) gives an account of experiments on albino mice where the influence of potentised Agaricus muscarius L was observed on the cataleptic effect of subsequently administered haloperidol. If the homoeopathic remedy was placed on the tongue, the effect of haloperidol was reduced, while injecting this remedy into the peritoneum had no effect. Sukul surmises that a homoeopathic remedy acts via the taste bud receptors. However, it would just be as likely that the organism regards something placed on the tongue as coming from outside and therefore gives it more attention. Regarding the manner in which a homoeopathic remedy needs to be ingested for optimal effect – or for any effect at all – further research is needed. There are several indications that direct contact is not crucial at all. Endler (1998) devoted his attention in many animal experiments to changes in duration of metamorphosis in tadpoles triggered by potentised thyroxin. The preparation was usually dripped into the water in which the tadpoles lived, but Endler also describes experiments in Ch.2.3 where thyroxin was placed in the water in closed glass vials. The effect was comparable in both experiments.

This closes the circuit. In the section on electro-acupuncture (Ch.6.1), we talked about the medicine being placed within the electrical circuit in remedy testing. But here, too, there is no real electrical contact. The test gives analogous results whenever the remedy is near the patient (van Wijk & Wiegant 1994); cf. Ch.6.1. Just as in kinesiology, it suffices to place the substance in contact with the subject. Which mechanisms are responsible for these effects is still largely unclear. From a physical perspective, primarily electromagnetic interactions come to mind, but perhaps there will be some surprises in this field, too.

Chapter 7

Traditional Chinese Medicine
and its Roots

7.1. Yin and Yang, Deficiency and Excess

Chinese medicine is thought to be between 3000 and 4000 years old. Within three centuries after the first unification of the Chinese empire in 221 B.C. , this medicine system changed appreciably (Unschuld 2002 & 2003, Part VI), and developed into what is now known as *Traditional Chinese Medicine* (TCM). We will call the older one *ancient Chinese medicine* and come back to it later in this chapter. In contrast to Western medicine, TCM has continued to be used in the traditional way up to present times and, compared with the recent ever-growing developments of the former, has changed very slowly over the centuries. Even the political changes in China after World War II (the People's Republic of China from 1949 onwards) left the essence of TCM untouched. However, processes of standardisation and simplification took place.

In the West, acupuncture is the best known facet of TCM. In one way, it accords with our Western way of thinking since it is a reproducible technique, which consists of inserting needles into certain points on the body. The meridians, on which this technique is based, are, however, more foreign to us. We are aware of the anatomical systems of nerves, lymphatics and blood vessels that traverse the whole body and form networks. However, these are verifiable, while the meridians appear to be only a construct, with which one can work and heal but which do not 'really' exist. We shall come back to this point in Ch. 7.4.

TCM is based on a complete system of natural philosophy. In China, acupuncture only comprises a small part of a wide range of therapeutic measures, of which the most important is prescribing medicinal herbs. Thus, if we want to look at TCM, we need first to understand a few fundamental terms. The central theme is the polarity of yin and yang. Some of their characteristics are listed in Table 7.1. According to Chinese understanding, yin and yang are equipollent – not opposites but two mutually complementing and dependent poles. A corresponding one-dimensional representation is given in Figure 7.1. In a situation or in a person, either yin or yang can be predominant at certain times. A complete yin or yang situation corresponds to a point far to the left or far to the right, respectively; the midpoint of the 'scale' denotes an exact balance in yin and yang. This, of course, does not give any indication of whether yin and yang are weak or strong, but just that they are balanced.

A two-dimensional representation can give more detailed information about yin and yang. It can be likened to antagonists in the organism, which complement each other in their effect: for example in muscles (flexors and extensors) or in the vegetative nervous system (sympathetic and parasympathetic system). A corresponding representation is given in Figure 7.2a. The arrows on the yin and yang axes denote the direction of increasing yin or yang respectively. At each axis, there are three specific points corresponding to the following values: (theoretical) minimum, neutral middle and maximum. Values below and above the neutral middle correspond to deficiency and excess, respectively. In TCM, the terms vacuity (emptiness) and repletion (fullness) can also be found. As to the TCM terminology in English, see Wiseman & Feng (1998), Unschuld (2003) and Tian & Lachner (2006). In the following, we distinguish between deficiency and vacuity, the latter being the extreme of the former. In an analogous manner, we distinguish between excess and repletion.

Now we come back to Figure 7.2a. In the spirit of TCM, the centre is called earth, which will become clear in the discussion of Table 7.3 and Table 9.2. The triangular regions in Figure 7.2a (two grey and two white) define four cases or types:

Table 7.1. Some characteristics of yin and yang

Yin	Cold	wet	deficiency	internal	dark	below	structure	feminine
Yang	Hot	dry	excess	external	light	above	dynamics	masculine

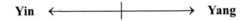

Figure 7.1. Yin/yang polarity in one dimension.

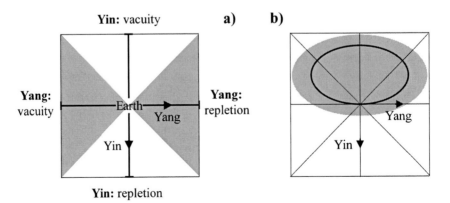

Figure 7.2. Yin/yang polarity drawn in two dimensions. **a)** The four triangular regions around the directions towards vacuity and repletion of both yin and yang. **b)** The displayed grey and black ellipses are explained in the text.

Yin deficiency (mixed type)   (7.1a)

Yang deficiency (YIN type)   ━┼━   Yang excess (YANG type)   (7.1b)

Yin excess (mixed type)   (7.1c)

The types are characterised by their dominating deviation of yin *or* yang from the neutral value. An overall assessment of YIN and YANG is included in parentheses (YIN, YANG and mixed types). In order to explain this, we start with the example on the left in (7.1b). Yang deficiency means *too little yang,* a circumstance corresponding to *yin* in the representation of Figure 7.1. Furthermore, in TCM deficiency itself is one of the properties of *yin*, cf. Table 7.1. Thus, both arguments strengthen each other, resulting in the overall assessment YIN for yang deficiency. By analogous arguments, yang excess yields the overall assessment YANG.

Thus, the two cases of (7.1b) can be interpreted easily, the corresponding triangular regions being displayed in grey in Figure 7.2a. The cases (7.1a&c) are more complicated. For example, yin deficiency (7.1a) is characterised by *too little yin* and thus is *yang* in the representation of Figure 7.2a. On the other hand, deficiency is assigned to *yin*, cf. Table 7.1. Thus, yin deficiency, which is characterised by *deficiency*, results from this viewpoint in *yin*. The two arguments come to different conclusions, cf. Kaptchuk (1996, p.217f). For this reason, the expression 'mixed type' has been used in (7.1a). An analogous situation can be found in (7.1c).

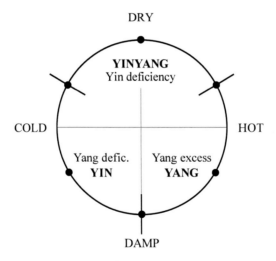

Figure 7.3. Circle representation of Chinese types YIN, YANG & YINYANG corresponding to yang deficiency, yang excess and yin deficiency.

In general, yin tends to *deficiencies*. According to Jarmey & Mojay (1995, pp.132-134) yin excess is, in practice, very rare, and this has been confirmed by an experienced acupuncturist (Jochen Gleditsch, personal communication). Thus, for simplification we can neglect the corresponding case (7.1c) for now but will return to it later on (see Chs.8.4, 9.2 & 13). For the time being, we restrict ourselves to the upper half of the square displayed in Figure 7.2b. More precisely, we shall consider the black ellipse as a representative of typical states.

When using a formal transformation (vertical stretching by a factor $3^{1/2}$, the square root of 3), the black ellipse turns into a circle (Figure 7.3). In later chapters, we will extend our field of attention to the shaded ellipse of Figure 7.2b, which transforms to a circular disc (health disc; Figures.8.4, 9.4 & 13.3).

Considering the black ellipse of Figure 7.2a or the resulting circle of Figure 7.3, the three types of (7.1a&b) remain. They are described in more detail by Jarmey & Mojay from the perspective of shiatsu. For example,

Yang deficiency: cold – always and everywhere   (7.2a)

Yang excess: hot – always and everywhere   (7.2b)

Yin deficiency: hot – sometimes and in certain parts of the body; otherwise cold.   (7.2c)

Here, too, it is immediately obvious that yin deficiency is a mixed type. Temperature, apparently, relates primarily to *yang*. It stands to reason that the second pair wet/dry listed in Table 7.1 primarily relates to *yin*. Then the yang axis in Figure 7.2b can be interpreted as the temperature axis, and the yin axis as the moisture axis, which relates to the ideas of Greek Antiquity (see Figure 2.1 and Kaptchuk 1996, p.218f). Following on from this, we can see that *yang* covers the range of *cold* (vacuity) to *hot* (repletion) and *yin* the range of *dry* (vacuity) to *damp* (neutral).

To round things off, we can look at a classification into three TCM constitutions modelled after Badelt (1983, p.109). Following the sequence of (7.2a-c), we have three constitutions:

Yin constitution: deficiency symptoms, chronic diseases,   weak stimulus.   (7.3a)

Yang constit.:   excess symptoms,   acute diseases,   strong stimulus.   (7.3b)

Mixed form: mixed symptoms,   subacute diseases, moderate stimulus.   (7.3c)

The interesting point here is the relationship between the character of disease and the strength of the stimulus. The latter is subject to the Arndt-Schulz Law (Table 5.1): weak stimuli activate ('tonify'), strong stimuli weaken ('sedate') and medium stimuli equilibrate ('create eutony or harmonise'). It is important to note that the types or constitutions also appear in healthy people where they indicate a predisposition to yang deficiency, yang excess or yin deficiency in times of stress.

Thus, the two-dimensional yin/yang representation finally leads to a ternary typology, analogies of which can be found worldwide. The three types can also be characterised by the general terms YIN, YANG and YINYANG (mixed type). This same classification can also be found in Kubny (1995, p.170f), who considers the combined effect of yin and yang to be a third type and the human being to consist of all three factors. Ternary typologies are often characterised by two pure types and one mixed type, which, in a certain respect, also contains the other two (for example: the miasm *psora* in homoeopathy). We shall come back to these ideas frequently.

Figure 7.3 demonstrates this in the form of the above-mentioned circle. The three types correspond to circular arcs of 120° each, which are delineated by intersecting axes. The six black dots indicate the centres of, and the boundaries between, the three arcs or regions. In addition, the vertical moisture or yin axis and the horizontal temperature or yang axis are shown in grey. They already hint at the planned extension from *circle* to *disc*, which we shall address in the following chapters. This will lead to a cross-cultural graphical representation.

7.2. Elements and Meridians

It is also possible to equate these types that we have discussed with Chinese *elements*. In ancient Chinese medicine, there were six elements. The usual number in TCM is five. However, as we shall see below, a memory of the former number 6 remains. As we have already noted, the Ancient Greeks had first three, then four, and at last five elements – the opposite poles of water and fire, earth and air with ether in the centre (see Figure 2.2). The six black dots in Figure 7.3 can now be interpreted as Chinese elements. In Figure 7.4, the Chinese elements are assigned to the three types YIN, YANG, and YINYANG. This will become clearer in Ch. 8, especially (8.4a-c). First, however, we need to concentrate on the names and the interrelation of the Chinese elements.

In Figure 7.4, the Chinese elements – shown outside the circle – are indicated by curly brackets. These will be used in the future in order to avoid confusion with elements that occur in other healing traditions. The effective range of each element extends one sixth of the way around the circle (as shown by the arcs with arrows). In the middle of each section, the name of the corresponding element is given and a black dot marks the exact location. From now on, whenever an *element* is mentioned, the context will reveal whether it refers to the whole region or only to its centre.

In the more detailed discussion of elements, which now ensues, axes that pass through the point of origin and intersect the circle at opposite points will be mentioned. For the moment, while we are using the circle representation, only these two points will be considered. Later we shall look at the whole axis.

Axes: {water} – {ruling fire}, {earth} – {metal}, {wood} – {minister fire}. (7.4a)

The distinction between {ruling} and {minister fire}, which can still be found in TCM, reminds us of the earlier system of six elements. However, {ruling fire}, which is sometimes called {master fire}, is thought to be 'true fire'. If {ruling} and {minister fire} are subsumed under a single element {fire}, five elements result, cf. Unschuld (2003, App.). In Tibetan medicine, the sixth element is attributed to *water*. To avoid confusion when developing a cross-cultural medicine, we have given the sixth element a completely different name. In the spirit of ancient Chinese medicine, this is {flora}. Thus, (7.4a) turns into:

Axes: {water} – {fire}, {earth} – {metal}, {wood} – {flora}. (7.4b)

Now, let us look at these axes as shown in Figure 7.4. On one axis, {water} and {fire} are at opposite ends as was the case with the elements *water* and *fire* of the Ancient Greeks. This suggests that the Chinese elements may have something to do with the Greek elements of the same name, but they cannot be presumed to be identical. The pair {earth} and {metal} at opposite ends of another axis suggests that {metal} might have something in common with the *air* of the Ancient Greeks and, indeed, there is a relationship. {Metal} is assigned to the lung meridian and also to the large intestine meridian (Table 7.2a). The former has to do with *air*, the latter fits in with the interpretation of {metal} as *hard earth*, which can also be found in the literature. These two opposite aspects reflect the ambiguous nature of yin deficiency (mixed type); cf. (7.1a) and (7.2c). One can also find the following polarity of metals in {metal}: as unsightly ore and as a smoothly polished metal surface, where the solid metal recedes, becomes 'airy' and reflects its surroundings.

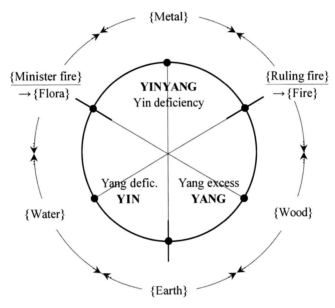

Figure 7.4. Circle representation of the Chinese elements. Those located at human legs and arms at equivalent sites (Table 7.2) are shown on opposite sides of the circle. '*Back*': {water} – {ruling fire}, '*front*': {earth} – {metal} and '*middle*': {wood} – {minister fire}. For the types YIN, YANG and YINYANG (yang deficiency, yang excess and yin deficiency), see Figure 7.3. As to the renaming of two elements, see the text.

There is also a third axis in Figure 7.4, which connects {wood} with {flora} and which was not recognised by the Ancient Greeks since {wood} has no counterpart in the Greek system of elements. In TCM, one often speaks of a system of *five* elements, but there are also indications of a *sixth* element, which plays a special role (Connelly 1995, p.47) and also has various names (Kratky 2000a). Badelt (1983) discusses the six elements in detail. In Tibetan medicine, the sixth element is assigned to *water* (see Ch.7.5) and, as we have already mentioned, in TCM it is frequently associated with *fire*. Stressing the difference between Tibetan and Chinese attributions, the name 'waterfire' would be fitting for the sixth element, too. Comparison with Ayurveda, on the other hand, reveals a relationship to the Greek-Indian element *ether* (see Ch.8). The name {flora} was suggested in Kratky (1997b&c). In ancient Chinese medicine, it was called *grain* or *stone*; see Wilhelm (1998, p.6) and Lo (2002), respectively. The findings of Hertzer (1996, p.71f) suggest that {flora} was also given the name *grass* (*plant*). The name *rice* was also used in ancient Chinese medicine (Gerhard Wenzel, personal communication).

Table 7.2a. Systematics of meridians, each of them having two names. For instance, kidney is also called foot *shaoyin* if one refers to the bottom / top (foot / hand) relationship, cf. Table 7.2b. Based on Kubiena (1995, Ch.5).

Meridian	Back	Front	Middle
Interior (yin) Bottom (foot)[b] Exterior (yang) Bottom (foot)[b] **Element**[c]	Kidney Foot *shaoyin* Bladder Foot *taiyang* **{Water}**	Spleen Foot *taiyin* Stomach Foot *yangming* **{Earth}**	Liver Foot *jueyin* Gallbladder Foot *shaoyang* **{Wood}**
Interior (yin) Top (hand)[b] Exterior (yang) Top (hand)[b] **Element**[c]	Heart Hand *shaoyin* Small Intestine Hand *taiyang* **{Fire}**	Lung Hand *taiyin* Large Intestine Hand *yangming* **{Metal}**	PC [d] Hand *jueyin* SJ [d] Hand *shaoyang* **{Flora}**

Table 7.2b. Explanations to Table 7.2a

[a] Foot and hand- meridians	They have their endpoints in foot and hand, respectively.
[b] Associated foot/ hand pair	e.g. in posterior position: * interior: *shaoyin* – foot: Kidney, hand: Heart * exterior: *taiyang* – foot: Bladder, hand: Small Intestine
[c] Associated inte- rior/ exterior pair	e.g. in posterior position: * foot: **{water}** – interior: Kidney, exterior: Bladder * hand: **{fire}** – interior: Heart, exterior: Small Intestine
[d] Meridians PC, SJ	* PC: Pericardium (Circulation/Sex, *yang* or *fire* kidney) * SJ: *Sanjiao* (Triple Heater, Burner or Energiser)

Now, let us look at the relationship between meridians and elements In Table 7.2a&b you can see that each of the elements is associated with two of the twelve regular meridians. The meridians vary greatly in length and each is named after the internal organ with which it is associated, such as the kidney(s) or bladder. The regular meridians are bilateral, i.e. they have counterparts in both the left side and the right side of the body. In the following, meridians are written with a capital letter to distinguish them from the corresponding organs. The abbreviation of all meridians consists of two capital letters (see below, Table 7.5), the notation of Wiseman & Feng (1998, p.XII) being used with one exception: *sanjiao* (SJ). There are several English translations of this Chinese expression (see Table 7.2b), which are all somewhat misleading. Nowadays, *san* and *jiao* mean *three* and *burning*, respectively. In Ancient Chinese, however, *jiao* meant *body cavity*; see Meng (1997, p.203). In fact, SJ is the only meridian that is not associated with a single organ, but is understood to be a generalisation of functions of the organs in the three body cavities (*upper jiao*: chest, *middle jiao*: upper abdomen, *lower jiao*: lower abdomen).

At certain sites, the meridians come close to the surface of the skin (at the location of the acupuncture points) and are thus accessible to therapy by way of acupuncture needles. Six meridians run through the *leg* ('bottom') and six through the *arm* ('top'). Within these two groups, the meridians are further divided into pairs associated with their location: 'back', 'front' and 'middle'. Within each of these pairs (corresponding to the elements), one meridian is *yin* or 'interior' and the other *yang* or 'exterior'. Thus, the topology of the meridians is mirrored in Table 7.2a&b (see also Figure 7.5). For example, the *Heart* and *Small Intestine* meridians are the yin and yang meridians of the element {fire}. In the arm, they are close to one another (in the *back* position). It is also possible to associate meridians at corresponding locations in leg and arm ('foot/hand pair', sometimes called *meridian* axis). In the back interior position, these are the *Kidney* (foot) and *Heart* (hand). Both these meridians are known by the Chinese name, *shaoyin*, so the *Kidney* and *Heart* meridians are also called foot and hand *shaoyin*, respectively. The other meridians can be considered in the same way.

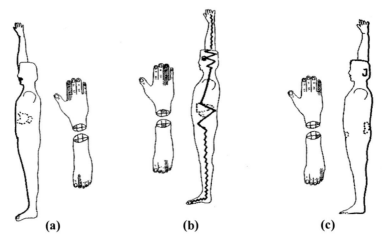

Figure 7.5. Location of the six *yang* meridians in the body, detailed in foot and hand.
a) Front: *yangming* (foot: Stomach; hand: Large Intestine). **b)** Middle: *shaoyang* (foot: Gallbladder; hand: SJ). **c)** Back: *taiyang* (foot: Bladder; hand: Small Intestine), cf. Table 7.2a&b. This Figure is based on Gleditsch (1988a, Figure 1).

Now we come back to the axes of the elements, see Figure 7.4 and (7.4a&b). Two elements in a foot/hand relation form such an axis, cf. Table 7.2a. All in all:

{Water} – {fire}:	back	(esp. water: *Bladder*);	connection to P2;	(7.5a)
{Earth} – {metal}:	front	(esp. earth: *Stomach*);	connection to P3;	(7.5b)
{Wood} – {flora}:	middle	(esp. wood: *Gallbladder*);	connection to P1/P4.	(7.5c)

The three yang meridians *Bladder*, *Stomach*, and *Gallbladder* are particularly long, traversing a large part of the body. According to Gleditsch (2001), there is a cross-link to the psychological characteristics assigned to the elements (see Table 7.3). {Water} ('back') stands for security and trust, as long as one is protected and supported from behind, and for fear if one feels threatened from behind. {Earth} ('front', free range of vision) stands for making contact. As we shall see in the next chapters, this is also true for {metal} in a special way, {metal} being on the same axis as {earth}. {Wood} ('middle'): the Gallbladder meridian runs in a zigzag down the side of the body. It stands for needing space, implementing the 'elbow technique' and for anger. Thus, there is a connection between elements and emotions (see Table 7.3).

In this table, one can also find the *sensory functions* that are attributed to the elements. These will give us the opportunity of assigning the perspectives P1-P4 introduced in Ch.2.2; see (7.5a-c) regarding the results. The axis {water} – {fire} corresponds to *hearing – speaking* (here speaking is considered a sensory function). It is about communication, which can only be successful when somebody is listening to the speaker and which is only complemented by the feedback loop, where both conversation partners can speak in turn. This gives a close connection to P2.

Table 7.3. Correspondences of the Chinese elements;
based on Kubiena (1995, Ch.3.3), supplemented

Yin/yang pair of Meridians	Back	Front	Middle
Element (foot) Emotion Sensory function	**{Water}** Fear Hearing	**{Earth}** Brooding Taste	**{Wood}** Anger Seeing
Layer, tissue Taste Climatic influence	Bones Salty Cold	Muscles Sweet Dampness	Tendons Sour Wind (gusty)
Element (hand) Emotion Sensory function	**{Fire}** Joy Speaking	**{Metal}** Sadness Smelling	**{Flora}** Equanimity (Inner) vision
Layer, tissue Taste Climatic influence	Hypodermis Bitter Heat	Epidermis Pungent, acrid Dryness	Outmost / inmost Harsh /astringent; bland Calm (draught)

Now to the axis {earth} – {metal} that corresponds to *taste – smell*. {Metal} is also assigned to touch (or, more precisely, to all sense organs of the skin: pressure, temperature and pain). In general, touch is not mentioned explicitly. However, due to the assignment of {metal} to the epidermis (see Table 7.3), it finds its natural place with this element.

Taste and touch – associated with {earth} and {metal}, respectively – are contact senses, which fits in with Gleditsch's argument. Furthermore, we have already mentioned the ambivalent relation of {metal} to *air* and to its polar opposite, *hard earth*, which reflects the double meaning of yin deficiency. This recalls P3, in which mirroring plays an important role and whose motto is: "Everything is a symbol and stands for something else". This is also confirmed by the sensory functions: we often confuse smell and taste. When the nose is congested, we notice that we cannot 'taste' anything. In Swiss German, the sentence "Da *schmeckt* es aber gut! (Something *tastes* good here!)", 'schmecken (*taste*)' actually means *smell*. Furthermore, the German word 'tasten' does not mean *taste* {earth}, but *touch* {metal}.

The axis {wood} – {flora} and P1&4 remain to be considered. The sensory function *seeing* is assigned to the element {wood}; for {flora} I have added 'inner seeing'. This fits in well with the paradoxical nature of {flora} (which we shall mention frequently) of being able to get in touch with the 'entire world' most readily by seemingly withdrawing from it (e.g. in certain forms of meditation). It is seeing with the inner eye. In addition – also due to the proximity of {flora} to {water} in the circle representation – the sense of equilibrium related to the ear is a possibility (see Badelt 1983, p.33). Here it is true, too, that someone is aware of his location relative to his surroundings, even if he withdraws from them (the force of gravity coming from outside is felt internally). Because of its connection to meditation, the suggested emotion here is 'equanimity' (see Table 7.3).

P1 stands for *separation* but also battle and hierarchy, P4 for *union*. P1 finds its place with {wood} but is also an aspect of {flora}, where P4 also finds its place. Thus, we encounter a transition between perspectives P1 and P4, which, at first glance, seem to be those that are farthest apart. The internal solidarity of a group (P4) is often accompanied by battling or ignoring other groups (two variants of P1). An extreme example of this is: I do not know anything about others anymore, everything (namely I) is a union with everything (namely me). The clearly recognisable P1 from an outsider's perspective can be described (internally) as P4. This different internal/external perspective is also reflected in the body layer (tissue) of {flora}. The sequence from {water} to {metal} in Table 7.3 corresponds to more and more superficial body layers. In the graphical representation of Figure 7.4, this corresponds to a counter-clockwise movement. Closing the circle again at {flora}={minister fire} results in tipping over from the outmost to the inmost body layer.

One more thing should be noted concerning the remaining entries in Table 7.3, regarding the characteristics of {flora}. In TCM, generally the five tastes *salty, sweet, sour, bitter,* and *pungent* are considered. They are attributed to the usual five TCM elements (see Table 7.3). In Ayurveda, the traditional Indian medicine, *astringent* taste, in addition to the five tastes we have mentioned, is also known and therefore takes its natural place with {flora}. Furthermore, as well as the customary five tastes, occasionally two others are mentioned in TCM: *harsh/ astringent* and *neutral* (Heise 1996, p.15), also called *flavoursome* and *bland*, respectively (Badelt 1983, p.33). There will be more on this in Ch. 8.3, where the equivalent tastes of umami and glutamate are also explained. It is especially interesting that the graphic character for *tan* (bland taste) is a combination of *huo* (fire) and *shui* (water); see Fisch 1994, p.30. Thus, the connection between {flora} and '*waterfire*' comes up again.

In Table 7.3 climatic influences are also given, which result in polar characteristics on the axes (cold – heat, dampness – dryness). Since {wood} is generally associated with *wind* (gusty wind or draught) and by its nature fits in better with a *gusty* wind, it stands to reason to assign the *draught* or also *calm* to {flora}. Badelt (1983, p.33) associates wind with {wood} and change in pressure or weather with the sixth element. Calm and change in weather can be summarised by the term 'calm before the storm', which fits in well with the seasonal aspect of {flora}, *late winter* (Kratky 2000b, Ch. 1), where nature is about to start a new life cycle. We shall come back to this in Ch. 11.1.

Let us return to the axis {earth} – {metal} and look at a few inconsistencies with the aid of some examples. In Figure 7.4, we recognise that there are two types of transitions between YIN and YANG: the element {earth}, which connects the two, and the region YINYANG. {Earth} in TCM is traditionally seen as *centre*, or neutral element, to which all processes keep returning. YINYANG (yin deficiency) is only rarely mentioned in this connection, but it presumably concerns an *unstable* connection between YIN and YANG, as opposed to a stable {earth}; see also (7.2c). Since {metal} is the central element of YINYANG, it would have to be neutral like {earth}. In TCM, however, {metal} is generally treated as *yin*. There is also an inconsistency regarding moisture: the element *air* of the Ancient Greeks is *damp*, but in TCM {metal} is *dry*.

In order to solve this puzzle one has to delve deeper into TCM. Then one realises that subjects are often simplified in books and a more in-depth knowledge can only be acquired by seeking it in a more deliberate fashion – often inspired by another healing system. First of all, {metal} stands for external matters, for the surface of the human being (epidermis, see Table 7.3) and external is assigned to *yang*, (Table 7.1). From this viewpoint {metal} also has a yang character. In addition, the eight so-called trigrams, which play a role in daoism, are very instructive (see Kratky 2000a, Ch.3). Six of those trigrams belong to the human realm and are assigned to the Chinese elements. In addition, there are the trigrams 'heaven' (highest yang) and 'earth' (highest yin). However, 'heaven' and 'earth' also affect the human realm. In comparison to the usual elements, 'earth' is assigned to the element {earth}, and 'heaven' to the element {metal}. Thus, {metal} represents the highest yang! In addition, the usual trigram for {metal} translates as 'sea', which does not quite fit in with the dryness of {metal}.

There are books on TCM, however, that reveal more in-depth information. An exemplary contribution is the following quote from Heise (1996, p.11), where *fèi* stands for {metal}: "... the system *fèi* is easily irritated by deficient fèiqi – e.g. in form of coughs and sneezes with extreme paleness or reddening of the skin and a lack of or excessive sweat – or in a rigid inability to adapt quickly to a new situation." This again demonstrates the ambivalence of {metal}, where temperature and moisture now also come into play. The pale or reddened skin refers to cold and hot, respectively, (lack of) sweat to dry and damp, respectively. Overall, {metal} presents a dazzling picture. According to Figure 7.3, {earth} has a medium dampness. Thus, it depends on whether the damp or dry side of the ambivalence of *air* or {metal} is emphasised. Depending on this outcome, the axis {earth} – {metal} is either damp – wet or damp – dry. In the first case, moisture increases on this axis (the view of Greek Antiquity), in the second case, it decreases (TCM). This point will be illuminated further in Ch. 13. It is an example of how an intercultural approach can be fruitful and help prevent prejudices.

At last, we come to the traditional yin and yang properties of the other elements. According to Figure 7.4, The elements {fire} and {wood} are on the right (or YANG) half of the circle; {water} and {flora} on the left (or YIN) half. This may be compared with the usual TCM attribution of {fire} and {wood} to *yang* and of {water} to *yin*. {Flora} lies on the same side as {water}, which is in the spirit of Tibetan medicine. We shall come back to that several times.

7.3. The Cyclic Flow of Qi

Now we turn to the Chinese concept of *qi,* often translated as *life force or energy*. It is thought to be generated by a cooperation of yin and yang. Since one of the literal translations of qi is *vapour,* this may be utilized for the following allegory: burning wood (*yang*) heats a kettle containing water (*yin*), the result being vapour (*qi*). The symbol of *yin* and *yang* (monad, *taiji* symbol) shows how to create a third (cooperation, unification); see Figure 7.6a. In Figure 7.6b, the translation of *taiji* as 'high roof ridge' is used, *qi* and *ji* being different words.

In Ch. 7.1, the result of the interaction of *yin* and *yang* was called *yinyang*. Thus, *qi* and *yinyang* may well be compared, and Figure 7.6b is just another version of Figure 7.3 displaying the three types in another way. There is another triad in TCM, the so-called treasures or gems: *jing* (essence), *shen* (vitality) and *qi,* where qi has the usual meaning. As to *jing* and *shen,* since material structure is the central aspect of *jing,* and energy that of *shen,* they resemble *yin* and *yang,* respectively; see Heusser-Buchs (2002). Again, the consequence is that the treasure *qi* resembles *yinyang*. Table 7.4 summarizes the correspondences. The Western triad matter – energy – information fits quite well, so it is also included, together with the worldwide division body – mind – soul. Finally, the three doshas, the Indian regulatory principles, are added to the table. They will be treated in detail in Ch. 8. For the moment, the Western triad is the most interesting. Everything has material, energetic and informational portions. The question is where the focus is. As to *qi,* it is clear from Table 7.4 that the informational content is central. Similarly, the term 'energy medicine' that one frequently hears should in most cases be replaced by 'information medicine'.

Table 7.4. Comparison of YIN, YANG and YINYANG with other ternary typologies

Chinese triad	YIN	YANG	YINYANG
Characterization	Yang deficiency	Yang excess	Yin deficiency
Treasures (gems)	Jing/ essence	Shen/ mind *	Qi
Western triad	Matter	Energy	Information
Worldwide triad	Body	Mind	Soul
Indian triad	Kapha	Pitta	Vata

* Other translations of the Chinese 'shen': vitality, spirit.

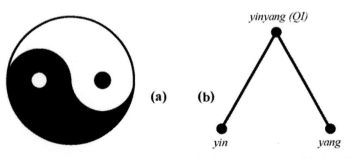

Figure 7.6. *Yin, yang* and *yinyang* (or *qi*) are symbolized in two ways. **a)** *Yin* (black, with a white dot) and *yang* (white, with a black dot), yielding the *taiji* symbol. **b)** *Taiji* as 'high roof ridge'.

Table 7.5. Diurnal qi cycle ('meridian clock') from 3:00 am to 3:00 am,
see Richter & Becke (1989, Ch. 4.4)

Qi Circuits	1st Circuit	2nd Circuit	3rd Circuit
Thorax → Hand	LU = Lung	HT = Heart	PC (see Table 7.2c)
Hand → Head	LI = Large Intestine	SI = Small Intestine	SJ (see Table 7.2c)
Head → Foot *	ST = Stomach	BL = Bladder	GB = Gallbladder
Foot → Thorax	SP = Spleen	KI = Kidney	LR = Liver

* These are the especially long meridians ST, BL and GB, see (7.5a-c).

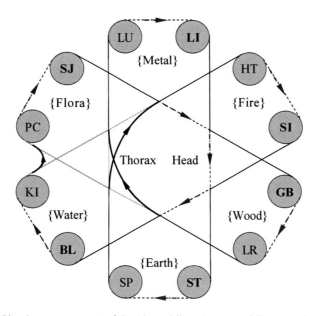

Figure 7.7. Circular arrangement of the 12 meridians (yang meridians are shown in bold type). Each pair of meridians belongs to the {element} specified between them. The arrows indicate the direction of flow of qi, resulting in the meridian clock.

The next question is: how does *qi* flow in the human body? In order to study this, we need to return to the 12 meridians. Table 7.5 gives their names, abbreviations and *qi* circuits, which we shall address shortly. Six meridians run through the leg and six through the arm (see Table 7.2a&b), and their first (or last) acupuncture points often lie in proximity to a toe or finger nail, respectively. Such an end point corresponds to the traditional point 'source' (*jin*); see Kubiena (1995, Ch. 4.8). For example, the end points of the *Heart* (HT9) and *Small Intestine* (SI1) meridians are located at the inner and outer corners, respectively, of the nail of the little finger. HT9 is the last and SI1 the first point of the respective meridians. This corresponds to the idea that *qi* flows into the finger from inside the body along the Heart meridian HT, and from the finger to the inside of the body along the Small Intestine meridian SI. In order for qi congestion to be avoided, qi must be able to flow from SI1 to HT9 somewhere around the nail.

In total, qi flows in three successive circuits (see Table 7.5). The first circuit contains the four 'front' meridians (see Table 7.2a). According to the latter table, these four meridians form the interior/exterior pairs {metal} and {earth} or the hand/foot pairs *taiyin* and *yangming*. The other two circuits, which correspond to the 'back' and 'middle' axes, result in an analogous manner. They all are characterised by the fact that qi flows first from the thorax into the hand, from there into the head, from the head to the foot and finally back to the thorax. The circuits are presented in chronological order. After the third circuit the first begins again, namely at 3:00 am. Since it is a cyclic succession, the numbering of the circuits is not unique. Kubiena (1995, Ch.5.4), for example, begins the first circuit with HT and correspondingly the second with PC and the third with LU. Each meridian in succession exhibits its highest state of activity for two hours. Completion of one cycle takes 24 hours (three circuits of four meridians each). This diurnal qi cycle, which is also called the Chinese *organ* or *meridian clock*, forms a circadian rhythm and is a TCM contribution to chronomedicine. In Ch.11, we shall compare this to Western results. Incidentally, there are also other possible successions of the five or six elements; see Kratky (2000b) for more details. For our current considerations – and with respect to interlinking with other systems of healing – the meridian clock, above all, will be of interest to us; see also Kubiena (1995, Ch.5.4).

Figure 7.4 reveals some of the relationships between the meridians (cf. Table 7.2a&b). The interior/exterior pairs have already been combined into elements there. The elements indicated on bottom and top of the figure belong to the bottom and top meridians, respectively. Two opposite elements together form the four meridians of one of the three circuits: {metal} – {earth} being the first, {fire} – {water} the second and {flora} – {wood} the third circuit. The arrangement of elements corresponds to that in Figure 7.4. Now, let us render the representation more precise and distribute the twelve meridians over the circle. The horizontal yang axis of Figure 7.4 serves as a guide for splitting each element into its two associated meridians; see Kratky (2000b, Figure 4). The yin meridian of each element is thus located at the left of its yang partner.

The result can be seen in Figure 7.7, with the yang meridians in bold type. Throughout this scheme, the yin and yang partners are located exactly opposite each other. The connecting lines in Figure 7.7 (rectangular 'conveyer belts') correspond to the circuits. The meridian clock emerges by a threefold change-over from one conveyer belt to the next via the curves printed in bold. The figure can also be interpreted as a stylistic representation of a person with his head turned to the right in the sense of Table 7.2a, with one hand held up and one foot dangling. The lower and upper six grey circles symbolise the end points of the meridians at the toe and finger nails, respectively. In addition, the direction of flow of qi is indicated by arrows. The solid lines denote the meridians (designated by their respective end points). Because of the two-dimensional representation, they appear to be crossing each other but in reality they run on different planes. The three transitions at hand, head and foot (see Table 7.5) are marked by dashed lines.

If the three circuits were separated, each of them would be closed by one of the three thin lines (meridian transitions in the thorax). Instead, the transitions are located at the thick curves, which results in the diurnal qi cycle (meridian clock). We shall, from now on, use the arrangement of meridians of Figure 7.7 also for the circle representation (Figure 7.4).

7.4. Modern Methods of Confirmation and Application of TCM

One important point for Western scientists is whether these meridians really exist. They have been described, precisely and consistently, for centuries by TCM and have been used in diagnosis and therapy, although apparently they are a concept that has resulted from thorough observations of healthy and ill individuals. To us they are inaccessible at first. Conversely, some structures and functions that are very important to us hardly play a role at all in TCM. If we were to pick out two TCM books, the word 'nervous system' would appear once in Porkert (1992) and not at all in Maciocia (1994). What seems obvious to us remained hidden to TCM or just has not inspired any interest there. In any case, the complementary nature of the European and Chinese viewpoints is rather striking.

As far as objectifying meridians is concerned, much has been done in the West in recent years. Heine was able to discover a morphological characteristic (Heine 1997, p.62) and a French group employed radioactive substances (tracers) in order to make the meridians visible (de Vernejoul et al. 1985, Darras et al. 1987). In this procedure, the substance is injected into various sites on the skin, at 'common' sites and acupuncture points. A diffuse dispersion of the tracer in all directions (hemispherically into the body) is expected, which looks like a growing circular region of radioactive rays around the injection site. However, injection into acupuncture points results in an additional phenomenon: a part of the tracer moves along the corresponding meridian. This can be observed for a while until the radioactivity is exhausted or the meridian dives into the depth and renders the tracer undetectable from outside due to absorption by the tissue. The trajectory leaving the injection point keeps growing paler but intermittently flares up, which means that the meridian comes to the surface, i.e. reaches an acupuncture point. In this way, the sections of the TCM meridian system that are not too deep in the body, including the acupuncture points, can be examined.

The French group's experiments confirmed TCM repeatedly. The tracer traversed the meridians with a velocity of a few cm/min and only in the direction indicated by TCM (see Table 7.5 and Figure 7.7). In this respect, it is now possible to establish a connection to essential claims made by TCM with Western methods as well. Thus, the meridians are not just a mere mental construct. The main problem with this is that, so far, they cannot be detected anatomically. The tracer substance does not traverse the blood vessels and lymphatic pathways, and there is no obvious connection to the nervous system. Perhaps there are inconspicuous structures that correspond to the meridians by the principle 'small causes – large effect'. Doepp (1998) believes that the meridian system is located at the internal surface between the cellular and extra-cellular regions. The latter has been called 'fundamental system' by its discoverer, Pischinger, and has attracted growing interest in recent years (Pischinger 2004, Heine 1997).

Another approach to acupuncture has resulted from the development of the Prognos device, a further development of EAV, (see Ch.6.1). The problems with objectifying EAV inspired a Russian group to develop a better device for the space station, Mir, (Zagriadskii et al. 1996). This device follows the same principle of measuring the electrical resistance between a 'relevant' electrode placed on an acupuncture point and a 'neutral' electrode remaining constant. However, the electrical (alternating) voltage used is much lower, the electrodes are larger and only 24 standardised terminal points of the meridians are measured (on the fingers and toes on the right and left). A cleverly devised system also ensures that the pressure on the acupuncture points is independent on the pressure applied to the point by the tester. In any case, instead of requiring a month-long training, this technique can be learned in a few hours and the results are reproducible (Treugut et al. 1998). One could say that because of a high-tech effort it will be possible to measure a simple parameter (the electrical resistance R between two points on the body) in a simple fashion.

The body's resistance R is generally quite high, but relatively low in the meridians (Zagriadskii 1996). It is analogous to an electric current finding its way through the cables in a circuit and, in normal circumstances, not passing through the neighbouring air. The detected changes in resistance, therefore, are primarily the result of changes in those meridians at whose end points the 'relevant' electrode is placed. An increase in resistance indicates a lack of qi or a blockage. The experiential values from the Prognos device, together with the Chinese interpretation of the significance of meridians, makes possible a quick check of a person's state of health, according to TCM standards. In addition, something needs to be said about the 'neutral' electrode as well. In EAV, an electrode with a large surface is held in one hand, in Prognos it is a strap, which is loosely wound around the wrist. It has been discovered that the resistance R in healthy people is about the same from all end points.

This is quite remarkable form a physical perspective, since the distance between the strap and a finger of the same hand is about 15-20 cm, and to a finger of the other hand or even a toe about ten times that. A usual conductance process would result in a tenfold value for R. This observation allows structural statements about the meridian system. The current first runs from the end point along the meridian deep into the body and then across a fractal surface-like network to the neutral electrode. This network, which is the same for all measurements, presumably provides the main resistance, modulated by the contribution of the relevant meridian. Indications of this can be found in TCM, where, aside from the qi circulating in the known (regular) meridians, defensive qi, which is responsible for defence against illness, is also recognised. It flows outside of the meridians in a network traversing the entire body (Fisch 1994, p.150). In any case, Prognos not only offers the opportunity of bringing TCM closer to application in the West but promises new insights into the meridian system.

Another possible way of approaching TCM with Western technology consists in the detailed determination of functional changes in the organism because of needling. The methods developed for this procedure were very elaborate, for example the transcranial Doppler sonography for measuring the velocity of blood flow in the cranial arteries (Litscher & Cho 2000, Litscher 2001). Nevertheless, the results make the effort worthwhile. For example, after needling acupuncture points responsible for sight, according to TCM, an increase in blood flow in the relevant arteries could be detected, while neighbouring blood vessels did not show any change. In a further publication, laser acupuncture was analysed scientifically (Litscher & Schikora (2003).

Another remarkable point for the West is pulse diagnosis, which is usually performed by hand and gives information about a person's overall condition. This is a much more informative and detailed process than our well-known method of assessing a pulse. A more in-depth insight into various versions will be given shortly. First, let us attempt an objective understanding of pulse diagnosis. For this purpose, electronic devices have been developed which allow automatic pulse registration by means of sensors placed on pulse points. The substitutability of a person by a device lets this phenomenon seem more plausible to our Western way of thinking, even if an experienced pulse diagnostician must interpret the curves on the monitor or printout. I was able to observe the electronic pulsograph of Paik & Yoo (1979, Ch. III) in use on several occasions and was surprised at how many different pulse curves result on the six TCM pulse sites. Reichle (1997, pp.152-5 & 223-5), incidentally, describes a Buryatian pulse palpation device based on Tibetan pulse diagnosis. We shall now discuss this in more detail.

7.5. Chinese and Tibetan Pulse Diagnoses

There are several ways of ascertaining the organism's momentary state of health. In TCM, as well as in Tibetan medicine and in Ayurveda, *pulse diagnosis* plays a central role. At first, it is surprising that this 'detour' via the blood is made. From the detail of the pulses, however, the state of the meridians can be deduced. In principle, the pulse can be felt at several sites on the body (Maciocia 1994, p.174) but feeling the pulse at the wrists, which is also the preferred method in the West, has proved to be the most effective. In TCM, the doctor places index, middle and ring fingers on the patient's radial artery (arteria radialis), 1 *cun* or fingerbreadth – ca 1.6 cm – apart, the middle finger being located above the styloid process of the radius (processus styloideus radii) near the wrist. This results in six pulse palpation sites on each arm, which are assigned to the six interior/ exterior pairs (elements).

One of the TCM schools holds the view that statements can only be made about the interior (=yin) meridians, another recognises a superficial and a deep pulse at every site in order to distinguish between interior (=yin) and exterior (=yang) meridians. Yet another school recognises three different pulses at different depths. We shall use the version of superficial and deep palpation. However, there are also other views concerning the question which meridian and which organ should be assigned to which pulse. According to Maciocia (1994, p.175), however, this does not lead to confusion, since essentially the same results are achieved by all the methods. The yin meridians are the more important and so feeling the pulse at just a single depth to examine the yin meridian, will be enough to make an adequate diagnosis.

From now on, I shall refer to a version that is described, e.g., in Paik & Yoo (1979, Ch. II). It is represented in the upper half (I) of Table 7.6a&b. In every case, the quality of pulse must be ascertained, and this requires much practice. This quality of pulse can be different at different sites and depths. The resulting diversity of combinations allows a detailed diagnosis of the patient's present condition. This goes far beyond Western pulse diagnosis, which, in essence, merely determines heart rate and – with the aid of an apparatus – blood pressure.

Table 7.6a. Chinese (I) and Tibetan (II) pulse diagnoses: Pulse positions, location and meridians. Specific Tibetan expressions are shown in square brackets

Posi-tion [a]	Site [b]	Left arm of female patient [c]		Right arm of female patient [c]	
		Yin	Yang	Yin	Yang
I/1	0.0	Heart	Small Intestine	Lung	Large Intestine
I/2	1.6	Liver	Gallbladder	Spleen	Stomach
I/3	3.2	Kidney	Bladder	PC	SJ
II/1	4.2	Lung	Large intestine	Heart	Small intestine
II/2	5.8	Spleen	Stomach	Liver	Gallbladder
II/3	7.4	[Left] kidney	[Testis, ovaries]	[Right] kidney	Bladder

Table 7.6b. {Chinese} and [Tibetan] elements corresponding to Table 7.6a. Where the Tibetan name does not differ from the Chinese one, no bracket is used

Pos. [a]	Site [b]	Left arm of female patient [c]	Right arm of female patient [c]
I/1	0.0	{Fire}	{Metal}
I/2	1.6	{Wood}	{Earth}
I/3	3.2	{Water}	{Flora}
II/1	4.2	[Iron] = {Metal}	Fire
II/2	5.8	Earth	Wood
II/3	7.4	[Water] = {Flora}	Water

Table 7.6c. Explanatory notes to Table 7.6a&b

[a]	Pulse position (1, 2, 3: index, middle and ring finger of the physician). I: TCM palpation sites near the wrist. II: Tibetan pulse palpation sites, from there toward the elbow.
[b]	Location of pulse positions, given in cm away from the index finger I/1 (estimation).
[c]	The Tibetan fire and [iron] pulses are on opposite sides in a man, all other pulses are independent of gender.

Table 7.6a&b shows, for example, the element of {fire} for the pulse palpation site nearest the left thumb (1st pulse position: I/1, doctor's index finger, I stands for TCM) and the associated meridians. It lists first the *yin* meridian (Heart) and then the *yang* meridian (Small Intestine). The yin meridian is examined with a greater pressure or palpation depth than the yang meridian. This corresponds to interior= yin and exterior=yang. One could say that the yin pulse corresponds approximately to the systolic and the yang pulse to the diastolic pressure (Paik & Yoo 1979, p.10).

Tibetan medicine also uses pulse diagnosis. Yin and yang pulses are not distinguished here by depth of palpation but by turning the fingers from side to side. The interior meridians of TCM can be felt on the proximal side of the artery relative to the examining finger and the exterior meridians on the distal side. (*Proximal* is closer to the elbow, *distal* is closer to the fingers.) The classification of pulse sites is given in the lower half (II) of Table 7.6a&b (see Asshauer 1993, p.107). Expressions specific to Tibetan medicine are marked with square brackets. {Metal}, for example, is called [*iron*] in Tibet, {flora} is assigned to [*water*]. Instead of *Kidney*, for example, we have [right] kidney. Presumably, this refers to the right kidney position being palpated.

The deviations regarding {flora} are the most interesting aspect: instead of PC we have [*left*] kidney, instead of SJ [*testicles, ovaries*]. Moreover, yin and yang seem to be interchanged in comparison with TCM. The exterior meridian [testicles, ovaries] – which is sometimes translated as semen bladder, due to its sexual nature – has a clear relation to PC (whose alternative name is Circulation/ sex meridian!), the interior or *yin* meridian of {flora}. Admittedly, there is also some confusion in the Chinese tradition (see Kratky 2000a, Chs.1 & 2 and Maciocia 1994, pp.46f, 103-6, 126-9, 174f). Furthermore, *mingmen* (meaning *gate of life*) is closely connected to {flora}; see Kratky (2000a&b). *Mingmen* is located close to the kidneys and is identified by Meyer (1988, p.155) with PC, the yin meridian of {flora}, while Maciocia (1994, p.175) also suggests a close connection between the two.

An important difference between Chinese and Tibetan pulse diagnoses consists in the fact that the pulse palpation sites in the two systems are in essence interchanged left to right. *Wood*, for example, is felt with the middle finger in both systems but in TCM on the left and in Tibetan medicine on the right arm. The pulses felt with the index finger show another peculiarity in the Tibetan system: the assignment to left or right depends on the patient's gender. In order to keep confusion to a minimum, we shall only consider the case of a female patient, as in Table 7.6a-c. In this case, all sites are interchanged right to left when we compare TCM with Tibetan medicine. The solution to this puzzle is that the pulse palpation sites are not the same!

The Tibetan palpation sites, (II/1-3), come directly after the Chinese sites (I/1-3): The position of the index finger (II/1) is ca 1 cm further away from the ball of the thumb than the Chinese position of the ring finger (I/3). One can then determine the other positions by measuring fingerbreadth of roughly 1.6 cm between each pair. Assuming that the two methods are consistent, one can speak of six palpation sites on each arm, each of which represents one of the six elements. This results in 24 available sites, although this does not mean that Liver at I/2 on the left will give the same result as at II/2 on the right. A possible interpretation is that the 24 sites give information about 24 meridians if we distinguish between the left and right Liver meridians, for example. In Ch. 8, we will look at another interpretation and will continue with our comparison of different medicine systems.

7.6.* More on Pulse Diagnosis and the Sixth Element

In Western acupuncture, van der Molen has found an analogue of Tibetan pulse diagnosis (Gerhard Bujak, personal communication). Adjacent to the usual Chinese positions I/1-3, he found, after a small gap, a further three positions that lie closer to one another. The positions are not identical to the Tibetan ones, II/1-3, but only for the first position is the difference appreciable (more than 1 cm). In fact, van der Molen's interpretation differs from the Tibetan only in that position. In addition, for male patients he measures {metal} and {fire} on the left and right arm, respectively. In total, all the attributions of Table 7.6a&b are valid gender-neutral. Thus, it is possible to palpate all 12 meridians at one arm, which is important if one arm is in a plaster cast or has been amputated.

In addition, the correlation between palpation site and depth is also interesting. The varying distance of the radial artery from the surface of the skin must be taken into consideration. Proceeding from the styloid process of the radius, it travels deeper and deeper into the body. This means that site and depth are linked. Now the Chinese elements are assigned to body layers or tissues of varying depth anyway (see Table 7.3). Indeed, this succession – getting deeper as one travels from {metal} to {water} – is compatible with the assignment in Table 7.6b. In particular, from Tibetan diagnosis we can establish the depth of body layer for {flora}, which had to be left open in Table 7.2b (inmost or outmost or both?). {Flora} is about as deep as {water}, which is palpated at the corresponding site on the other arm. According to Tibetan medicine *semen*, which is assigned to {flora}, lies even deeper than *bone*, which is assigned to {water}. Now let us look at the Chinese pulse position of {flora} in Table 7.6b. There we see that [iron] / *metal* (in men) or *fire* (in women) is palpated immediately after this. Both elements correspond to the skin (epidermis and subcutis, respectively; compare Table 7.3). Thus, there is a chasm in between, which presumably corresponds to the gap found by van der Molen.

Within the realms of ear acupuncture (see Ch. 3.3), there is another variant of pulse diagnosis. One of the patient's wrists is used to test (often with two fingers) whether he or she reacts to the relevant points in the ear being stimulated. The RAC (réflexe auriculocardiaque, also called Nogier reflex), discovered by Nogier, corresponds to a change in pulse in the region of the wrist which can be detected by an experienced physician. This, allegedly, can be traced back to a shift or expansion of the (alleged) standing pulse wave at this site (Bahr 1981, pp.28-31) although there is no scientific evidence for this. In RAC, the human pulse diagnostician is not (yet) replaceable by a machine, but the meaningfulness of the results has been confirmed (Nogier & Bricot 1978, Moser et al. 1998). Whatever this phenomenon is based on, a variant uses just the index and middle fingers placed immediately above and below the styloid process of the radius – exactly between the Chinese pulse positions (I/1 and I/2)! When I asked whether this is the only site where the RAC can be palpated, the answer was that there is another site about 5 cm from the styloid process of the radius (Peter Gründler, personal communication). Interestingly, this corresponds roughly to the shift from Chinese to Tibetan pulse positions (from I to II; see Table 7.6a, which also specifies estimated values in cm). It is possible, then, that there is a deeper connection between Oriental pulse diagnosis and the independently discovered European Nogier reflex.

Finally, we return to a time before the development of TCM. In China, during the second half of the 20th century, several graves were found that contained old texts, presumably originating from the time before 221 B.C. , the date of the first unification of the Chinese empire. Especially interesting are the medical texts, which describe a form of medicine quite different from TCM as we know it. Only 11 vessels or channels were described rather than the 12 meridians. On the other hand, six elements and not five were recognised. The meridians were named according to foot-hand pairs (see Table 7.2a&b). The only meridian of the sixth element was hand *shaoyang*, also called *sanjiao* (SJ), a name not associated with a recognized organ but indicating that it is a higher-order meridian, which connects all the body functions. The missing meridian was hand *jueyin*, the meridian that was later called Pericardium (PC) in TCM. Acupuncture points and needles were not mentioned. At that time, cuspidal stones were used to treat meridians. This may be the reason why the sixth element was called 'stone', (see Lo 2002).

After the discovery of the twelfth meridian (hand *jueyin*) and the reduction to five elements, the question arose as to which element the meridians hand *jueyin* and SJ should belong. The Chinese answer was *fire*, the Tibetan answer (about 1000 years later) was *water*. Accordingly, in China the association was made with *Heart* (yin meridian of *fire*) and in Tibet with *Kidney* (yin meridian of *water*). Thus, in China a name that is usually translated *Pericardium* was chosen. In Tibet, the fact was utilized that we have two kidneys, so the additional meridian could be named after the second kidney. However, in China the two kidneys are also occasionally split into a *fire* and a *water* kidney (see Table 7.2b). Interestingly enough, in the Western hemisphere, the name *circulation/ sex* is often used for that yin meridian. This means that no particular organ is attributed to this meridian, like its yang counterpart SJ.

The question of the reduction from six to five elements is still open. Granet (1993, p.113f) suggests a possible answer – in ancient China, the numbers 6 and 10 were attributed to *heaven*, 5 and 12 to *earth* and a human being has a share in both. Thus, he or she should have 6+5 meridians. The 'heavenly' element was the sixth. After 221 B.C., there was obviously a loss of spiritual attitude and a tendency to emphasise *earth* and the body. Thus, the numbers 12 (meridians) and 5 (elements) have been chosen in spite of the fact that it would have been more natural to distribute the 12 meridians over 6 elements. In fact, TCM seems to be less spiritual than, for example, Ayurveda. This has its advantages for TCM: out of all the Eastern medicine systems, TCM is the most readily accepted in the West.

Finally, it should be mentioned that the development of Chinese medicine was discussed in Kratky (2005a), and the question of its transmission to the West was treated in Hsu (1999).

Part II:
Integration into a Complete Picture

Chapter 8

Ayurveda and Tibetan Medicine

8.1. The Three Regulatory Principles

Now, we shall get acquainted with *Ayurveda* (which means 'knowledge of life') and *Tibetan medicine*, which will offer interesting comparisons to *Traditional Chinese Medicine* (TCM). Tibetan medicine will serve as a bridge, since it contains elements of both TCM and Ayurveda. First, we shall look at the three Indo-Tibetan *regulatory principles,* which, among other things, are based on an individual's fundamental modes of reactions to stress. They are called *doshas* in Indian and *nyepas* in Tibetan (we shall refer to them in general as doshas). The names of the three regulatory principles can be found in Table 8.1. Since the transcription is not consistent in Tibetan, we shall, in future, use the *Indian* names – *vata, pitta* and *kapha*. Life force or *prana* (corresponding to *qi*) is in all the doshas, but primarily in *vata*. The doshas are also called *humours*. As the English translation of the corresponding Tibetan names (Table 8.1) suggests, there is indeed a close connection to the three Greek elements and humours, which were recognised before the introduction of the fourth element, earth (humour: black bile); cf. Ch.2.3 and Kratky (2002).

These three predispositions or fundamental modes of behaviour can be described according to their positive (+) and negative (–) characteristics (see Table 8.2, modelled after Schrott 1994, pp.18-21). It shows how all three doshas have their good and not so good sides, where the latter can be either an exaggeration of the former or, sometimes, the opposite. Every human being is characterised by his individual mixture of dosha proportions. The starting point is his inborn constitution (*prakriti*). This is his ideal reference point for his entire life. In addition, there are deviations (*vikriti*) specific to time of day and season, as well as age and illness; see Schrott (1994, p.17) and Chopra (1993, p.111f). In order to enable disturbances or illnesses to be assessed, comparisons must be made with the individual's constitution. Chopra (1993, Part I.2-4) gives detailed information on the doshas. A brief characterisation follows:

Vata: changeable,   *pitta:* intense,   *kapha:* constant.   (8.1)

The *temperature* and *moisture* axes are also relevant here:

Vata (V):   dry   & cool (neutral temperature);   (8.2a)

Pitta (P):   damp & hot,   (8.2b)

Kapha (K):   damp & cold.   (8.2c)

Table 8.1. The names of the three basic regulatory principles
(doshas, nyepas) in Ayurveda and Tibetan medicine.
Comparisonwith equivalent Chinese terms

Indian	Vata	Pitta	Kapha
Tibetan [a] Tibetan [b] Translation	rLung LUNG Wind	mKhrispa TrIPA Bile	Badkan BEKAN Mucus
Chinese	Yin deficiency	Yang excess	Yang deficiency

[a] cf. Qusar & Sergent (1997, Ch.16)   [b] cf. Sachs (1997, Ch.1).

Table 8.2. The three doshas in Ayurveda broken down into the typical
predispositions (+) and their negative aspects (−)

Characteristics	Vata (V)	Pitta (P)	Kapha (K)
Mind (+) (−)	flexible overly sensitive	critical intolerant	persevering unyielding
Life style (+) (−)	fond of travelling unsettled	athletic daredevil	enjoying luxurious
Feeling (+) (−)	elated anxious	humorous wrathful	content gloomy

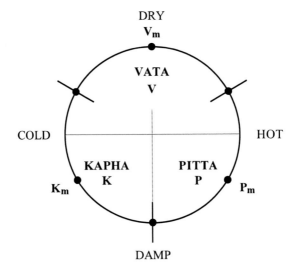

Figure 8.1. Circle representation of Ayurvedic doshas vata, pitta and kapha. Each of them dominates a circular arc of 120°. The centre of each arc is designated V_m, Pm and K_m, respectively, where *m* stands for *mean* or *middle*. Compare the analogous Figure 7.3 for the Chinese case.

More precisely, vata is described as 'inherently' neutral in temperature but this dosha has a tendency of toppling over to hot or cold; see Qusar & Sergent (1997, pp.82, 184 & 205). This resembles yin deficiency, cf. (7.2c). The 'mucous' kapha is understandably damp. That hot pitta is also damp might be surprising; we shall return to this in Ch. 8.2. In any case, with the aid of the temperature and moisture characteristics we can make a connection to Figures 7.3 & 7.4 and smoothly integrate the doshas into the circle representation. This results automatically in the following assignments of Chinese and Indian terms:

Vata: yin deficiency, *pitta*: yang excess, *kapha*: yang deficiency; (8.3)

See Table 8.1. This assignment also fits in with the other characteristics of the Chinese terms discussed in Ch. 7.1. If we look at (8.1) and Table 8.2 we can see that this assignment is plausible: the ambivalence of yin deficiency is reflected in the *vicissitude* of vata, yang excess in the *intensity* of pitta, the cold, calm yang deficiency in the *constancy* of kapha. Figure 8.1 results from replacing the Chinese terms in Figure 7.3 with the analogous *Indian* ones. In this circle representation, the centres of the corresponding dosha regions are now called V_m, P_m, and K_m.

To continue with this cross-cultural comparison, we need a more elaborate diagram. Inside the circle, the three doshas are split up into six two-dosha regions (see below). On the outside, there are the Chinese elements (in curly brackets) and meridians. The definite configuration of meridians was adapted from Figure 7.7 (see Table 7.5 for their full names). Unlike Figure 7.7, they now represent the *entire* meridians and not just their *end points*. Further evidence for the dosha assignment of Figure 8.2 can be found in Tibetan *pulse diagnosis*. It not only contains the relation to the Chinese elements (Table 7.6a-c) but also to the *regulatory principles*:

1st Pulse position: {metal} and disturbances in *vata*, (8.4a)

2nd Pulse position: {wood} and disturbances in *pitta*, (8.4b)

3rd Pulse position: {water} and disturbances in *kapha*; (8.4c)

see Asshauer (1993, p.107) and Reichle (1997, p.172). Here again, the Indian names for the Indo-Tibetan regulatory principles have been used.

(8.4a-c) refer to the *right* arm in male patients. For female patients, (8.4a) holds for the *left* arm. There is no change of sides, however, with respect to (8.4b&c). In Ayurveda vata, pitta and kapha are also palpated one after the other, using the index, middle and ring fingers. The pulse positions are slightly shifted toward the wrist compared with the Tibetan positions. In Ayurveda, however, a man's pulse is only felt in the *right* arm and a woman's in the *left* (Chopra 1993, p.175). As in TCM, the pulse is felt at two depths. In TCM, strong pressure (a deep pulse) corresponds to the *yin* and gentle pressure (a superficial pulse) to *yang* meridians (see Ch. 7.5). Ayurveda, which is ignorant of the Chinese meridians, interprets these pulses differently: a deep pulse indicates the *inherent* constitution and a superficial pulse the *current* situation brought on by illness (Chopra 1993, p.177). The assumed compatibility of TCM and Ayurveda allows the following conclusion: The deeper pulses relate to *long-term* and the superficial pulses to *short-term* fluctuations in the patient's state of health. The former is indicated by *yin*, the latter by *yang* meridians. This also explains the greater importance of the yin meridians – as indicators of long-term disturbances – in TCM.

Now, let us take a closer look at the *type assignment of Ayurveda*. Each dosha covers a third of the circle (or, more precisely, an arc of 120°). A 'pure' dosha type would be exactly in the *centre* of the corresponding arc: {metal} in case of vata, {wood} in case of pitta and {water} in case of kapha. According to Ayurveda, however, pure types are very rare. A person usually exhibits a mixed form, in which one dosha dominates and another is in second place (two-dosha types). The least dominant dosha is neglected. This, then, results in a total of six combinations V-K, V-P, P-V, P-K, K-P and K-V, where the capital letters stand for the respective doshas, see (8.2a-c). In V-K, for example, *vata* dominates and *kapha* is in second place. In Figure 8.2 such a two-dosha type corresponds to one sixth of the circle (arc of 60°), whose midpoint is marked by a white dot, where the name of the corresponding type is also shown. For example, V-K is represented by the arc from *{flora}* to *{metal}*. This half of vata is in closer proximity to kapha. As we travel from *{metal}* in direction of *{flora}*, we encounter an increasing portion of kapha until we reach {flora}, where we find an equal portion of vata. Ayurveda, incidentally, also acknowledges the so-called three-dosha type, where the doshas are represented in (almost) equal portions. This can be thought of as being at the centre of the circle. The latter, however, is not part of the circle, which suggests that the circle representation with which we have worked so far is not elaborate enough.

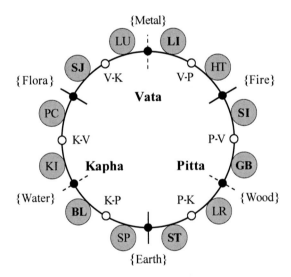

Figure 8.2. Circle representation of Indian and Chinese terms. The three doshas and six two-dosha regions V-K, V-P, P-V, P-K, K-P and K-V are shown *inside* the circle. The Chinese elements and the meridians assigned to them are placed *outside* the circle.

The Tibetan system also offers seven types (including the three-dosha type in the centre) but the six on the circle are rotated by 30° compared to the Ayurvedic types; see Schwarz & Schweppe (1998, pp.81ff) and Kratky (2000b, Table 8). The Chinese elements thus lie at the *borders* of the Ayurvedic elements but in the *centre* of the Tibetan types. This distribution is just as useful as the one for Ayurveda. The difference in the Tibetan and Indian classifi-cations presumably goes back to the fact that the Chinese elements are known in Tibetan medicine and it orients itself according to these elements. Strictly speaking, in Ayurveda as well as in Tibetan medicine both variants of classification can be found, but with widely differing frequency. For this reason, we shall continue to speak of *Ayurvedic* and *Tibetan* classifications.

From the doshas, a bridge to the *miasms or diatheses* of homoeopathy can be built (see Ch. 5.4). Ayurveda and Bach Flower Remedies have already been compared in Table 5.2. The connection will now become clear. The term 'deficiency' for psora indicates a condition of deficiency (vata), the expressions 'loud' and 'overabundance' relate to one of excess (pitta). The four indicated modes of reaction there (5.2b-d) correspond to the ambivalent behaviour of *vata*, the expenditure of energy in *pitta* and the unresponsiveness of *kapha*, respectively. The subsequent succession of reactions can be translated for the doshas in the following way. If communication is unsuccessful (vata), the organism (over-)compensates (pitta). Once this no longer works, a *decompensation* (kapha) or *unresponsiveness* follows. The latter is a term from TCM; the diathesis corresponding to the dosha kapha is also described as *rigid* (Table 5.2). In agreement with this sequence, Ayurveda usually sees vata as the origin of illness, since it gets out of balance more easily than the other two (Chopra 1993, pp.98 & 113). If we look at homoeopathy, we find that Hahnemann saw the miasm psora, which is equivalent to vata, as *prime evil;* see Kratky (2000c, Ch.3.1).

Individuals are especially susceptible to certain challenges according to their dominant dosha. In Tibetan medicine, reference is made to the *three poisons*. These may be equated with the three doshas in the following way:

Vata: greed (attachment, craving, zest for life); "I want everything!" (8.5a)

Pitta: hatred (anger at hindrances, aversion, dislike);
"Woe betide anyone who gets in the way!" (8.5b)

Kapha: illusion (ego-delusion, ignorance);
"I've had enough! You can all go to hell!" (8.5c)

See Reichle (1997, p.166). The expressions are *my own* interpretation. We see here con-nections with ideas that we have already covered and the suggestion of a natural sequence. Vata is characterised by the ambition of attracting everything to itself. A vata type 'never has enough'; moderation or letting go is a problem. Whenever there are hindrances or limitations, the energy reserves are mobilised for battle (pitta). Once there is no energy left, the vata type goes into exhaustion (kapha) and shuts itself away from its surroundings (comparable to 'playing dead'). From the characteristics (also positive) of the doshas listed in Table 8.2, the vicious circle that has just been described can be surmised. It is also mirrored in the progres-sion of illness. This field of tension of constitution (dosha) and emphasis of negative impacts can be compared to diathesis and miasm. One more thing should be said about delusion (8.5c). The philosophy underlying Tibetan medicine and Buddhism is the same – indeed, Tibetan medicine is often referred to as Tibetan Buddhist medicine because the spiritual aspects of the religion play such a large role in it. According to Buddhist beliefs, the ego is impermanent and – ultimately – a delusion. While we remain unenlightened, the ego seems all too real and plays a role especially in kapha conditions, where the individual wants to separate himself from his surroundings and withdraw.

Here, too, in (8.5a) the ambivalence of kapha is evident: 'there is never enough' indicates a deficiency, although from an external perspective there *is* enough. The tension between expectation and fulfilment, between subjectivity and objectivity is especially great in vata. Furthermore, the statement "*I want everything!*", which at first is an indication of strength, needs to be clarified. The potential failure of this demand is not only based on those who would undermine this desire but also on the weak-mindedness of vata itself. It could just as well say: "*I want everything, but ...*" Greed is just one side, blocking this greed another. Irregular eating together with irregular digestion, which is attributed to the vata type, fits well into this picture. In the extreme case we have bulimia, where vomiting immediately follows the satisfaction of greed for food. Ayurveda's experience with vata could thus be useful in the treatment of bulimia. According to Ayurveda, pitta has a strong, quick digestion, while it is slow in kapha – with a tendency toward gaining weight.

The division into vata, pitta and kapha is comparable to *yinyang* (neutral), *yang* and *yin*, see Figure 7.3. This division can be made again and again on many levels, which resembles the branching out of fractals. Thus, the metabolism or digestion in particular can be assigned, at first glance, to *pitta* (heat and energy production). From a closer perspective, however, the metabolism is divided among all three doshas as follows:

Vata:	metabolism	(in general), as well as accumulation of energy;	(8.6a)
Pitta:	catabolism	(decomposition, energy production);	(8.6b)
Kapha:	anabolism	(composition, substance synthesis).	(8.6c)

This allocation can be found in Schwarz & Schweppe (1998, p.39) and in Qusar & Sergent (1997, p.73). The idea of accumulation of energy is taken from a reference that does not encompass the Indian or the Chinese body of thought and thus – as an independent source – supports our connections. This is to say, Warnke (1999, pp.19ff) is involved with those partial systems of the human being that deal with *accumulation of energy*: the skin, lungs and large intestine. From a Chinese perspective, the element *{metal}* immediately jumps into view: the associated meridians are Lung and Large Intestine, the associated layer is (superficial) skin, (see Table 7.3). In fact, {metal} lies in the centre of *vata*, see Figure 8.2.

Another cross reference to Western thinking is the pulse-respiration quotient (PRQ; number of heartbeats per breath), which we shall meet again in chronobiology (Ch. 11.3). The various doshas are characterised by the following values (see Sachs 1997, p.37):

Vata: PRQ from 5 to 6,   *pitta:* PRQ towards 7,   *kapha:* PRQ below 4.   (8.7)

On average we expect a PRQ of 5 to 6; see Qusar & Sergent (1997, p.182). In Kratky (2000b, Table 6) a formula can be found which states the pulse-respiration quotient as a function of the location on the circle and where PRQ=4 corresponds to {earth}. This can be reconciled with experiences from pulse diagnosis in TCM, Ayurveda and Tibetan medicine. It should be mentioned here that, from a modern perspective, a PRQ of 4 is especially beneficial (Hildebrandt et al. 1998, p.25, 42 & 76). This, then, exactly coincides with the element *{earth}*.

Now we come to an essential aspect of the circle representation (Figures 8.1&8.2). As can be seen on the axes cold – hot and damp – dry, types and elements located on *opposite sides* (same *axis*) belong to the same category and are characterised by polar properties. The fact that P·V corresponds to heat has the following meaning: Someone who is inherently P·V or who tends towards P·V because of age, time of day or season will like moderate heat, which corresponds to him anyway. An 'ideal' neutral temperature is not aspired to here. On the other hand, too much heat would strengthen P·V to such a degree – and thus bring it out of balance – that it would have a harmful effect. This is not only true for heat but also for many other things assigned to or 'related' to the doshas or elements in sequences by analogy. With regard to the *tastes*, see Qusar et al. (1997, pp.34-36). Such considerations can also be found in TCM. There, according to Porkert (1992, p.127), we have the fundamental rule that related things in moderate intensity support but, in excess, harm the organism. This, in the end, resembles in practice the useful rule of *hormesis* and the Arndt-Schulz Law (see Table 5.1), where a connection to *homoeopathy* can be found. This is not surprising, since a common axis relates complementary characteristics. Ebert (1992), incidentally, points out a different relationship between homoeopathy and TCM (homoeosiniatry). He draws the conclusion that sometimes a homoeopathic diagnosis is easier than a TCM diagnosis and sometimes it is the reverse. By way of a 'translation table', it is possible to use a TCM diagnosis, for example, as an aid to determining the simile.

If an individual is a P·V type, he should be careful with temperature, one way or another. The moisture axis on the other hand is perpendicular to him. This means he should not be at risk from wetness or dryness. A dosha can get out of balance in two ways: it gets either too strong or too weak (Chopra 1993, p.91). Nonetheless, many books – including this one – consider a disturbance in a dosha to be an *overabundance*. Since on the other side of the axis the complementary aspect of the same characteristic can be found, the overabundance of P·V (overabundance of *heat*), for example, is very similar to a weakness in K·V (i.e. lack of *cold*), the type on the opposite side of the axis. Thus, a large part of Ayurveda can be covered by only considering *one* type of disturbance (overabundance or deficiency, relative to the other doshas). The suggested circle representation, which of course is only a model, gives a clear illustration and interpretation of experiences from TCM, Ayurveda and Tibetan medicine and allows useful prognoses to be made.

Table 8.3. Relationships between meridians and the psyche modelled after Doepp (1998, Table 5). Elements: {wood}, then {flora}

Meridian	Attribute	Exaggeration	Opposite
LR	*sensitive*	*sorrowful*	**vindictive**
GB	pensive	feeling guilty	angry
PC	motivated	**pushy**	fearful
SJ	ambitious	hating	*begrudging*

One field of application would be the characteristics of the psyche in connection with the meridians. There are various systems. Doepp (1998) looks at attributes including their exaggeration and opposite, which fits in with our prior considerations. Let us look at the axis {wood} – {flora}, where in Table 8.3 first the *yin* and then the *yang* meridian is listed (see Table 7.2a&b). We shall not go into the problems arising with the nomenclature chosen by Doepp. In any case, the characteristics listed under 'exaggeration' turn out to be closely connected to those under 'opposite' of the other element (crosswise strengthening). This is in alignment with our expectations for elements lying at opposite ends of the same axis. Closer inspection of these terms yields an especially close relationship between the two meridians of the same polarity (yin, yang). The pairs of terms associated in this way are marked by the same font (normal, bold, italic, underlined). An analogous situation arises for the other two axes. This illustration is, of course, just a first step, but it points out how to tackle the partly contradictory statements in literature and gives an idea of which direction further research could take.

8.2. Comparison of Indo-Tibetan and Chinese Elements

Now to the *elements*: In Greek Antiquity the four elements were assigned to the same number of humours (see Table 2.3). In the Far Eastern tradition, assignment of regulatory principles (three doshas or 'humours') to elements (five or six Chinese elements) is not quite as clear, as can be seen from Figure 8.2. The circle representation serves to establish a correlation, which automatically yielded a sixth Chinese element. Now we want to tackle the *Indian* elements as well, which are also considered in Tibetan medicine but in addition to the Chinese elements. These five elements are (English and Sanskrit); see Bäumer (1996):

Table 8.4. Assignment of Indo-Tibetan elements to the three regulatory principles. Comparison of three variants

Source reference	Vata	Pitta	Kapha
Ayurveda [a]	Air, Ether	Fire	Earth, Water
Ayurveda [b]	Air, Ether	Fire, Water	Earth, Water
Tibetan medicine [c]	Air	Fire	Earth, Water

[a] Dash (1980, p.19);   [b] Chopra (1993, p.75f);   [c] Qusar et al. (1997, p.7).

| Water, | fire; | earth, | air (wind); | ether (space); | (8.8a) |
| Ap (jala), | tejas; | prthivi, | vayu; | akasha. | (8.8b) |

By name, they are the same as the Greek elements, including the last addition of *ether*. The elements are assigned to the doshas, but the literature is not consistent here (see Table 8.4). Sometimes they are classified according to the first variant depicted there. What stands out is that only pitta is represented by a single element. Perhaps in order to ease this asymmetry, the assignment of *water* can sometimes be found with pitta and not only kapha. This probably has something to do with the fact that pitta is hot as well as damp – see (8.2b), which is not ensured by (dry) fire. In Tibetan medicine, on the other hand, ether is not assigned to any dosha, since it permeates everything and can be found everywhere. The assignment of the remaining four elements to the doshas can be deduced, for example, from the information in Qusar et al. (1997, p.32). They are:

Water: amplifies K, diminishes P;   *earth:* amplifies K, diminishes V;   (8.9a)

Fire: amplifies P, diminishes K;   *air:* amplifies V, diminishes K.   (8.9b)

V, P, K stand for vata, pitta and kapha. Amplification in general means aggravation, while diminishing (weakening) means an easement or calming. Since *earth*, for example, amplifies kapha, it must be located somewhere in kapha (see the considerations of Ch. 8.1). The elements listed vertically in (8.9a&b) show opposite behaviour, just as the elements of the same name in Ancient Greece (see Ch. 2.3). For this reason, they are located on opposite sides in the circle representation. More precisely, *earth*, for example, is in the region of K but opposite V. However, since P is not involved, *earth* must not be in too close proximity to P. Similar considerations lead to the assignment of all four elements shown in (8.9) to positions on the circle (see Figure 8.3). There, the Indo-Tibetan elements are shown inside the circle, in angle brackets to distinguish them from the Chinese elements that have partly the same names. From now on, angle brackets will be also used in the text for Ayurvedic elements in their English translation. Each element covers one sixth of the circumference of the circle (60° arc length). Their respective *centres* are located most probably at the locations indicated by the white dots. The grey areas (±15° arc length) reflect the imprecision of the Tibetan information. In order to keep the model as simple as possible, we shall only refer to the *most probable* locations of elements from now on.

Figure 8.3 shows that after assigning the four elements we have discussed (dark grey) two opposite places on the circle remain empty, one in vata and one in pitta. Now Ayurveda offers us a way of solving this problem. There, the element ether (space), which can be placed coherently in the empty vata position (light grey), is located in *vata*. In the second variant of Table 8.4, water also appears in *pitta* so that the remaining empty position can be filled on a trial basis. However, as can be seen from the position of water in *kapha*, it does not border on pitta and a double assignment of *water* to quite distant locations seems peculiar. Therefore, we reject this version. To a certain extent, this is a similar problem to the one in TCM, when a sixth element was suggested by the structure. Here, too, a position for a sixth element remains open.

There are two common words for *fire* in Sanskrit: *tejas* and *agni*; see Bäumer (1996, Chs. 5-6) and Dash (1980, p.16f). Usually, the element of fire is equated with *tejas*; see (8.8a&b). Tejas, among other things, is associated with light, sun and rays. The second word, agni (Lat. *ignis*), is an important term in Ayurveda, and is closely related to pitta but is not usually considered an element. I filled in the remaining open position with ⟨agni⟩ as an element (see Kratky 1996c&d), since (jathar-)agni also means *fire of digestion*. We shall refer to this element in this sense. Indeed, digestion is characteristic of pitta, compare the TCM meridians located there (see Figure 8.2). Furthermore, digestion occurs in a watery atmos-phere and thus contains as 'damp fire' moisture, which is contained in pitta, see (8.2b).

Tejas as light is often interpreted as coming from above, while agni is earthbound. Agni also means ritual fire and is the earthly counterpart, which combines with divine fire. In the Indian tradition there are also two complements fire – water that are sometimes seen as separate: tejas – ap and agni – soma. The first pair of terms corresponds to the usual ⟨fire⟩ – ⟨water⟩, which results in the horizontal axis in Figure 8.3. This suggests then that the other complement agni – soma corresponds to the axis ⟨agni⟩ – ⟨ether⟩. Indeed this premise can be substantiated (see Ch. 8.5).

In any case, the axis ⟨agni⟩ – ⟨ether⟩ enjoys an exceptional position. ⟨Ether⟩ distinguishes itself substantially from the other four elements, at least in the Tibetan tradition, and ⟨agni⟩ is the complemented sixth Indian element. We now assume that the centre of each of the six elements is located directly at the midpoint of the respective region of the arc marked in grey and that its influence covers one sixth of the circle, just as in the case of the two-dosha types and the Chinese elements. Now all the gaps in the circle have been filled and a direct com-parison with Figure 8.2 is possible. The following correlations result:

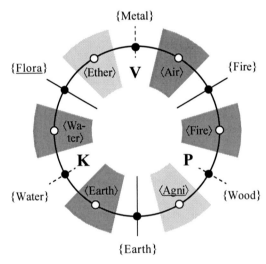

Figure 8.3. Relationship between the doshas (vata **V**, pitta **P**, kapha **K**) and the six ⟨Indian⟩ and {Chinese} elements. The special role of the underlined elements {*flora*} and ⟨*agni*⟩ is explained in the text.

⟨Air⟩ ≜ V-P,	⟨fire⟩ ≜ P-V,	⟨agni⟩ ≜ P-K,	(8.10a)
⟨Earth⟩ ≜ K-P,	⟨water⟩ ≜ K-V,	⟨ether⟩ ≜ V-K.	(8.10b)

Now we shall tackle the comparison with the *Chinese* elements specified in curly brack-ets in Figures 8.2-3 on the *outside* of the circle. This situation is also not clear in the literature. Around the most probable location, there is an uncertainty of about ±15° corresponding to the white regions in Figure 8.3 located between the grey regions. We shall use the centres of these regions again as the best estimate (black dots). Accordingly, the Indian and Chinese elements are placed equidistant to each other (white and black dots). In Figure 8.2 this means, for example, that the successive meridians *Heart, Small Intestine, Gallbladder* and *Liver* are associated with the elements {fire} and {wood}, but the overlapping Indian elements lead to the *Small Intestine* and *Gallbladder* meridians being associated with the Indian ⟨fire⟩. The *Small Intestine* meridian is the one associated with {fire} / ⟨fire⟩. Thus, the same name is used for the Chinese and the Indian element. If you take every second meridian as a representative of an element (see Figures 8.2-3), then this is also the case for *earth* and *water*:

$$\text{LI: } \{\text{metal}\} \mid \langle\text{air}\rangle, \qquad \text{SI: } \{\text{fire}\} \mid \langle\text{fire}\rangle, \qquad \text{LR: } \{\text{wood}\} \mid \langle\text{agni}\rangle, \qquad (8.11\text{a})$$
$$\text{SP: } \{\text{earth}\} \mid \langle\text{earth}\rangle, \qquad \text{KI: } \{\text{water}\} \mid \langle\text{water}\rangle, \qquad \text{SJ: } \{\text{flora}\} \mid \langle\text{ether}\rangle. \qquad (8.11\text{b})$$

From this, we can conclude that {metal} and ⟨air⟩, {wood} and ⟨agni⟩ as well as {flora} and ⟨ether⟩ enjoy a special relationship. LI – SP stands for the polarity or complement *metal / air – earth*, SI – KI for the one of *fire – water*. LR and SJ remain. *Liver* stands for *life* and *vitality*, the complementary *SJ* connects the three bodily regions and is a {flora} meridian. Also, the opposite positions of ⟨agni⟩ and {flora} corresponding to the polarity of LR – SJ is interesting: Ayurveda does not regard the former, TCM not the latter as an element in general, although (or because) something special is hidden behind it. This brings to mind how some individuals in self-assessment are particularly unaware of their worst characteristics. Gienow (2000, p.35) points out in connection to a missing name of a colour in homoeopathy that emphasising a fact by concealing it has a name in Hebrew: *rechem* ('grace').

8.3. Tastes and Nutritional Guidelines

With similar considerations to those in Ch.8.2, the elements and types can also be assigned to *tastes* (*rasas*), which play an important role in Far Eastern healing methods. While the *chemical* composition of foods is central to our culture, the Far Eastern traditions have a sophisticated doctrine on nutrition, which focuses, aside from temperature and moisture, especially on these *rasas*. The boundary between food and remedy is fluid; appropriate nutrition is an important contribution to staying healthy. As is the case in our culture (although for other reasons), the rules for diets and nutrition are confusing. In the West, partly contradictory diets that claim to be beneficial for everyone compete with each other. First, we were told to avoid meat, now meat is said to be essential in a balanced diet. Statements such as 'yoghurt is healthy' suggest that the same food is beneficial or harmful for everyone. The Eastern approach is quite different; see Chopra (1993, p.65): an ideal combination of tastes is determined depending on the individual's constitution and current condition. For healthy individuals there is the general rule, however, that the tastes should be present in a balanced proportion in every meal (Qusar & Sergent 1997, p.119).

From an Eastern perspective, the Western diets may well be beneficial for some types but for others are considered counterproductive. In the West, we could learn much from this model since we concentrate on the statistical average, its response being determined by costly tests. For example, we ascribe a certain diet or therapy to a significant healing effect. However, the fact that this particular situation is especially harmful to, let us say, a K-V type is overlooked. As one of the seven Indian types, it does not assert itself statistically against the other six. This results in a certain percentage of individuals being treated incorrectly due to this tunnel vision. Conversely, the positive effect of a diet or a remedy is neglected, if it only benefits one or two types and thus is drowned in the sea of statistics.

In Eastern healing modalities, on the other hand, there is at least a guiding light despite the differences between Ayurveda, Tibetan medicine and TCM. These differences start with the number of tastes. We know *four* (sweet, salty, sour, bitter), TCM *five* (with the addition of *pungent*), Ayurveda and Tibetan medicine *six* (with the addition to TCM of *harsh* in Ayurveda and *astringent* in Tibetan medicine). In following, we will use the term *astringent*. Sometimes TCM also includes *neutral/ bland* (Fisch 1994, pp.29f & 56) and *harsh/astringent* (Heise 1996, p.15) as tastes. From a Western viewpoint, only the four tastes known to us seem meaningful. However, a fifth type of gustatory papillae has been discovered of late called *Umami* ('good') by its discoverers and presumably can be equated with *astringent*. In the West, there had been talk about *glutamate* as a fifth taste for some time, but the discussion ran along the lines of it just being an enhancer of *other* existing tastes.

The numbers five and six naturally bring to mind the Eastern five and six elements. Table 7.3 immediately confirms this insight. In TCM the five tastes are directly associated with the five usual TCM elements, which leaves astringent ($\triangleq$ *Umami* or *glutamate*) automatically for *{flora}*. This also makes sense for the very reason that {flora} meridians are attributed a supporting function (see the yuan points in acupuncture corresponding to {flora}), which fits in with the function of the {flora} taste as *taste enhancer*. The neutral taste, by the way, is located at the centre of the circle. Now we come to the position of tastes with regard to the *Indo-Tibetan* elements. Since the latter are shifted on the circle with respect to the *Chinese* elements (Figure 8.3), one would expect every taste to be assigned to those two *Indo-Tibetan* elements, between which it is located. This is indeed the case, even if it leads to occasional disagreements between Ayurveda and Tibetan medicine. The literature referred to in this process includes Chopra (1993, pp.258ff), Dash (1980, pp.60ff); Schrott (1994, pp.68ff); Asshauer (1993, pp.118ff), Qusar & Sergent (1997, Ch.2) as well as Qusar et al. (1997, pp.33ff). For *two* tastes, there is agreement in all the literature:

Pungent: $\langle$fire$\rangle$ & $\langle$air$\rangle$,   i.e. {fire},   (8.12a)

Sweet: $\langle$earth$\rangle$ & $\langle$water$\rangle$,   i.e. {water}.   (8.12b)

The Chinese element that results from this, according to Figure 8.3, is given in curly brackets. An interesting point is the two tastes to which $\langle$agni$\rangle$ contributes. Since Ayurveda does not usually regard $\langle$agni$\rangle$ as an element, there should some indication that it is missing. Indeed this is the case (see Sathaye & Nadkarni 2000). They show the following attribution for the two tastes concerned:

Sour: $\langle$fire$\rangle$ & $\langle$earth$\rangle$,   i.e. {wood},   (8.12c)

Salty: $\langle$water$\rangle$, $\langle$fire$\rangle$ & $\langle$earth$\rangle$, i.e. {earth}.   (8.12d)

In order to discriminate between these two tastes, it is no longer sufficient to state only two of the usual five Ayurvedic elements. Moreover, (8.12c&d) indicate that the missing element lies between ⟨fire⟩ & ⟨earth⟩, which is true (see Figure 8.3).

The direct relation of the tastes to the doshas is also fruitful. There are some slight variations as well, but overall we get the following result; see Schrott (1994, p.72):

Astringent: ↑ V, ↓ P, ↑ K {flora};   sour: ↓ V, ↑ P, ↓ K {wood}.   (8.13a)

Pungent: ↑ V, ↑ P, ↓ K {fire};   sweet: ↓ V, ↓ P, ↑ K {water}.   (8.13b)

Bitter: ↑ V, ↓ P, ↓ K {metal};   salty: ↓ V, ↑ P, ↑ K {earth}.   (8.13c)

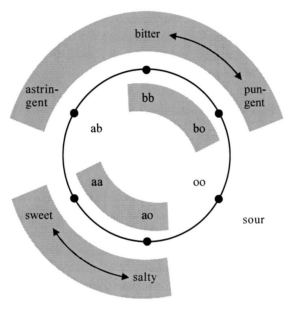

Figure 8.4. Tastes (rasas) and allele pairs of the blood types in the circle representation. Rasas with the same 'aftertaste' (vipak) are in the same grey region. The same is true for allele pairs with the same blood type. Location of rasas according to Ayurveda. Arrows signify an exchange of locations in the case of TCM. Note: alleles are concrete gene formations.

In this scheme ↑ means *amplifying (aggravating)* and ↓ *diminishing (calming)*; see (8.9a&b). The opposite directions of the arrows immediately indicate that the tastes located side-by-side form polar pairs, the resulting Chinese elements being in agreement with (8.12a-d). These pairs, then, are placed on opposite sides of the circle, where the assignment to the Chinese elements can be found easily with the aid of this information (arrows). *Astringent* comes to rest at *{flora}*. Comparison with the direct Chinese classification of tastes, Table 7.3 (with *astringent* at *{flora}*), shows a similar, but different picture: in TCM, the same polar pairs appear. The axis *astringent – sour* remains unchanged, while the axes *pungent – sweet* and *bitter – salty* are interchanged (see Figure 8.4). A simple interpretation of this situation is that *{fire}* and *{metal}* as well as *{water}* and *{earth}* are very similar to each other. There are indications of this fact: the TCM assignment of *damp* to *{earth}* instead of the expected *{water}*, Table 7.3, but also the gender-specific assignment of {fire} and {metal} pulses in Tibetan medicine (Table 7.6a-c).

There is yet another reference. D'Adamo (1997) introduced the concept of (diet) types dependent on blood types. In Kratky (2000b, Ch.3.3) an attempt was made to establish a correlation to the Chinese elements and the circle representation. There are six combinations of pairs of gene forms (alleles a, b, 0), which lead to the four known blood types (8.14a-c). Homozygous pairs correspond to the dosha *centres*, heterozygous pairs to the dosha *transitions*. Both {water} and {earth} correspond to blood type A, {fire} and {metal} to blood type B. One interesting point is that the blood type AB automatically falls on *{flora}*. It is by far the rarest of all the blood types, (about 4%). This fits in with the *moon* type, which is assigned to {flora}, being the rarest of the seven Tibetan regulatory types (Schwarz & Schweppe 1998, p.91). But according to D'Adamo the blood type AB has only been in existence for about 1000 years.

Elements:	{wood};	{earth} & {water};	{fire} & {metal};	{flora}.	(8.14a)
Alleles:	oo;	ao & aa;	bo & bb;	ab.	(8.14b)
Blood type:	0;	A;	B;	AB.	(8.14c)

In this light, it makes sense that the element *{flora}* is usually not taken into account in TCM, while the *moon* type in Tibetan medicine does come into play. In short: TCM is considerably older than 1000 years but Tibetan medicine is not. More precisely, in the spiritual/philosophical early phase of China, there was talk about six elements or types. When TCM was developed about 2000 years ago, the {flora} type was not found among individuals, which presumably led to a reduction to five elements. In comparison: the main work of Tibetan medicine, the rGyud-bzhi (or Gyüshi, the four tantras), was written – based on forerunners – in the 12th century A.D. and received its current form in the 17th century (Reichle 1997, p.157; Schwarz & Schweppe 1998, pp.26ff; Überall 2000, pp.47ff). At this time, AB was already in existence and accordingly the moon type was adopted. TCM, however, maintained its system of five elements. It is possible that TCM experiences difficulty healing individuals with blood type AB. The lengthy experience and persistence of TCM might be a disadvantage in this case, because the human race *has* changed with regard to blood types. However, since this only affects about 4% of the population, it is only obvious if you look for it. More research needs to be done in this area in order to clarify this point. From my perspective, these considerations are one more reason for reintroducing the element {flora} into the Chinese system.

Let us now go back to the six tastes (rasas). They do not all possess the same curative effectiveness. In decreasing order of healing powers, we have:

$$\text{Astringent} > \text{pungent} > \text{bitter} > \text{salty} > \text{sour} > \text{sweet}; \qquad (8.15)$$

see Schwarz & Schweppe (1998, p.115f) and Qusar & Sergent (1997, p.97). It stands out that the taste that does *not* appear in TCM (*astringent*) has the highest curative effect from the Tibetan perspective! This has to do with the fact that it can hardly be overdosed. Moreover, a glance at Figure 8.4 reveals that the tastes with the higher curative effects lie in the *upper* half of the circle representation. The rasas only relate to the (short-term) effect during digestion. According to Qusar & Sergent (1997, p.117), the *sweet* component of a meal is primarily responsible for digestion from *mouth to stomach* (upper region, *kapha*), the *sour* component primarily for the *small intestine* (middle region, *pitta*) and the *bitter* component for the *large intestine* (lower region, *vata*), compare with the meridians of the same name in Figure 8.2. These three tastes then also appear as so-called post-digestive tastes ('aftertaste' *vipak*, see Chopra 1993, p.281), which are responsible for longer-term effects such as cell metabolism. Since they do not represent actual tastes, the nomenclature is unclear. The typical 'aftertaste' [bitter] is called ⟨pungent⟩ in the Indian system. In any case, the following rule applies (with the Tibetan nomenclature):

Rasa:	astringent, pungent & bitter;	sour;	salty & sweet;	(8.16a)
→Vipak:	[bitter] ... *vata*;	sour ... *pitta*;	sweet ... *kapha*.	(8.16b)

See Figure 8.4, where rasas with the same vipak can be found in the same grey zone, which is also true for pairs of alleles with the same blood type (take note of the similarity). This has the following important consequence: The disagreements we have noted between TCM on the one hand, Ayurveda and Tibetan medicine on the other with respect to the rasas are only of secondary importance. The discrepancies disappear in relation to the more important vipaks: {Water} and {earth} have the same 'aftertaste'; the same is true for {fire} *and* {metal}.

8.4. Cycles of Life and Digestion

Traversing the circle – from *{flora}* via kapha, pitta and vata back to *{flora}* – also corresponds, in the symbolic thinking of Ayurveda, to the following two cycles:

a) *Digestion cycle*, from the *ingestion of food* via the passage of nutrients through the digestive system to *elimination*. Kapha (top): mouth to stomach, pitta (middle): stomach to small intestines. Vata (bottom): large intestine and descending colon.

b) *Life cycle,* from birth via childhood, adulthood and old age (kapha, pitta and vata) to death. The critical transitions (birth/death, puberty and the midlife crisis) are characterised by dosha transitions and thus by the corresponding Chinese elements {flora}, {earth} and {fire}.

Both processes have been mentioned in other contexts. They have in common that on the one hand, one talks about *cycles* (return to the same point) but on the other hand food ingestion and elimination and birth and death are as far apart as is conceivable. These two points of view correspond to the representation of Figure 7.4 and Table 7.3 ({flora} as the *linking* or *separating* element). The idea that time is linear in one direction is expressed better in the *table*. If one thinks of time as cyclically recurrent, the *circle* representation is more fitting. Nevertheless, even the circle with six two-dosha types complemented by its centre (three-dosha type) is only a simplified model. In order to be able to represent every possible combination of the three doshas the entire circular *disc* must be utilised, which we shall call the health disc. Starting at the centre of the disc (with equal parts of vata, pitta and kapha) and proceeding in the direction of {fire}, for example, the components of vata and pitta increase by the same amount. Kapha on the other hand decreases and becomes negligible at the boundary of the disc. From now on, we shall utilise this *disc* representation (see Figure 8.5). If, however, in a given case one can work well with the two dominating doshas, then consulting the simpler circle representation is preferable.

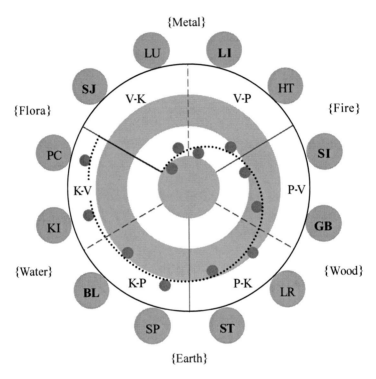

Figure 8.5. (Circular) disc representation with concentric regions and life spiral. The six two-dosha types and the three-dosha type (circular region in the middle) correspond to Ayurveda. Small dark grey discs on the spiral: location of the twelve meridians. Their names are indicated outside the disc (as seen from the centre in the same direction), and so are the names of the Chinese elements.

Let us take a closer look at the disc representation in Figure 8.5 (disc radius R). At first, we shall ignore the grey ring and focus on the Ayurvedic expressions. The six two-dosha types (V-K...) are placed at their respective locations and separated by radial lines. The seventh type – the three-dosha type, where the doshas are represented in almost equal proportions – has now its own region (the light grey disc in the centre), which makes the two-dosha regions a little smaller. The radius $r=(1/4)R$ of this seventh region was chosen in such a fashion as to ensure the weakest dosha a portion of at least 1/4, the strongest dosha no more than 1/2 (the sum of portions is 1). We shall say more on this in Ch. 8.5. For comparison: in the centre, all doshas have a portion of 1/3, whereas at the boundary of the disc, the respective dosha located on the opposite side is not represented (allotment: 0). In proceeding from the boundary at {wood} towards {water}, for example, the portion of vata remains 0, while the proportion P:K shifts from 1:0 to 0:1. At {earth} they have the same portion of 1/2 each.

As in Figure 8.2, the Chinese elements and meridians are indicated at the boundary corresponding to the *circle* representation. Now we need to go one step further and also fully utilise the *disc* representation with regard to the meridians. To accomplish this we shall first deal with the spiral ('life spiral') in Figure 8.5 (see Kratky 2002). In order to explain the concept, we shall proceed from the question of where a 'halfway healthy' two-dosha type would be located on the disc. To put it in a different way: How far from the centre is an individual dependent on the angle still just healthy (angle: {earth} 0°, {Fire}: 120°, for example)? Answer: not on a (concentric) circle, but on the life spiral. On the outside of the spiral, we find the ill, on the inside the healthy states with the following progression: towards the boundary *more and more ill*, towards the centre *healthier*.

So how did the spiral come about? Since vata *itself* is characterised by instability, an individual in this region must have a relatively large portion of the other doshas for stabilisation. For this reason, the spiral is especially close to the centre there. This is particularly true for V-K, which was deduced in the following way. The Indo-Tibetan element ⟨ether⟩ (corresponding to V-K, cf. the circle representation in Figure 8.3) is the only one in Tibetan medicine that is *not* assigned to *any* dosha – in contrast to Ayurveda. According to Qusar et al. (1997, p.7), ⟨ether⟩ permeates everything and can be found everywhere. Within the frame of the disc representation this seeming discrepancy can be dissolved: ⟨Ether⟩ must lie *near* or *in* the three-dosha type, which unites all doshas. In Figure 8.5, this was reconciled by the spiral going to the boundary of the three-dosha type.

Additional clues can also be found in Ayurveda itself. If you make a rough division into the three regulatory types vata, pitta and kapha (the three corresponding arcs in Figure 8.2) and then, after some contemplation, cannot decide which one of the three types you are, you are most likely a *vata* type. Vata and the centre of the disc have a close connection. Furthermore, it is true in Ayurveda that vata types fall ill twice as often as pitta, and pitta twice as often as kapha (Chopra 1993, pp.98ff). This corresponds semi-quantitatively to the *spiral*, which leaves on the outside *little* room around kapha and *a lot of* room around vata. On the other hand, if one crosses the spiral in a direction away from the centre, one reaches the boundary of the disc much sooner at kapha than at vata. This agrees with the statement that ailments and states of distress are much more common in vata, while in pitta acute and in kapha, chronic illnesses predominate. Thus, a pattern emerges where from vata to kapha (*clockwise*) the frequency of illness *de*creases but its severity *in*creases.

At this point, we can interpret the concentric regions in Figure 8.5 as representing an illness getting more severe as one moves from inner to outer regions, or the tendency of an illness to change characteristics from inside toward the boundary: and that from latent via functional to acute and finally chronic; see also (7.3a-c). In Ch.11 & 12, we will readdress questions of illness dynamics. Now let us return to the life spiral, which indicates the boundary of health. In vata, the latency region is left behind outside the spiral: first, a sense of malaise and functional illnesses appears, and only in approaching the boundary do acute illnesses and finally chronic illness emerge. Now in pitta the area outside the spiral constitutes acute, and in kapha chronic illnesses. As to the characteristics of illnesses, the life spiral makes a connection between the distance from the centre and the angle on the circle.

According to Hering's Law (Table 5.3), increase in the severity of an illness is given by symptom progression from *outside to inside*. For reasons of consistency, it follows that *outside* for the organism corresponds to *inside* on the disc representation – and vice versa. This is indeed the case, as can be seen by comparison with Table 7.3 and Figure 8.5: Going from {water} to {metal}, i.e. from kapha to vata in a counter clockwise direction, one gets closer and closer to the surface of the body, but the spiral goes deeper and deeper towards the centre of the disc. Therefore, a particularly high integration of the doshas should be found on the *surface* of the body (the skin). Since inside and outside are interchanged in the organism relative to the disc representation, in Figure 8.5 the *interior* or *yin* meridians are marked *outside* and the *exterior* or *yang* meridians *inside* the spiral. Thus, the spiral also functions as a template with respect to being able to locate the meridians precisely within the frame of the disc representation. Incidentally, the Chinese *SJ* (sanjiao, the triple energiser, which connects the three body cavities) comes to rest at the Indian three-dosha type – one more case of consistency.

We can also use this to specify the assignment of {flora} to the different perspectives. In Ch. 7.2, we talked about an overlap of P1 and P4, of unity and separation, see especially (7.5c). For PC (the first meridian after birth) this is true in the sense that birth is a dramatic separation on the one hand, but the bond with the mother is also very strong in the first months of life. SJ with its integration of all doshas corresponds to meta-perspective MP4, which we introduced in Ch. 2.2 as a synthesis on a higher level.

The meridians PC and SJ are unusual inasmuch as they belong together but are noticeably far apart in the disc representation. In this region, the spiral splits open. Inside and outside meet here, being separated by an 'abyss'. We have already met this gap with the digestion and life cycle (see the layer depth of {flora} in Table 7.3 and the considerations in Ch. 7.6). The cycle is closed *beyond* the human organism. In the process of digestion it is closed by natural bacteria utilising the products of elimination to produce new food, in the life cycle by the stay in the *beyond*, (at least if one assumes rebirth, which is prevalent in India). In this context, we remember the 'gate of life' *mingmen*, which is closely connected to {flora}; see Ch. 7.5. This expression acquires a very concrete meaning now.

The life spiral offers a correlation between the path (on the disc from inside to outside) and a clockwise movement (*outward spiral*). For this reason, a disease progression from vata via pitta to kapha is expected because of Hering's Law. The normal path of life is *counter*-clockwise and corresponds again to an *inward spiral*, an increasing integration of the three doshas. This is the ideal development during the course of life, which started with {flora} and ends in {flora} with a 'healthy' death (the beginning and end of the life spiral). The disc representation thus allows us to distinguish the two terminal points *birth* and *death* (both in {flora}) by their distance from the centre. In a certain sense, the spiral combines the different statements of table and circle representations, which emphasise the *separation* or *connection* in {flora}. In conclusion, we should point out that in Ch. 9 further generalisations of the circle representation will be introduced.

What about *top* and *bottom*? Let us look at the *digestion* cycle. According to this, movement takes place from kapha to vata, from *top* to *bottom*. In TCM the assignment, however, is reversed. In order to understand this we must take a closer look at the meridians and assume for simplicity's sake a close relation between the names of the *meridians* and the *organs*. Let us start in vata, more precisely, with *{metal}*, with Lung LU and Large Intestine LI. The corresponding organs are very distant, lungs – *top*, large intestine – *bottom*. It is typical for TCM to consider the *yin* meridians as being more important. Thus, for vata a correlation to 'top' suggests itself. From an Ayurvedic perspective, the doshas are present everywhere but for vata the *large intestine* in particular is characteristic, i.e. 'bottom'. For the meridians in pitta, stomach to small intestines, there is no discrepancy. The combined assessment is 'middle'. In kapha, it becomes more difficult again. What is missing at first is the corresponding TCM relation for the kapha relation, head and chest ('top') while kidney and bladder in {water} indicate 'bottom'. In Porkert (1992, p.121), however, we find an indication that *{water}* is closely connected to the nervous system and the brain, which was also true for the Ancient Greeks (see Table 2.3). Overall, the (apparent) inconsistencies should have to do with the fact that in TCM the structural *yin* aspect is central. In Ayurveda, however, this is the case for the energetic *yang* aspect, and therefore the focus differs.

Mittwede (1998, p.96f) offers an interesting insight regarding this situation. One would expect that which is heavy ($\langle$water$\rangle$, kapha) to be on the bottom and that which is light ($\langle$air$\rangle$, vata) on top. In the living human being, however, this must be permanently interchanged in order to keep the digestive fire (middle) functioning. Air must kindle the fire from below so that the pot on the fire (with food and water) can be heated up. Therefore, the inanimate order must be reversed in order to enable life. This argument resembles the Lorenz equations discussed in Ch.4.2. There, it is not about animate versus inanimate but about the preliminary question of complex versus simple. Only when the 'unnatural' reversal of temperature (below hotter than on top) has developed to a sufficient degree, interesting structures will form, namely the air coils.

Thus, Mittwede (1998) enables us to achieve a more profound perspective. From this point of view, Rhyner (2001) and Ranade (1994) are also recommended.

8.5.* More on Soma, the Health Disc and Ayurvedic Literature

In Ch.8.2, we talked about the fact that there is another complementarity, *agni* and *soma*, apart from the usual $\langle$fire$\rangle$ – $\langle$water$\rangle$. The assumption was that the former corresponded to the axis $\langle$agni$\rangle$ – $\langle$ether$\rangle$. In this case, the meridians SJ and LU can be considered as soma. Thus, now we need to look at the meaning of soma. This is not water in the usual sense but is often translated as *nectar*, which is related to immortality. Sometimes soma is also thought of as a plant or rather the essence of a plant, which is closely related to water. Another interpretation is that *agni* relates to eating (digesting) and *soma* to that which is eaten (digested).

The reference to plants as well as to immortality points to {flora}. Then for soma, TH would result as a common meridian for {flora} and $\langle$ether$\rangle$. From the point of view of its function, it connects the organism. Fisch (1994, p.91) points out that the ancient Chinese ideograph representing the *SJ* originally consisted of three ideograph, which correspond to the word stems for *plant*, *herbal essence* and *net*. The first two expressions bring to mind soma and {flora}, the third the connecting function. Thus, {flora}, ⟨ether⟩ and soma can be seen as being closely related and the polarity *agni – soma* and LR – *SJ* results automatically. It might be surprising from the point of view of TCM that {flora}is related to water, but it corresponds to the Tibetan viewpoint (Table 7.6a&b).

The next point is a more precise characterisation of the four concentric regions in Figure 8.5 of the previous subchapter; see Tab. 8.5. R is the radius of the disc, the r's are the radii of the circles defining the concentric regions. The relevant variable is $\zeta=r/R$ with the five boundaries of the regions given by:

$$\zeta=r/R: \quad \zeta=0, \ \zeta=1/4, \ \zeta=1/2, \ \zeta=3/4, \ \zeta=1. \tag{8.17}$$

A characterisation of the four regions relative to the states of illness can also be found in Table 8.5, in addition to the minimal and maximal dosha components. The corresponding formulae are given in the in-depth section of the next chapter (9.5).

Table 8.5. Characterisation of the four concentric regions in Figure 8.5

Region of ζ		Illness	a_{min} interval *	a_{max} interval *
$0 \leq \zeta \leq 1/4$	g	latent	$1/4 \leq a_{min} \leq 1/3$	$1/3 \leq a_{max} \leq 1/2$
$1/4 \leq \zeta \leq 1/2$	w	functional / light	$1/6 \leq a_{min} \leq 1/4$	$3/8 \leq a_{max} \leq 2/3$
$1/2 \leq \zeta \leq 3/4$	g	acute / medium	$1/12 \leq a_{min} \leq 1/6$	$5/12 \leq a_{max} \leq 5/6$
$3/4 \leq \zeta \leq 1$	w	chronic / severe	$0 \leq a_{min} \leq 1/12$	$11/24 \leq a_{max} \leq 1$

ζ: $\zeta = r/R$ g, w: grey and white concentric regions in sequence.
* Smallest and/or largest dosha component, a... From a_{min} we get thecorresponding
   a_{max} interval: $a_{min} \leq a_{max} \leq 1-2\,a_{min}$.

In conclusion, one more remark concerning Ayurvedic literature. Ayurveda has a long-standing tradition in India but it was introduced into the West only a few decades ago in the form of Maharashi-Ayurved. This is distinguished from traditional Ayurveda mainly because it is associated with transcendental meditation, an invention of the founder, Maharishi Mahesh Yogi. Some swear by this system, others consider it a sect. In accordance with my attempt of avoiding judgement, I should only point out that for a considerable time the vast majority of books available in the West were those on the Maharashi system, which helped to make Ayurveda popular in the West. Furthermore, from the perspective of medical principles, there appears to be little difference at first glance.

In the last decades, though, traditional literature has also been readily available. There are three books in particular I would recommend: Rhyner (2001), Ranade (1994) and Mittwede (1998). All three give in-depth information and orient their terminology in Sanskrit. The book by Rhyner is the most comprehensive and despite its title, 'A Practical Guide', contains a considerable amount of theory. In the section on pulse diagnosis, the reference on p.172 to scientific research is remarkable. In Ch.14, Ranade describes, among other things, the treatment of common clinical pictures, and in Ch.16 the author compares the traditions of yoga and Ayurveda. In Mittwede the historical reference, which prevents a dogmatic way of thinking, deserves mention. The author reveals that many of today's seemingly established theses have undergone changes over the centuries, especially when the therapy was in its early stages. For example, on p.74 the development of the elements with regard to name and number is discussed. All three books are recommended for more in-depth information.

Chapter 9

Advancement of the Cross-Cultural Model

9.1. The Basic Circle Representation

We have spent most of our time with the circle representation, and in Ch. 8.4 we developed a step from the circle to the disc. In the following section, we want to take a systematic look at this and start again with the circle. In Figure 8.1 the centres of the arcs of vata (V), pitta (P), and kapha (K) have been called V_m, P_m, and K_m, respectively. Now, we come to more elaborate considerations (see Figure 9.1a&b). The axes of coordinates are formed by the vertical *yin* axis (variable x, from top to bottom, points on the circle X_m^- and X_m^+) and the horizontal *yang* axis (variable y, from left to right, points on the circle Y_m^- and Y_m^+). Every point on the circle can be described by the pairs (x, y) or (r_c, α), see Figure 9.1b. r_c is the radius of the circle (*c* stands for *circle*), and α is the angle measured counter-clockwise from the x-axis, $0° \leq \alpha \leq 360°$. Thus,

$$\text{Yin: } x = r_c \cos\alpha; \quad \text{yang: } y = r_c \sin\alpha; \quad 0° \leq \alpha \leq 360°. \tag{9.1}$$

The circle can be divided into six arcs around the *Chinese* elements (from one *white* dot to the next) and the same goes for the *Indo-Tibetan* elements (from one *black* dot to the next). In Ch. 8.1-2, we concentrated on the Indo-Tibetan elements, resulting in (8.10a&b). In order to do something analogous for the Chinese elements, we must first compute the respective arcs. It would seem sensible to specify the arcs around the centres of the doshas by V^+, P^+, K^+ and the respective arcs on the opposite side by V^-, P^-, K^-. In the latter, the arcs in Figure 9.1a are explicitly marked as arrows. Overall, this yields in a clockwise direction:

$$\{Metal\} \triangleq V^+, \qquad \{fire\} \triangleq K^-, \qquad \{wood\} \triangleq P^+, \tag{9.2a}$$
$$\{Earth\} \triangleq V^-, \qquad \{water\} \triangleq K^+, \qquad \{flora\} \triangleq P^-. \tag{9.2b}$$

Compare this with (8.10 a&b) for the Indo-Tibetan elements. The centres of the arcs contain the additional index m (m stands for *middle* or *mean*), i.e. V_m^+, P_m^+, K_m^+ and V_m^-, P_m^-, K_m^-. The following identities are valid (cf. Figures 8.1 & 9.1a):

$$V_m^+ = V^+, P_m^+ = P^+, K_m^+ = K^+. \quad (9.3)$$

Now let us look at the meaning of x and y. In Kratky (2000b, Ch.2.3) the information available for yin and yang was used to define the values for *moisture* (yin dependency) and *temperature* (yang dependency) on the circle. For simplicity's sake *neutral*, middle values were set to zero. Since we want to take a closer look at the available yin and yang *strength* (in the following called v and w, respectively), the *minimal* value must be at least zero. The neutral value is now set to 1. This gives a representation in v and w equivalent to Kratky (2000b).

$$v = 1 + p\ (\cos\alpha - 1), \quad \text{maximum at } X_m^+\ (\alpha = 0°); \qquad (9.4a)$$
$$w = 1 + 3^{1/2}p\sin\alpha, \quad \text{maximum at } Y_m^+\ (\alpha = 90°). \qquad (9.4b)$$
$$\text{In general:} \qquad 0 \le p \le 0.5. \qquad (9.4c)$$

For more details, see Ch.9.5. The maximal yin strength v is the neutral value 1, cf. (9.4a). This is consistent with the considerations in Ch.7.1, where it was argued that with a good approximation there is no yin excess.

The selectable parameter p is a measure for the differences of the values on the circle: for p=0, v=w=1 on the entire circle, i.e. the elements do not differ in their values. The other boundary case is p=0.5, where for X_m^- ($\alpha=180°$, {metal}) the value for v=0, which according to the above is the smallest value possible. The following concrete values refer to p=0.4. For X_m^+ ($\alpha=0°$, {earth}), v=w=1, independent of p; both variables have a neutral value. The *minima* of v and w are located exactly opposite their *maxima*, i.e. at X_m^- and Y_m^-, respectively, cf. (9.4a&b) and Figure 9.1a.

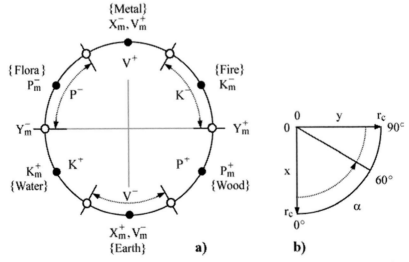

Figure 9.1. a) Circle representation of the Chinese {elements} and the six Tibetan regions V^+, K^-, P^+, V^-, K^+, P^- as well as their centres $V_m^+,..,P_m^-$. The vertical yin axis (from X_m^- to X_m^+) and the horizontal yang axis (from Y_m^- to Y_m^+) are light grey. **b)** In detail: quarter circle ($0 \le \alpha \le 90°$) with positive x- and y-axes.

The variable v stands for *yin strength* and *moisture*, w for *yang strength* and *temperature* or *warmth*. There is also a connection with the autonomic or vegetative nervous system. v has a close relationship to the *parasympathetic*, w to the *sympathetic* nervous system. The two are most often antagonists (Schmidt et al. 2000, Ch. 19). The sympathetic nervous system, for example, is responsible for *speeding up* the heartbeat, the parasympathetic for *slowing* it *down*. The two-dimensional considerations in Ch. 7.1 regarding yin and yang will now find a correspondence: There are, in principle, four types of possibilities: to activate or calm the sympathetic or the parasympathetic nervous system. The vagal (or parasympathetic) activity v stimulates digestion, thus we will use it as a measure for *digestion*. It reaches its maximum at {earth} and its minimum at {metal}. There, it would come to a complete stop with the boundary value of p=0.5. At a value of p=0.4, the maximal strength of digestion (at {earth}) is five times that of the minimal.

The metabolism related to digestion also consists of two parts: *synthesis* (anabolism) and *decomposition*, which produces energy (catabolism). Anabolism concerns the synthesis of substances and the replacement of old cells, which uses up the energy of nutrients ('cold' in the sense of TCM). Catabolism concerns the production of heat and the release of energy, e.g. in muscle power ('hot'). According to (8.2.b&c) and (8.6.b&c), anabolism has its focus in *YIN* (kapha), catabolism in *YANG* (pitta). To simplify matters, we will assume anabolism to be proportional to v and catabolism proportional to w. Estimations for anabolism and catabolism then result from the proportions (adding up to 1), $v/(v+w)$ and $w/(v+w)$ of digestion, v. These proportions must be multiplied by the digestion v, on which they both depend. The final result then is $v*[v/(v+w)]$ and $v*[w/(v+w)]$ as estimates for anabolism and catabolism.

In general, sympathicotonic reactions (sympathetic system dominates, w−v>0) have to do with 'flight and fight', vagotonic reactions (w−v<0) with relaxation, regeneration and recuperation. One also speaks of ergotropic and trophotropic phases, which should be kept in balance. Sympathicotonic reactions are useful in urgent cases and emergencies, but in the long run the system must be balanced by vagotonic phases (rest, sufficient sleep). However, this is just the way it is in professional life: If (in the short run) something urgent and (in the long run) something important must be achieved, the important thing usually has to take a back seat. This works well for a while, but at some point the system breaks down and the organism gets its rest by falling ill.

The sum $\Sigma = w+v$ represents a measure of total 'energy', the difference $\Delta = w-v$ shows the dominance of one of the two components. From (9.4a&b) it follows:

Sum: $\Sigma = w + v$,   max. at P_m^+ ($\alpha=60°$);   neutral value: $\Sigma = 2$.   (9.5a)

Difference: $\Delta = w - v$,   max. at K_m^- ($\alpha=120°$);   neutral value: $\Delta = 0$.   (9.5b)

Y_m^+ ($\alpha= 90°$), the point of the maximum of w, is located exactly between the maxima of Σ and Δ. If Σ is a measure of total energy, then $\Sigma<2$ means energy deficiency (extreme value: {flora}), and $\Sigma>2$ energy excess (maximum: {wood}). $\Delta<0$ on the other hand means *yin* surplus, $\Delta>0$ *yang* surplus (maxima: {water} and {fire}). Minima and maxima are located on *opposite* sides on the circle representation. There will be more on this in Ch. 9.5, where you will also find tabulated results of v, w, Σ, Δ, v^2/Σ and vw/Σ for important points on the circle with p=0.4. The last two values stand for *anabolism* and *catabolism*.

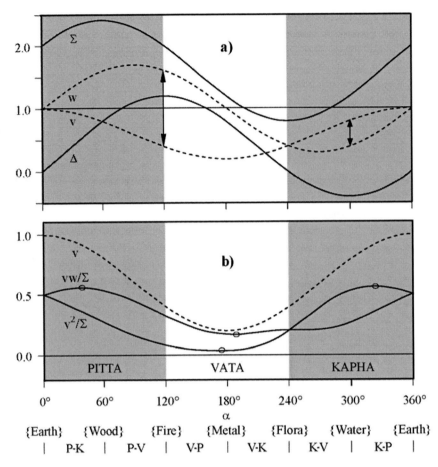

Figure 9.2. a) The variables v, w, Σ=w+v and Δ=w−v as functions of the angle α in the circle representation. The first third (pitta, grey) corresponds to $\Sigma \geq 2$ and $\Delta \geq 0$, the second third (vata, white) to $\Sigma \leq 2$ and $\Delta \geq 0$ and the last third (kapha, grey) to $\Sigma \leq 2$ and $\Delta \leq 0$. This is valid for all p; see (9.4a&b). The specific curves are based on p=0.4. **b)** The variables v, v^2/Σ and vw/Σ as functions of the angle α; v stands for the entire metabolism. It is divided into a catabolic (vw/Σ) and an anabolic (v^2/Σ) component (maxima in pitta and kapha, minima in vata). p=0.4.

Now these parameters are represented graphically (see Figure 9.2a&b). Let us first look at v (*yin*) and w (*yang*), the dashed curves in Figure 9.2a. Remember that the neutral value is 1 in both cases. {wood} is slightly under the neutral value with respect to v but strong with respect to w, corresponding to yang excess of *pitta*, Table 8.1. {Metal} is weak with respect to v and neutral with respect to w, corresponding to the yin deficiency of *vata*. {Water} is slightly below the neutral value with respect to v but w is still smaller, corresponding to the yang deficiency of *kapha*. The transitions are given by the elements {earth}, {fire} and {flora}. The solid curves for Σ and Δ give us further information. The neutral value Σ=2 occurs at {fire} and {earth}, the neutral value Δ=0 at {earth} and {flora}. {Earth}, then, is neutral with respect to both values Σ and Δ, (and also with respect to v and w). This corresponds to the TCM statement that {earth} is located in the *middle*. No matter how *neutral* this element is (Kubiena 1995, pp.17 & 50f), it is also considered to be *extremely yin* (Porkert

1992, p.126). What at first looked like a contradiction can now be reconciled. Only at {earth} is *yin* is not below the neutral value.

Comparing the curves in Figure 9.2a reveals more information concerning the possibilities of the organism. From {earth} to {flora} (pitta and vata, yang excess and yin deficiency) yang is above yin except at the endpoints, where it is equal to yin (thus w≥v, Δ≥0). Thus, activity dominates over recuperation (ergotropic region), being strongest at 120°, {fire} (Δ=max, see left double arrow). However, pitta is much more energetic (Σ is maximal in {wood}) than vata. Vata tends to exhaustion, which we find repeatedly in vata's lack of stability. At {flora}, the location of least total energy, *yin* deficiency goes into *yang* deficiency. From {flora} to {earth} (kapha, yang deficiency) yang lies below yin and is only equal to it at the endpoints (thus Δ≤0). Now recuperation dominates over activity (trophotropic region), being strongest at 300°, {water} (Δ=min, see right double arrow). This fits in with kapha types sleeping longer, and childhood, which is assigned to kapha, is a period marked by prolonged sleep. The statements of this paragraph are valid for all p, 0≤p≤0.5, the concrete curves of Figure 2a relate to p=0.4.

If we move on to Figure 9.2b, v now stands for intensity of digestion, a measure for the entire metabolism. It also shows the division of v into catabolism and anabolism (decomposition and synthesis). As expected the maximum point of *catabolism* lies in pitta (more precisely, P-K) and the maximum point of *anabolism* in kapha (more precisely, K-P). This corresponds roughly to the position of the Indian elements ⟨agni⟩ and ⟨earth⟩, see Figure 8.3. Both minima lie in vata, in the region of {metal}. The minimum point of *catabolism* lies in V-K, that of *anabolism* in V-P. Figure 9.2b relates again to p=0.4. The maxima only shift slightly in the entire p-region.

The basic statements relating to Figure 9.2a&b are also mirrored in behaviour and appearance (*physique* types by Kretschmer). Most vata types are asthenic (leptosomes) and give an impression of frailness. In pitta types athletes dominate; strength and athleticism are in the foreground. They also eat heartily without gaining weight. Not so kapha, where only a small amount of digestion goes into strength and more into body mass and regeneration. If kapha types become too calm or do not exercise enough, they need to reduce their food intake considerably in order not to gain weight. This relates, therefore, to the pyknic type. One more thing should be said about the term *digestion* in Ayurveda: pitta is associated with strong digestion, kapha with weak and vata with medium, variable digestion. Since it is associated with the fire of digestion *(jathar-)agni*, it stands to reason that in Ayurveda *catabolism* is central, having its maximum in pitta. However, Figure 9.2b shows that this is not the whole truth, because kapha is still stronger than vata with respect to catabolism. If one considers the strength of the sympathetic system alone on the other hand (yang, represented by w in Figure 9.2a), then its maximum lies in *pitta* (at Y_m^+, ⟨fire⟩), the minimum in *kapha* (at Y_m^-, ⟨water⟩) and the neutral middle value in *vata* (at V_m^+). Since the variable w also stands for temperature, the fire of digestion in the sense of Ayurveda apparently refers to the last step of heat and energy production (see Rhyner 2001, pp.211-4).

Much can also be said with regard to susceptibility to illness. The circle representation can be seen in such a way that the organism tends to that location on the circle where it can best cope with the moment-to-moment demands. According to Figure 9.2a, a range of reaction modes is available. For acute threats from outside, it is beneficial to be in the proximity of {fire}, since the ergotropic reaction is especially strong there (Δ especially high). If that is not sufficient, the organism will go into a tailspin at the location of {fire} ($\alpha=120°$). In Ch. 11.1&4, we shall see that this is indeed the case. In the long run, if one has not been able to recharge one's batteries often enough (at {water}, $\alpha=300°$), it may no longer suffice to go to {water} for a trophotropic reaction to occur. Then chronic exhaustion, for example, may result. Indeed, kapha types are considered very healthy, but severe disorders can arise in the long run. Connections to analogous statements in homoeopathy can be found in Ch. 12.4.

9.2. Life Spiral, Health Disc and Health Cone

The circle only reveals a limited view of the organism's possibilities. For this reason, the step to the *disc* representation was initiated in Ch. 8.4 (see Figure 8.5, where the keyword is life spiral). This corresponds to a transition from a *one*-dimensional to a *two*-dimensional approach. A point on the health disc is characterised by the pair (r, α), where α is defined as before and r is the distance of the considered point to the centre of the disc (origin). The disc has radius R. We have:

$$x = r\cos\alpha, y = r\sin\alpha, \quad 0 \le r \le R, \ 0° \le \alpha \le 360°. \tag{9.6}$$

This is a generalisation of (9.1). The variables v and w are now also dependent on r. A simple rule can be stated that all trigonometric functions in (9.4a&b) must be multiplied by $k=r/r_c$. This yields the following new relations:

$$v = 1 + p(k\cos\alpha - 1), \quad \text{max. at } \alpha = 0°; \ k = r/r_c; \tag{9.7a}$$
$$w = 1 + 3^{1/2}pk\sin\alpha, \quad \text{max. at } \alpha = 90°. \tag{9.7b}$$

Thus, the angles for maxima remain unchanged with respect to (9.4a&b). The relations (9.5a&b) are still valid for Σ and Δ but a more complicated formula results from substitution (see Ch. 9.5). At the centre of the disc, we have:

$$r = 0: \ x = y = 0; \quad v = 1 - p, \ w = 1; \quad \Sigma = 2 - p, \Delta = p. \tag{9.7c}$$

For the purposes of comparison we need to make circle and disc representations as equivalent as possible. Where on the disc, then, should the circle ($r=r_c$) of the circle representation be inserted? The angle α remains the same, but which radius should be chosen? The following approach seems appropriate: Dosha centres of the circle representation (Figure 8.1) need to maintain their meaning as centres (V_m, P_m and K_m) on the *disc* as well. 'Centre' now refers not to an arc, but to a sector ('third of a pie'), see Figure 9.3. Angle α of this centre is evident. To calculate the distance r, a small strip or, to be more accurate, sector, is considered. A brief computation yields $r/R=2/3=0.667$ (see Ch. 9.5). The resulting circle and the dosha centres V_m, P_m, and K_m can also be found in Figure 9.3. The results of the circle representation are then embedded in the disc accordingly. Incidentally, the circle intersects the life spiral just at P_m. This means that in a counter-clockwise direction, the spiral lies *outside* between {flora} and {wood} and then *inside* (between {wood} and {flora}). The spiral divides the circle with radius r=(2/3)R into two equal parts.

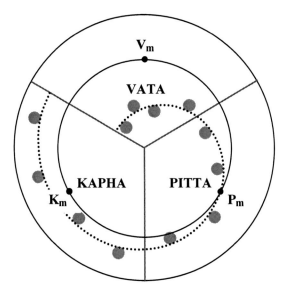

Figure 9.3. The three doshas and their centres on the disc, compared to the meridians and the life spiral. The centres V_m, P_m and K_m are located on the circle with r=(2/3) R, R being the radius of the disc.

The disc can just as well be cut into six pieces of pie instead of three. The resulting six centres are then located again on the circle r=(2/3)R. There are two versions of this. In the *Ayurvedic* arrangement the six regions V-K, V-P, P-V, P-K, K-P, K-V are preserved by cutting each third of the pie in half – compare with Figure 8.2, now generalised to the disc. The *Tibetan* regions V^+, K^-, P^+, V^-, K^+, P^- are now shifted by 30° with respect to the Ayurvedic regions (generalisation of Figure 9.1a to the disc). The two are in comparison (clockwise with correct interleaving):

Ayurveda:	V-K	V-P	P-V	P-K	K-P	K-V	(9.8a)
Tibetan:	V^+	K^-	P^+	V^-	K^+	P^-	(9.8b)
Centres:	V_m^+	K_m^-	P_m^+	V_m^-	K_m^+	P_m^-	(9.8c)

(9.8c) gives the centres of the Tibetan regions (cf. Figure 9.1a). In addition to the six regions exhibited in (9.8a&b), it is customary to consider the three-dosha type, as was illustrated for the first time in Figure 8.5 and Table 8.5. In Figure 9.4a, this seventh type is represented again as a grey disc with radius R/4. This limits the scope of the six other types but to an equal extent for the Ayurvedic and the Tibetan versions. Accordingly, their centres are shifted slightly outwards; they are now at r/R= 7/10 = 0.700 instead of 0.667 (see Ch.9.5). It is a matter of taste as to which of the almost identical circles is more suitable for the embedding into the disc. Since the arrangement of the seven types is the more common, we shall from now on assume $r_c/R=0.7$ for conversion from health circle (r_c) to health disc (R). See Ch.9.5 as to further possibilities to choose r_c.

There is one more point to be made concerning notation. The Tibetan types and the Chinese elements have their centres in V_m^+, K_m^-,..., P_m^-; see (9.8c). The corresponding points at the border of the disc will be denoted by V_e^+, K_e^-, ..., P_e^-, see Figure 9.4a (*e* stands for *external* or *extreme*, i.e. *outermost*). Accordingly, Y_m^- and Y_m^+, Figure 9.1, yield the boundary points, Y_e^- and Y_e^+.

Now it is possible to expand the arrangement of the TCM regions of Figure 7.4 to the disc. The result is also shown in Figure 9.4a. The boundaries of the regions are given by two straight lines, which go through V_m^-, K_m^- and P_m^- with $r/R=0.7$, corresponding to the 'transition elements' {earth}, {fire}, and {flora}.

Line through P_m^- and V_m^- :   to the left $\Delta < 0$, to the right $\Delta > 0$.   (9.9a)

Line through K_m^- and V_m^- :   to the left $\Sigma < 2$, to the right $\Sigma > 2$.   (9.9b)

On the lines, $\Delta=w-v=0$ and $\Sigma=w+v=2$, which corresponds to their neutral values, see (9.5a&b). This results in the following four regions, cf. (7.1a-c):

Yin deficiency (white)   (9.10a)

Yang deficiency (light grey)   Yang excess (light grey)   (9.10b)

Yin excess (dark grey   (9.10c)

The regions and their boundaries are valid independent of the parameter p, see (9.5a&b) and (9.7a&b). Because of the expansion into the disc representation, a small gusset (dark grey) appears at the bottom corresponding to *yin excess*. At the intersection of the two lines, the 'doubly neutral' {earth} can be found. It is also consistent for the spiral and the two {earth} meridians to be very close. However, only *one single* meridian, namely Small Intestine, is located directly on one of the lines ($\Sigma=2$). This means that it is the only one with a neutral total energy. The three-dosha region is located within the region of yin deficiency. This is also true for the majority of *vata* as a whole (see Figure 9.3). Yang excess corresponds largely to *pitta*, yang deficiency to *kapha*. Nevertheless, the regions of TCM and Ayurveda are no longer congruent in the disc representation. However, it is possible to convert from one medicine system to the other.

A further point should be made about the parameter p, see (9.4a-c) for the circle and (9.7 &b) for the disc: on the circle (r/r_c), the condition $0\leq p\leq0.5$ holds. Since on the disc there are also r-values *outside* r_c (corresponding to $k=r/r_c>1$), v and w can now be negative near the disc border for $p<0.5$. Since we want to exclude this situation, the range of p must be restricted for the disc, compared to (9.4c):

Disc: $0 \leq p \leq 0.7/3^{1/2} = 0.4041$.   (9.11)

Thus, the transition to two dimensions has brought a few new insights. Now we will tackle the generalisation to *three* dimensions (x,y,z) and expand the disc into a cone. For the sake of simplicity, let the cone be on its tip (at z=0). At the level of z=1, let the radius of the horizontal disc (conic section) be R=1; it is to represent the disc we have been working with (R=1 $\triangleq$ 3.5 cm, r_c=0.7 $\triangleq$ 2.45 cm). Figure 9.4b gives a side view of the cone. At the level z, a respective variable radius R (R=z) results for the horizontal disc. More precisely:

Cone: $R = R_z = z$, $0 \leq z \leq z_{max}$.   Moreover, $r_c = 0.7\,R$.   (9.12)

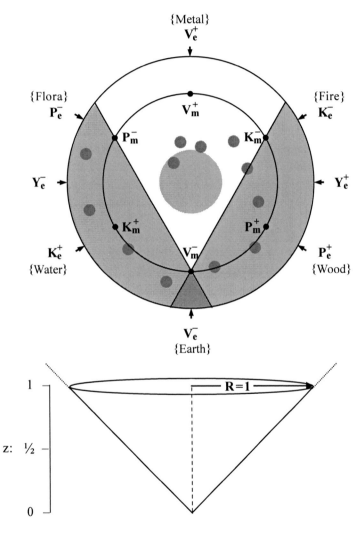

Figure 9.4. a) Disc representation of TCM regions of yang excess and deficiency, as well as yin deficiency and excess; r = 0.7R. **b)** Expansion of the disc to a cone.

The dotted lines indicate a continuation of the cone beyond z=1 in Figure 9.4b to an undetermined z_{max}, which will be at about 2 (see below). We already know the last relation in (9.12). It now holds for arbitrary z. What does z mean anyway? Let z be a measure of the power (*qi*) available to the organism. It is proportional to z and therefore disappears at the tip of the cone. Accordingly, the variables v and w are now related to z proportionally. This results in the following generalisation of (9.7a&b):

$$v = z[1 + p(k\cos\alpha - 1)]; \quad k = r/r_c = r/(0.7z);$$ (9.13a)
$$w = z[1 + 3^{1/2} p k \sin\alpha].$$ (9.13b)

As before, we shall only consider points for the disc *within* the cone. For V_m^- ($\alpha = 0$, $r = r_c$, cf. Figure 9.4a) now v=w=z holds in general, i.e. the neutral value 1 for {earth} is reached exactly at the disc representation, (z=1). Whether or not the values of {earth} for $z \neq 1$ are also considered neutral depends on whether one refers to the energy at the respective height of z or whether the height of 1 is used as a fixed measure.

An individual's changing state of health corresponds now to the movement of a point on the circle, disc or cone, depending on the dimension considered. In the three-dimensional representation, at first glance an arbitrary movement within the cone appears possible. If, however, one relates the height (variable, z) to the scope of reaction, which becomes more and more restrictive towards the tip of the cone, advancement in biological age can be connected with a movement towards the bottom. According to TCM, the level of original *qi* (*yuanqi*) cannot be regenerated and is used up at a rate that depends, to a greater or lesser extent, on lifestyle and nutrition. In this sense, we can only move downwards (on the cone). We begin with $z = z_{max}$ (birth). Even in a life without severe illness, the possibilities for reaction become more and more limited, because the individual moves to smaller and smaller discs. Once the available energy no longer suffices, death occurs.

The life spiral can therefore be interpreted in two ways – not only as an area, but also spatially: looking down on the cone everything is projected onto a plane. The path of life, then, not only leads further inside in the sense of Figure 9.3 but also gets narrower corresponding to the radius of the cone getting smaller (Figure 9.4b). In this respect, the model can be generalised further.

In an acute illness, the point on the health disc moving (almost horizontally) towards the boundary of P-V (towards the 'heat pole', see Figures 8.1&8.2) can to all intents and purposes mean fever. The border (the boundary of the cone) is reached when the fever can no longer rise or must not rise any further (otherwise, severe injury or even death might result). From then on, the battle against the bacteria that have triggered the fever is lost. The 'battle zone' is now restricted more and more over the course of time, the available leeway becoming less and less (radius R_z of the disc). Indeed, high fever is not as dangerous – and may even be desired in principle – in small children as it is in adults. If the health disc (R=1), considered so far, refers to an adult in midlife, then a value of R≈2 must be assigned for birth. The health disc, then, is located about halfway up the cone.

9.3. Assignment of Colours to the Three Principles

Since there are three regulatory principles and our ability to see colours is based on three different colour receptors, the above considerations can be easily depicted with colours. The topic of colours is however very diverse – it encompasses physical, physiological, psycholog-ical and symbolic aspects (see Kratky 2000c, Ch. 2). We shall just introduce a small part of it.

Every ray of light corresponds to a certain frequency, which is broken down into three *primary colours* by the receptors. Since the colours themselves are ambiguous, one talks about S-, M- and L-receptors. S stands for *short* (wave) and encompasses the range violet to blue-green. M stands for *medium* (wave) and encompasses green and yellow, L stands for *long* (wave) and encompasses orange and red. For the sake of simplicity, *blue, red* and *green* are said to be *additive primary colours*. If a spotlight of these colours is trained onto a black wall, the result is white as a superimposition (*addition*) of the three colours. More precisely, it is grey which, depending on the brightness of the spotlight, can range from almost black to dark grey to light grey and white. The primary colours can be varied within a certain frame and correspond mostly to indigo (violet-blue), green and orange-red. They are used in com-puters, television sets, video and other projectors.

Additive primary colours:	indigo,	green,	orange-red;	(9.14a)
Subtractive primary colours: (complementary to *additive*)	yellow,	magenta,	cyan;	(9.14b)
Other complementary pairs:	blue,	yellowish green,	red;	(9.14c)
	orange,	violet,	bluish green.	(9.14d)

Taking away one of the additive primary colours from white, results in the sum of the other primary colours as *complementary colour*. Yellow is complementary to *indigo*, magenta (purple) to *green* and cyan (greenish blue) to *orange-red*. The *subtractive primary colours* are used in painting and for colour printing. In this case, light is *taken away* from the white background by adding colours. A colour that absorbs indigo, for example, reflects its comple-mentary colour and thus appears yellow to the eye. Thus, to speak of the (subtractive) pri-mary colours as *red, yellow* and *blue* is not quite correct.

At night, it is mainly just our *rods* (black/white receptors) that function properly. Accord-ingly, then we can only differentiate between the brightness of objects ("all cats are grey in the dark"). In daylight, however, we primarily use the *cones* (three colour receptor types), which allow us to recognise three aspects of colours: hue, saturation and brightness. Hue refers to the pure spectral colour as observed in a rainbow (bright with maximal saturation). In the ideal case, it is monochromatic light – in other words, it consists of one frequency or wavelength. As far as saturation is concerned, if we take blue as an example, starting with the rainbow shade of blue, the colour turns pale or pastel with decreasing saturation, then closer and closer to grey or white. The latter depends again on brightness, the third aspect of colour.

These three aspects can be easily transferred to our *health cone*, where the angle α refers to the hue, r to the saturation and z to the brightness. Let us start with the disc (R=1), which contains hue and saturation. We start at the border of the disc, that is to say, with the circle ('colour circle', r=1) containing the points V_e^+, K_e^-, P_e^+, V_e^-, K_e^+, P_e^-, cf. Figure 9.4a. The colours correspond to the maximal saturation of (rainbow) colours. All points on the colour circle can be produced as mixtures of the neighbouring *additive* primary colours. The points V_e^+, P_e^+, K_e^+ (α: 180°, 60°, 300°) correspond to the additive primary colours, opposite points

$V_{\bar{e}}$, $P_{\bar{e}}$, $K_{\bar{e}}$ (α: 0°, 240°, 120°) represent their complementary *subtractive* primary colours, cf. Figure 9.1 and (9.14a&b).

Going towards the *centre* of the disc, the third additive primary colour becomes more and more apparent. True blue becomes paler and paler and finally, in the centre, white (or grey). The expression 'light blue' is sometimes used here, but it is confusing. The *brightness* of the colours is the same everywhere on the disc. Differences in brightness can only be represented in the third dimension (z-direction: axis of *cone*). The axis is white at the top, turning darker as one moves toward the tip of the cone and is black at the tip (z=0). As the brightness decreases, the ability to distinguish between the colours diminishes, which corresponds to the narrowing of the cone.

The frequency distribution can only be analysed to a certain extent, of course, with only three receptor types. Thus, we know orange as a pure colour of the rainbow as well as a – subtractive – mixture of red (or magenta) and yellow. From an additive perspective, orange can also be produced by mixing (orange-)red and green. All these can appear to be identical colours to us. We tend to interpret as monochromatically as possible, i.e. seeing rainbow colours, even if they are (possibly) mixed colours. This no longer works, when the third primary colour is also represented to a noticeable degree. Then, we see pastel colours, which deviate clearly from the rainbow colours. A point on the border of the disc can indeed correspond to one singular frequency but does not *have* to. A point on the inside of the disc, especially near the centre, corresponds to a broader frequency distribution. All this is based on a fixed total brightness, so that we only have to consider one *disc* instead of the entire cone.

As far as the colours are concerned, we have a visibility region corresponding to a quotient of about 2 (maximum/minimum) with respect to wavelength λ and frequency ν.

Visibility thresholds:	violet:	$\lambda \approx 385\,nm,$	$\nu \approx 780 * 10^{12}\,Hz,$	(9.15a)
	red:	$\lambda \approx 770\,nm,$	$\nu \approx 390 * 10^{12}\,Hz.$	(9.15b)

1 nm (nanometre) is one billionth of a metre, i.e. 10^{-9} m, 10^{12} Hz (Hertz) are 1 trillion oscillations per second. λ and ν are linked to the speed of light, $c = 3.0 * 10^8$ m/s, ($\nu = c/\lambda$). In sound, the quotient 2 corresponds to one octave, a half-octave (quotient: $2^{1/2} = 1.414$) is also called a tritone. We are able to hear about 10 octaves (from 20 to 20 000 Hz), i.e. a far greater range than seeing. A tone and the one an octave higher appear somehow equal to us. There is a similar phenomenon with seeing: Although the short-wave violet has a maximal distance to the long-wave red, it seems that violet reminds us of red; the colour circle closes psychologically from blue to violet to red, where it is bridged by purple (or magenta). This colour, however, is constructed by us; it is not a rainbow colour! However, because only two receptors (L and S) are activated, we interpret it as a pure colour and not as a mix. The colour circle (circle representation!) cannot be justified purely by physics, but it also contains a constructivist aspect.

Another peculiarity lies in the fact that from around 650 nm on only the L-receptor is activated. This means that for monochromatic light (from 650 nm on up to the visibility threshold at 770 nm), there is no change in the impression of red, except that it appears darker and darker. Thus, our range of distinguishing colours is *less* than an octave. In fact, it is almost exactly ¾ of an octave (quotient: $2^{6/8} = 2^{3/4} = 1.682$). This range was suggested in Kratky (2000c) as a candidate for closing the (subjective) colour circle. The colours on opposite sides of the colour circle are *complementary* (quotient: $2^{3/8} = 1.297$) and together result in white (grey), but this is not true for opposite 'tritonal' colours, which are separated by a full octave (quotient: $2^{1/2} = 1.414$, see above).

Many variants of colour receptors and pigments with respect to their number n and their typical sensitivity to frequencies can be found in the animal kingdom. Apart from extreme cases, such as n=1 or n>4, in general we have n=2, 3 or 4. Our mammalian ancestors fled into the night from the dinosaurs (n>3), which were active in daylight. Colour vision became less important and thus was severely reduced. Even today many primates have only n=2 (S and L). They are able to distinguish brightness and colour but not saturation. After the extinction of the dinosaurs about 65 million years ago, n=3 had to be 'reinvented'. The third colour receptor type developed a comparatively short time ago. It came about as a consequence of the doubling of the corresponding L-gene with a subsequent mutation on one of the two sites into an M-gene. In humans, the M- and L-genes are located on the X-chromosome. This mutation is not quite stable; there are also functionless variants. For this reason about 8% of men (who only have *one* X-chromosome) have colour deficient vision (mostly n=2). On the other hand, there are many well functioning variants. In women, since they have two X-chromosomes, this gene doubling can lead to n=4, if the X-chromosomes have two different mutations of the L-gene.

With n=4, colours can be broken down into finer divisions, especially in the region of red. In discussions between men and women concerning a shade of red, (which supposedly happens on occasion), one must take into account the possibilities for men being n=2, and women n=4, apart from the usual n=3. It is probable that a mutation of the L-gene does not bring about a wider range of visibility (which remains one octave) but a higher ability to distinguish between colours (up to one octave). This yields additional rainbow colours from 650 nm on, which perhaps only differ slightly from the current constructed shades of magenta and purple. Once the colour circle closes to a *complete* octave, the complementary colours correspond to the *tritonal* colours. This altered view can be tested easily with a complementary colour test. Such individuals should see, for example, red and blue or yellow and violet as complementary colours, see (9.14a-d).

Table 9.1. Suggested colour assignment of those six points on the border of the disc that correspond to the Chinese elements

Point	V_e^+	K_e^-	P_e^+	V_e^-	K_e^+	P_e^-
α	180°	120°	60°	0°	300°	240°
Element	{Metal}	{Fire}	{Wood}	{Earth}	{Water}	{Flora}
Colour	Indigo	Cyan	Green	Yellow	Orange-red	Magenta

The points V_e^+, P_e^+, K_e^+ (with the angles of 180°, 60°, 300°) are now to be assigned symbolically to the three additive primary colours. There are six possibilities. The assignment chosen in Kratky (2000c, Ch.2) can be seen in Table 9.1. Concerning the assignment of *magenta* to {flora}, this element stands for birth and death, the most far apart events in a person's life. This corresponds to the short and long wave end of the visible spectrum of light, which we subjectively bend to form a colour circle. This fits in with the life cycle starting with birth and closing with death. Magenta's neighbour, indigo, now lies in *vata* or in *kapha*. The other colours result automatically. The choice of indigo in *vata* is inspired by TCM inasmuch as then the colours *yellow* of {earth} and *green* of {wood} agree with the present choice. Considering the primary colours in terms of the border of the disc does not nearly utilise all the possibilities. The two-dimensional expansion to the disc allows the inclusion of saturation, and a three-dimensional expansion to the cone allows that of brightness. As the visible light can be analysed according to the three additive primary colours, the relative portions of doshas A(V), A(P) and A(K), can be computed for every point on the disc. More will be said on this in Ch. 9.5.

9.4. Strengthening, Weakening, Harmonising

The proportions of the doshas, as they are usually regarded in Ayurveda, naturally do not say anything about the third dimension (z-axis). If, for example, kapha dominates, but the point is located near the tip of the cone, kapha is also weak, but the other doshas are even weaker. In order (partly) to counter-balance a relative excess of kapha, the options are to weaken kapha or strengthen vata and pitta. Which of the versions is optimal depends on the third dimension, i.e. on whether the regulatory principles are weak or strong as a whole. Strengthening and weakening is called *tonifying* and *sedating* in TCM (Ch. 7.1). There, too, both variants can be implemented to balance qi. Interestingly, TCM tends to tonify, while in Ayurveda the strong dosha is weakened, in general, or in Chinese terminology, sedated.

Here, the question arises as to whether tonifying (of a meridian) refers to strengthening the entire system or whether it signifies strengthening at the cost of other meridians and, on the whole, results in balancing the overall energy. The first case would imply that it *is* possible to climb up the cone again (temporarily) during the course of one's life. In the second case (pure redistribution), there would be no significant difference between the Chinese and the Ayurvedic approach. In any case, this merits further investigation.

We shall tackle this battery of questions concerning strengthening (tonifying) – weakening (sedating) – harmonising (creating eutony), with the aid of Figure 9.5. It is based on Figure 5.1, where we considered dose-dependent reverse effects (hormesis, Arndt-Schulz Law). This is also known in acupuncture: light needle stimuli activate (tonify), strong needle stimuli weaken (sedate). In Ch. 7.1, a third type was introduced: medium strong needle stimulation is harmonising (creating eutony). In Ch. 5.2, the latter was addressed in a different way. We spoke of a neutral needle stimulus, which occurs with stimulation of medium intensity and corresponds to going through the origin in Figure 5.1a. There, the organism reacts in the appropriate manner. A neutral stimulus, therefore, is not an absence of stimulus.

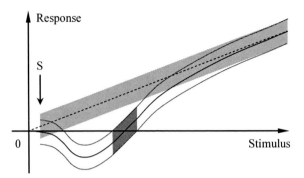

Figure 9.5. Linear and non-linear stimulus/response relationships. Around the specific effect, there is a region of nonspecific effect (grey strip), which takes place after a certain stimulus threshold S has been reached. The region of regulation at the zero crossing of the curve is indicated in dark grey.

These regulative effects cannot, however, be explained by Figure 5.1a alone – for this reason we have the expanded representation of Figure 9.5. Apart from the specific effect (linear and non-linear stimulus-response relationships), there is also a nonspecific effect, which is indicated by a grey strip around the specific effect. The organism has a certain bandwidth, through which it can react to the stimulus. The variation can go in both directions (up and down) and is – in our simple model – independent of the stimulus intensity, as soon as a threshold (minimal stimulus) is crossed. The dark grey area crossing the axis is particularly interesting. Here, the specific reaction is nil or very small such that the nonspecific reaction overcomes the specific one. For example, if in a patient suffering from high blood pressure, a medium strong stimulus is set (exactly at the zero crossing), the organism can change the blood pressure in the right direction with its own regulative ability. Further, away from the zero crossing, the specific effect establishes itself, and the stimulus intensity determines whether the blood pressure is raised or lowered.

This addresses self-organisation and organisation imposed by external forces again (see Ch. 5.2). There, we also talked about the importance of the alerting signal and the fact that it is not really crucial whether the organism is tonified or sedated. Similar considerations were discussed in Ch. 6.3 concerning two different settings for the Bioresonance device, in-phase and inverting feedback. According to Figure 9.5, the type of stimulus is not important only near the zero crossing, the regulative region. Other interesting consequences go beyond the scope of this chapter. We refer the reader to Ch. 12.3.

9.5.* Further Development
of the Geometric Model

We shall now supply some formulae that were left out of the main part of the previous chapter. We begin with the circle *representation*. The following hold:

$$x = r_c \cos\alpha = r_c \cos(\alpha - 0°), \quad \text{max. at } \alpha = 0°, \quad -r_c \le x \le r_c; \quad (9.16a)$$

$$y = r_c \sin\alpha = r_c \cos(\alpha - 90°), \quad \text{max. at } \alpha = 90°, \quad -r_c \le y \le r_c; \quad (9.16b)$$

Compare Figure 9.1a&b. x relates to yin and y to yang. In Kratky (2000b, Ch.2.3) values for *yin* (moisture ξ) and *yang* (temperature η) were defined on the circle. Now we get an equivalent representation in the variables v and w (instead of ξ and η):

$$v = 1 + p\,(\cos\alpha - 1), \quad 1 - 2p \le v \le 1, \qquad\qquad \text{max. at } \alpha = 0^\circ, \qquad (9.17a)$$

$$w = 1 + 3^{1/2}p\sin\alpha, \quad 1 - 3^{1/2}p \le w \le 1 + 3^{1/2}p, \ \text{max. at } \alpha = 90^\circ; \qquad (9.17b)$$

$$\text{with } v = 1 - p + p(r/r_c)x = 1 + p\xi, \qquad\qquad\qquad (9.17c)$$

$$\text{and } w = 1 + 3^{1/2}p(r/r_c)y = 1 + p\eta; \quad \text{parameter p: } 0 \le p \le 0.5. \qquad (9.17d)$$

This corresponds to an expansion of the Eqs. (9.4a-c). In the next step, we shall give a more exact version of (9.5a&b):

$$\Sigma = w + v = 2 - p + 2p*\cos(\alpha - 60^\circ), \quad \text{max. at } \alpha = 60^\circ; \qquad (9.18a)$$

$$\Delta = w - v = p + 2p*\cos(\alpha - 120^\circ), \quad \text{max. at } \alpha = 120^\circ; \qquad (9.18b)$$

Neutral values: $\Sigma = 2, \Delta = 0$; \qquad (of $v = w = 1$). \qquad\qquad\qquad (9.18c)

It should be noted that the variables Σ and Δ, utilised in Kratky (2000b), expressed the sum and difference of η and ξ, see (9.4c). Now Σ and Δ relate to v and w in an analogous manner, see (9.5a&b). We use the same symbols for the sake of simplicity. Conversion is easily done, if needed.

Table 9.2. Attribution of important points on the circle to yin (value v) and yang (w) for p = 0.4. Furthermore, sum $\Sigma = w + v$ and difference $\Delta = w - v$ are displayed together with measures of the strength of anabolism (v^2/Σ) and catabolism (vw/Σ). The centres of the doshas are displayed in bold type, which is also the case for the minimum, maximum and neutral values of the other columns

Point	α	v	w	Σ	Δ	v^2/Σ	vw/Σ
V_m^-	0°	**1.0**	**1.0**	**2.0**	**0.0**	**0.5**	**0.5**
P_m^+	**60°**	0.8	1.6	**2.4**	0.8	0.27 [d]	0.53 [d]
Y_m^+	**90°**	0.6	**1.69** [a]	2.29 [b]	1.09 [c]	0.16 [e]	0.44 [e]
K_m^-	120°	0.4	1.6	**2.0**	1.2	0.08	0.32
V_m^+	**180°**	**0.2**	**1.0**	1.2	0.8	0.03 [d]	0.17 [d]
P_m^-	240°	0.4	0.4	**0.8**	**0.0**	0.2	0.2
Y_m^-	270°	0.6	**0.31** [a]	0.91 [b]	−0.29 [c]	0.40 [e]	0.20 [e]
K_m^+	**300°**	0.8	0.4	1.2	−0.4	0.53 [d]	0.27 [d]
V_m^-	360°	**1.0**	**1.0**	**2.0**	**0.0**	**0.5**	**0.5**

[a] Exact values: $1.0 \pm 0.4*3^{1/2}$.
[b] Exact values: $1.6 \pm 0.4*3^{1/2}$.
[c] Exact values: $0.4 \pm 0.4*3^{1/2}$.

[d] 3.... and 6...., respectively (periodic).
[e] see v, w and Σ of the same row.
All other values are exactly displayed.

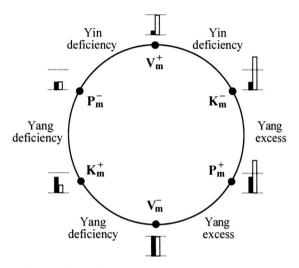

Figure 9.6. Yin and yang values of the six centres of the two-dosha regions (cf. Table 9.2 and Figure 9.4a). The values v for yin and w for yang are represented by the heights of the bars (black: yin, white: yang). The upper short dotted lines represent neutral (middle) yin and yang values and serve as reference lines. Where the bars are higher than these lines, there is excess; where they are lower, there is deficiency.

Table 9.2 lists the numerical values for those variables which are represented graphically in Figure 9.2 (p=0.4). The points on the circle in bold type and their angles α are located in the dosha *centres* and are therefore typical for the respective doshas – P_m^+: {wood}, V_m^+: {metal} and K_m^+: {water}. In Figure 9.6, the yin and yang values of the six Chinese elements on the circle are shown, characterised by the heights of the bars (black: yin, white: yang).

Now we move on to the *health disc*. First, let us look at a more precise version of (9.7a&b):

$$v = 1 + p(k\cos\alpha - 1), \quad 1 - (k+1)p \leq v \leq 1 + (k-1)p \; ; \; k = r/r_c; \tag{9.19a}$$

$$w = 1 + 3^{1/2}pk\sin\alpha, \quad 1 - 3^{1/2}pk \leq w \leq 1 + 3^{1/2}pk. \tag{9.19b}$$

This can be used to generalise (9.18a&b) to two dimensions:

$$\Sigma = w + v = 2 - p + 2pk*\cos(\alpha - 60°), \quad \text{max. at } \alpha = 60°, \; k = r/r_c. \tag{9.20a}$$

$$\Delta = w - v = p + 2pk*\cos(\alpha - 120°), \quad \text{max. at } \alpha = 120°. \tag{9.20b}$$

The trigonometric functions now contain the additional factor $k = r/r_c$. Now we tackle the optimal embedding of the circle coming from the circle representation (radius r_c) into the health disc (radius R). To do this, we shall first look at the centres of the doshas and their distance r from the point of origin (centre of the disc). From (9.21a) it follows k=(2/3)R. For the centres of the six Ayurvedic and Tibetan sectors, (9.8a&b), we also have k=(2/3)R. In the usual variant, where the three-dosha region (disc with radius R/4) represents its own seventh type, the remaining regions start with r=(1/4)R; cf. Figure 8.5. This increases the distance of the six centres from the point of origin from 0.667R to 0.7R, see (9.21b). The latter value is used for r_c.

$$\zeta=(r/R): \quad \int_0^1 \zeta^2 \, d\zeta \Big/ \int_0^1 \zeta \, d\zeta = \Big[(1/3)\,\zeta^3\Big]_0^1 \Big/ \Big[(1/2)\,\zeta^2\Big]_0^1 = 2/3 = \mathbf{0.667}. \qquad (9.21a)$$

$$\int_{1/4}^1 \zeta^2 \, d\zeta \Big/ \int_{1/4}^1 \zeta \, d\zeta = \Big[(1/3)\,\zeta^3\Big]_{1/4}^1 \Big/ \Big[(1/2)\,\zeta^2\Big]_{1/4}^1 = 7/10 = \mathbf{0.700}. \qquad (9.21b)$$

It should be pointed out that another choice of r_c would be the radius r_{M1} (radius of the median of the area). There, the disc of radius R is divided by a circle of radius r_{M1} into two equal areas:

$$[R^2 - (r_{M1})^2]\pi = (r_{M1})^2\,\pi, \qquad \text{thus } (r_{M1})/R = (1/2)^{0.5} = \mathbf{0.707}. \qquad (9.22a)$$

If not the *whole* disc is divided into two parts, but the three-dosha region with $r \le (1/4)R$ is excluded, then the radius of the median increases slightly:

$$[R^2 - (r_{M2})^2]\pi = [(r_{M2})^2 - (R/4)^2]\pi, \quad \text{thus } (r_{M2})/R = (17/32)^{0.5} = \mathbf{0.729}. \qquad (9.22b)$$

Thus, both solutions are comparable to (9.21a&b). For r_c we stick, however, to the value 0.7, (9.21b). – Now we move to the generalisation of the *health cone*. We start with a more detailed version of (9.13a&b):

$$v/z = 1 + p(k\cos\alpha - 1); \quad 1 - (k+1)p \le v/z \le 1 + (k-1)p, \qquad (9.23a)$$
$$w/z = 1 + 3^{1/2}pk\sin\alpha; \quad 1 - 3^{1/2}pk \le w/z \le 1 + 3^{1/2}pk \; ; \quad k = (r/r_c) = r/(0.7R). \qquad (9.23b)$$

From (9.18a&b), we get for Σ and Δ:

$$\Sigma = w + v = z\,[2 - p + 2pk*\cos(\alpha - 60°)]; \quad \text{max. at } \alpha = 60°, \qquad (9.24a)$$
$$\Delta = w - v = z\,[p + 2pk*\cos(\alpha - 120°)]; \quad \text{max. at } \alpha = 120°. \qquad (9.24b)$$

For the entire central axis of the cone (r=0), the following expansion of (9.7c) now holds:

$$r = 0: \quad x = y = 0; \quad v = z\,[1 - p], \quad w = z; \qquad \Sigma = z\,[2 - p], \quad \Delta = zp. \qquad (9.25)$$

Finally, we come to the calculations of the colour or dosha portions we discussed after Table 9.1. To do this, we shall look at a slice at a given height z (conic section). The variables r and α then are given by the following regions:

$$0 \le r \le R = z, \quad 0° \le \alpha \le 360° \; \text{ or } \; -180° \le \alpha \le 180°. \qquad (9.26)$$

The two equivalent intervals for the angle α we shall need later. The disc is composed of the following 'pie thirds' with the assignment of doshas (pitta P, vata V, kapha K):

P (around P_m^+): $\quad 0°\leq\alpha\leq 120°$, $\qquad$ V (around V_m^+): $120°\leq\alpha\leq 240°$,

K (around K_m^+): $240°\leq\alpha\leq 360°$; $\hfill$ (9.27)

Compare this with Figure 9.4a and Table 9.2. The angle α at the pitta/kapha boundary is set to $0°$ or $360°$, whichever is more suitable. Next we shall also need a division of the disc into thirds rotated $60°$, namely into the regions, P_{os}, V_{os}, K_{os} (in general: D_{os}), which are located on opposite sides of the doshas P, V, K (in general: D):

P_{os} (around P_m^-): $-180°\leq\alpha\leq -60°$, V_{os} (around V_m^-): $-60°\leq\alpha\leq 60°$,

K_{os} (around K_m^-): $\quad 60°\leq\alpha\leq 180°$; $\hfill$ (9.28)

Now the angle α at the boundary of P_{os} and V_{os} is set to $-180°$ and $180°$ as needed. (9.28) can now be reformulated:

$\alpha_{lo}\leq\alpha\leq\alpha_{up}$ ($\alpha_{up}-\alpha_{lo}=120°$): $\alpha_{lo}(P_{os}) = -180°$, $\alpha_{up}(K_{os}) = 180°$,

$\alpha_{lo}(V_{os}) = \alpha_{up}(P_{os}) = -60°$; $\quad \alpha_{lo}(K_{os}) = \alpha_{up}(V_{os}) = 60°$. $\hfill$ (9.29)

α_{lo} and α_{up} represent the lower and upper α-boundary of the respective D_{os}. They are the central angles of the doshas *bordering* on D_{os}, which will be called D_{lo} and D_{up} in the current context. Across from D_{os} we find D itself. Thus, for an arbitrary point (r, α) in D_{os}, the portions A_{lo}, A_{up}, A of the doshas D_{lo}, D_{up}, D result.

$A_{lo} = (1/3) - (r/R)/3 + (r/R)*(\alpha_{up}-\alpha)/120°$, $\hfill$ (9.30a)

$A_{up} = (1/3) - (r/R)/3 + (r/R)*(\alpha -\alpha_{lo})/120°$, $\hfill$ (9.30b)

$A = (1/3) - (r/R)/3$. $\hfill$ (9.30c)

The result is given here without proof. It is independent of z, if one considers r in relation to the maximal radius R=z. The sum of all portions automatically yields the correct value of 1, at the border of the disc (r=z), $\alpha=0$. For a concrete method of determining the portions, first determine in which of the thirds D_{os} the point is located and substitute this into the corresponding equation (9.30a-c). Thus, for a point in K-P, which must lie in V_{os}, we have: A(K) > A(P) > A(V). Let us look at a numerical example for r/R=2/3 and $\alpha=-30°$: the point lies in V_{os}, and therefore we have: $\alpha_{lo}=-60°$, $\alpha_{up}=60°$. This yields: $A_{lo}=A(K)=0.611$, $A_{up}=A(P)=0.278$, A=A(V)=0.111. A is the smallest of the three portions, more precisely: $0\leq A\leq 1/3$, see (9.30c). The larger A is, the less satiated is the corresponding colour. A=0 corresponds to a pure colour, A=1/3 at last results in white or grey (depending on the value of z).

Chapter 10

Western Type Assignments

10.1. Anthroposophical Considerations

Now our task is to interpret Western sources with the aid of the health disc. We shall begin with Anthroposophical medicine (see Fintelmann 2000, pp.40-61). This works with nested, fractal-like partitions of the organism into groups of three or four. For example, there is a partitioning of the body into four segments. This encompasses, in a wider sense, the whole organism but in a narrower sense is meant in terms of *material* or *physical* segments (and thus as part of the triad, body – mind – soul). If one considers the soul as a representative of the organism, a three-way partition results, namely in the form of the three *systems* or *functions* of the organism: the nervous-sensory, the metabolic-locomotor and the rhythmic system; see also Table 10.1 and Kratky (2002). The first two are polar principles and are connected or held in balance by the third principle. The wording in Fintelmann (2000, p.56) already suggests a (2+1) partitioning, where the rhythmic system (for example, respiration) plays the role of *vata*. Respiration is a rhythmic affair of inhalation and exhalation, where the former equates with taking *in* and is kapha-like, and the latter equates with going *out* and is pitta-like. Further characterisations such as unconscious/conscious and cold/heat lead to the dosha assignment given in Table 10.1.

It may seem astonishing that the nervous-sensory system is associated with *unconscious* processes. According to Anthroposophy, the natural way of thinking is the unconscious one, whereas conscious thinking eventually destroys the nerve tracts. It is presumably for this reason that the human being has such great need for sleep (deep sleep: kapha). Sleep allows regeneration and recuperation to such an extent that we are able to operate with waking consciousness during the day. Since we are usually *not aware* of our breathing but can bring it into *awareness*, this fits in well with the connecting ('semi-conscious') rhythmic system. There is an interesting cross-link, incidentally, from the partition into threes to the choice of homoeopathic *potencies* (see Table 10.1). According to Fintelmann (2000, pp.211f) the rhythmic system is again located in the *middle* with respect to this arrangement. The range of potencies for pitta still corresponds to strong chemical effects, that for kapha belongs to the higher potencies. In homoeopathy, acute diseases are often treated with *low* potencies, chronic diseases with *high* potencies. This in turn fits in with the statement in chapter 8.4 that pitta is characteristic for *acute* and kapha for *chronic* diseases. Incidentally, the correlation between Anthroposophical medicine and homoeopathy is something that is understood by Anthroposophical practitioners but is often not recognised by homoeopaths.

Considering the partition of the organism into four segments, one more column must be added which is located at the transition from kapha to pitta in Table 10.1. All in all, the four columns can be represented by coordinate axes (horizontal/ vertical). Accordingly, the characterisations of Table 10.1 can be found outside the disc in Figure 10.1. More information on this subject can be found in Kratky (2002). The Chinese elements are now located outside the disc as well. The location of the twelve meridians is specified on the disc in accordance with Figure 8.4. Taking all available data and selecting that information which is most typical for the four-part partition we get the assignment of meridians given in Table 10.1 and Figure 10.1. Consequently, a more precise position of the coordinate axes involves a slight rotation with respect to the horizontal and vertical axes. The resulting four sectors are marked grey and white in Figure 10.1.

To return to the three-part partition: the three systems of Anthroposophy are also assigned to different *ages*. The proportions of the *head* – which change during the course of a lifetime – reflect the life cycle from kapha via pitta to vata (Ch.8.4). This will serve as an example. According to Girke (1994) in a child the *upper* part of the head is more pronounced (corresponding to the nervous-sensory system), then the area around the *mouth* becomes more apparent (beginning of digestion, standing for metabolic-locomotor system) and finally the area around the *nose* comes to the fore (breathing: rhythmic system). In TCM (Table 7.3) smelling, connected to the nose, refers to {metal}, i.e. vata. In addition, it also stands for epidermis and thus for contact with the external world (compare the analogous Anthroposophical characterisation shown in the last column of Table 10.1). It is also about sensibility and sensitivity, typical vata characteristics. The body's reaction can be *insufficient* or it can *over*react, see (5.2). In the former case, we can expect a dynamic towards *kapha*, in the latter towards *pitta*. Fintelmann, incidentally, includes both possibilities in his terminology of allergy, where the *usual* allergy goes outward and is related to pitta. In the case of an *insufficient* reaction, on the other hand, the process continues *inward*, for example allowing parasites to enter the organism.

Table 10.1. Anthroposophical partitioning of the organism into groups of three or four. Comparison with other medicine systems

Organism	Substance	Life	Ego	Sensation
Characteristics	*Sclerosis, Auto-Aggressive Diseases*	*Tumour, Cancer*	*Inflammation, Outward Allergy*	*Contact: Allergies, Sensitivity*
State of Consciousness	Deep sleep	Sleep	Waking	Dream
Meridian	Kidney	Stomach	Small Intestine	Lung
Systems	Nervous-Sensory System	–	Metabolic-Locomotor System	Rhythmic System
Homoeopathic Potency	From D20 (20X) on	–	Up to D6 (6X)	D10-15 (10-15X)
Dosha	Kapha	Kapha/Pitta	Pitta	Vata

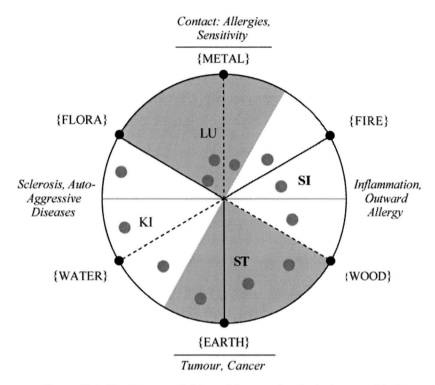

Figure 10.1. The four-part division of the organism in Anthroposophical medicine compared to TCM (cf. Figure 8.5).

As already mentioned, the Anthroposophical terms are nested in a self-similar fashion. Thus, the three systems are divided further into three aspects. This means dividing the thirds of the circle into thirds again (doshas, Figures 8.1 & 8.2). Each of these nine circular arcs now represents seven years of life, which starts at {flora} and continues counter-clockwise (Kratky 2002). After $9*7 = 63$ years the cycle is complete and according to Fintelmann (2000, p.51) life continues as a creative pause related to wisdom until death. In the sense of the disc representation, this path corresponds to the life spiral (Figure 8.5), where the final destination is SJ. The creative pause could relate to further steps in the three-dosha region, which does not appear in the circle representation.

Of these nine sections (circular arcs), the six near the dosha transitions correspond in reasonable approximation to meridians (e.g. SJ), the remaining three (those in the centre of a dosha) are located exactly between two meridians. Interestingly, at these sites polarities occur, according to Anthroposophy, marking important points in life (see Fintelmann 2000, pp.45, 53-55): in the kapha centre the polarity between *living* and *thinking*, in the pitta centre between *mind* and *heart*, in the vata centre between *past* and *future*. In addition, the *first* section in every dosha (counter-clockwise) seems to play a special role in this nesting, which closely corresponds to the meridians *PC, ST* and *HT*. For example, *PC* is in kapha, the realm of the body (see Figure 8.5). The first ninth corresponds to the material body, i.e. to the *physical* aspect of the body. Since zooming in from the third to the ninth does not change the aspect, one could speak of a fixed point (a counter example being *SP* as an *etheric body*).

Similar fixed points arise in *ST* with respect to the *soul* and in *HT* with respect to the *mind*. We shall come back to the 'constancy' of meridians in Ch. 11.4.

The first four ninths of the path of life (seven years each) are ordered as: material body, etheric body, astral (emotional) or soul body, ego-body. For this reason the sequence, deep sleep – sleep – dream – waking consciousness, is reflected in these four regions, which can be found on a greater scale on the entire circle (Table 10.1). The first three ninths still belong to *kapha*, the last already to *pitta* (at *ST*); parallel to this we also find the soul component 'emotional soul' (corresponding to the 'soul's soul' at *ST*, which has already been mentioned). The three-part and four-part partitioning overlap at this point. The Anthroposophical succession of states of consciousness from baby to young adult is interesting inasmuch as in this time period the frequency of brainwaves grows continuously as the duration of periods of sleep declines. Usually four ranges of frequencies are distinguished in the EEG. These frequencies are interlinked and depend on a person's age, degree of alertness, type and state of health; see Enne (2000 pp.70, 98-110, 146):

δ (below 4 Hz):	babies	Adult: deep sleep;	(10.1a)
ϑ (4-7 Hz):	children under 10 years	Adult: falling asleep, light sleep;	(10.1b)
α (8-13 Hz):	teenagers	Adult: relaxation, (day)dreams;	(10.1c)
β (over 13 Hz):	adults	Adult: eyes open, concentrating.	(10.1d)

1 Hz = 1 Hertz = 1 oscillation per second. When adulthood is reached first a slow shift from ϑ to β can be detected in the waking EEG. The waking state in an adult is characterised by β-waves but other frequencies depending on the degree of alertness also occur – which in turn fits in well with the Anthroposophical nomenclature. The resting EEG is usually dominated by α-waves but only in about 86% of adults (7%: β, 5%: ϑ). This brings to mind different types of individuals – for example expressed in terms of Chinese elements. The following connection results from (10.1a-d) and the life spiral (Figure 8.5), which links age to the Chinese elements:

$$\delta: \{Flora\}, \quad \vartheta: \{Water\}, \quad \alpha: \{Earth\}, \quad \beta: \{Wood\}. \tag{10.2}$$

β here represents the lower β-frequencies. According to this logic, {fire} and {metal} would correspond to even higher frequencies. In any case, the question of where the β-region ends is controversial at best in the literature. Assigning the various states of consciousness to the entire circle, Table 10.1, leaves the element *metal* related to the (day)dream (Table 10.1). From this perspective, we would expect α-frequencies for metal. This question must remain unanswered for now.

In conclusion, we should mention that in pathological cases, emotional situations and altered states of consciousness frequencies from the ϑ- and δ-regions are also possible. Rest and relaxation (α-waves) can already be viewed as light states of trance. These questions will be addressed again in Ch. 12.3. We should mention here that altered states of consciousness play an important role in ethnotherapy.

10.2. Dispositions

We shall now look at the so-called dispositions, a typology referring to the three germ layers, ecto-, meso- and endoderm. Incidentally, the denotation of the diatheses in homoe-opathy was based on this division (Dorcsi et al. 1991, p.162), even if this appears problematic upon closer inspection. The dispositions are based on research by Huter. They are also known by the name of psycho-physiognomy; see Aerni (2000). The following quotes (page numbers) are taken from an updated summary by Müller (2000). The author distinguishes three *primary* and three *secondary* dispositions, where the *secondary* dispositions represent transitions between the *primary* ones (pp.25-30). In addition, there are two *polar* dispositions sand-wiched in, which we shall discuss in more detail later. Müller's characterisation of types on pages 31-40 yields the following assignments to the primary types without difficulty:

Sensitive	disposition (ectoderm):	asthenic type/leptosome,	VATA;	(10.3a)
Movement	disposition (mesoderm):	athletic type,	PITTA;	(10.3b)
Nutritional	disposition (endoderm):	pyknic type,	KAPHA.	(10.3c)

Table 10.2a. Colour assignment of the *primary* dispositions (Müller 2000, p.41f). Compare the Chinese elements and the colour assignment suggested in Table 9.1 as well as the miasms (Gienow 2000)

Point	V_e^+	P_e^+	K_e^+
α	180°	60°	300°
Disposition	Sensitive	Movement	Nutritional
Colour	Yellow	Red	Blue
Element	{Metal}	{Wood}	{Water}
Colour	Indigo	Green	Orange-red
Miasm	Psora	Sycosis	Syphilis
Colour	Blue	Yellow	Red

Table 10.2b. Colour assignment of the *secondary* dispositions (Müller 2000, p.41f). Compare the Chinese elements and the colour assignment suggested in Table 9.1 as well as the miasms (Gienow 2000)

Point	K_e^-	V_e^-	P_e^-.
α	120°	0°	240°
Disposition	Sens.- Mov.	Mov.- Nutr.	Nutr.- Sens.
Colour	Orange	Violet	Green
Element	{Fire}	{Earth}	{Flora}
Colour	Cyan	Yellow	Magenta
Miasm	Tuberc. Miasm	Cancer Miasm	Parasitosis
Colour	Green	Orange	Violet

Comprehension again requires close examination of the individual words. According to Müller's description the nutritional disposition refers unambiguously to synthesis of substance (thus anabolism, KAPHA), not to energy production (catabolism, PITTA), which enables movement and expresses itself in the movement disposition. The sensitive disposition has to do with skin among other things, which fits in well with vata. Disregarding the two polar dispositions, a circle of six dispositions (three primary and three secondary) corresponding to the six Chinese elements can be formed. Indeed, Müller chooses a circle arrangement, e.g. on pp.41f. It also includes an assignment of dispositions to *colours*: the 'usual' colours yellow, red and blue as *subtractive* primary colours, orange, violet and green as the *additive* primary colours. In view of the difference from the colours displayed in (9.14a&b), this results in a slight deviation from the colour assignment of Table 9.1.

Disregarding these deviations one recognises that the two colour assignments are complementary to one another (see Table 10.1a&b). Müller justifies his choice based on the facial colours of the corresponding types, but he does concede the fact that they can only be recognised after lengthy practice. A yellow face colour means, for example, that the skin reflects yellow from the white daylight and accordingly absorbs the colour indigo. In this respect, there is a close connection. The colours of the miasms that can also be found in Table 10.2a&b will be discussed in Ch.12.4.

We shall return now to (10.3a-c) and discuss the obvious connection there between the dispositions and the germ layers, which play an important role in embryonic development. This is interesting inasmuch as the terms ecto-, meso- and endoderm refer to outer, middle and inner germ layer. The sequence from outer to inner corresponds exactly to the sequence vata, pitta, kapha (see the life spiral) – but a reverse order of inner to outer must be observed when comparing the body and the health disc (Ch.8.4). One point is still worth mentioning: the assignment regarding the head. The nervous system consists of ectoderm and is assigned to the sensitive type by Müller and thus in the end to vata. In Far Eastern medicine systems, this situation is different: in Ayurveda, the nervous system (actually the entire communication) is seen in vata, but the brain also has a place in kapha. In Tibetan medicine the head is the headquarters of kapha (Qusar & Sergent 1997, p.151), and in TCM, according to Porkert (1992, p.121), the brain and nervous system belong to the kidney meridian (i.e. kapha); see Ch.8.4. From this perspective, it is interesting that Müller makes an exception in germ layer assignment for the jaw and skull (but not for the brain and nervous system) on p.26: although they belong to the ectoderm, they are assigned to the nutritional disposition (i.e. kapha).

Table 10.3. The *polar* dispositions and their connection to their neighbouring dispositions as well as to the corresponding Chinese elements and trigrams

Disposition* polar	Mov.-Nutr. disharmon.		Mov.	Sens. harmon.		Nutr.-Sens.
Element Trigram	{Earth} Mountain	{Earth} 'Earth'	{Wood} Thunder	{Metal} Sea	{Metal} 'Heaven'	{Flora} Wind

* Abbreviations of dispositions as in Table 10.2b.

Now we can move on to the polar dispositions. They extend the six dispositions considered so far to eight (Müller 2000). From their position on the circle (see Table 8.3), the following connection can be deduced:

Harmonious   disposition (*white*) : V-K, ⟨ether⟩;   i.e. **SJ** or LU.   (10.4a)

Disharmonious disposition *(black)*: P-K, ⟨agni⟩;   i.e. **LR** or ST.   (10.4b)

In the circle representation, they are located on opposite sides. White and black, which do not fit in with the rainbow colours, already hint at an exceptional position. A similar case was examined in Kratky (2000a, Ch.3). There, an attempt was made to make them compatible with the six Chinese elements, in connection with the eight Chinese trigrams (see also Ch.7.2). Six trigrams were identified with the Chinese elements and arranged in a circle (horizontal plane). The remaining trigrams, 'heaven' and 'earth' were then drawn in above and below, respectively. The additional trigram, 'earth', means *in* or *under* the earth, which suggests associations with hell. Now the names *harmonious disposition* (white) for heaven and *disharmonious disposition* (black) for hell fit in with this interpretation. Since the disharmonious disposition is located in the region of the red movement disposition, we actually have a combination black – red, which again is reminiscent of devils or demonic figures. Incidentally, the expressions 'heaven' and 'harmonious disposition' suggest that this refers to sanjiao SJ, the union of all regions. Therefore, this meridian is bold in (10.4a). Accordingly, the Liver meridian LR, located at the opposite side, corresponds to the disharmonious disposition and is bold in (10.4b). In other words, SJ and LR are the best match for representatives of 'heaven' and 'earth' in the human realm.

In Kratky (2000a, Figure 3) an attempt was also made to fit the trigrams 'heaven' and 'earth', which lie in the third dimension, into a plane containing the six elements. The most sensible version turned out to be a circular arrangement corresponding to the so-called 'antemundane succession' by Fu Hi (Wilhelm 1973, p.247). This is how the extended circle representation finds its connection with ancient China. In addition, it turns out that this arrangement corresponds exactly to the one by Müller (2000). However, if we remain in the three dimensions, the health cone offers itself with 'heaven' as the centre of the base of the cone (top, white) and 'earth' as the tip of the cone (bottom, black). Projection onto the plane of the health disc, however, reveals by the 'colours' (white and black) that the two points located at opposite angles originate from somewhere else. This might have something to do with the special role of ⟨agni⟩, to which LR belongs – the Ayurvedic fire of digestion, usually not counted as an element. An analogous situation in the form of a mirror image arises in TCM with respect to SJ and {flora}.

Pitta, in whose region movement and disharmonious dispositions are located, is also characterised by dynamics, courage for risk-taking (risky sports), confrontation and anger. Pitta stands for midlife and in particular P-K, where LR is located, for young adult life. There the battle, the fullness of life, takes place; it is the generation that maintains both the older and the younger generation. There is no time for details, only for donkey work. Liver and life, incidentally, have a common ethnological root, which has to do with the word 'linger' (persist, survive). Related terms are: fat, salve, glue, paste, body (Kluge 2002). Over-defining pitta – more precisely: P-K, *LR* – leads to especially negative judgements. We shall come back to that in Ch. 14 in connection with Tibetan Buddhism. The positive side of SJ (in V-K) is, on the other hand, self-evident. Since SJ is located quite near the centre of the disc, it represents harmony – the doshas being represented in almost equal proportions. The colour assignment of the harmonious disposition (white) provides the best match (more precisely it should be a pale violet according to my colour interpretation – see Table 9.1).

A few more comments can be made about the poor image of the disharmonious disposition: Could one not just as easily see it as a 'poor devil', a scapegoat? The judging and hierarchical view, the proverbial thinking in black and white, the division into good and evil, are all part of perspective P1 (cf. Table 2.1). Harmony calls up visions of peace, disharmony visions of strife. Which is 'better'? The first term has to do more with statics (stagnancy), the second with dynamics (progress). Progress is a consequence of discontentment, 'something moves forward'. The fact that this progress is moving faster and faster is another matter altogether. The Tibetan types on the axis, {flora} – centre – {wood}, are called 'moon' – 'stillness' – 'clouds' (see Schwarz & Schweppe 1998, pp.81ff). Since SJ also belongs to ⟨ether⟩, which the Tibetans usually assign to the centre, SJ comes to rest somewhere between 'moon' and 'stillness'. The polarity of stillness and dynamics also plays a central role in Ayurveda; in particular, we refer the reader to the book 'Aufbruch zur Stille' ('Departure to Stillness', Bauhofer 1997). On p.47, the author describes the succession of dynamics (**R**) and arresting (**K**) with the aid of the central Vedic script, Rk Veda. All in all a pendulum motion results. Here, too, SJ fits in well as a pole of stillness. Since it is not located exactly in the centre, it still has some movement to it, which can then be amplified. It should be noted that the notation Rk Veda is not the norm; usually one talks about the Rigveda (Rg Veda), but this does not invalidate the argument of Bauhofer.

Of course, not only the pairs *content – discontent* and *stillness – dynamics* can be found but also the related pair *peace – war*. Assessment of these pairs is not as clear as it may seem at first. Heraclitos designated war to be the father of all things, and in the Old Testament we find the following in Ecclesiastes 3. 1-8:

> "To every thing there is a season, and a time to every purpose under the heaven: A time to be born and a time to die;... a time to break down, and a time to build up; … a time to keep silence, and a time to speak; A time to love, and a time to hate; a time of war, and a time of peace."

Here, the pairs of terms are placed side-by-side, without valuation. Instead of 'being blind in one eye', polarities are recognised as such. At this point, we might look at the position of the blacksmith – a manufacturer not just of horseshoes and ploughshares, but also of weapons. He used to enjoy a special position in many societies, where awe (fear!) and disdain for this profession walked a thin line. The dirty work in the dark (caves, coal) and at the same time in heat and light (fire) was somewhat eerie. Here, too, the colours black and red come together. Whenever a volcano erupted, the Ancient Greeks would attribute this to Hephaistos, god of the smiths, working too hard again. Other cultures relate the volcano to {wood}, ⟨agni⟩ and pitta as well. The Chinese trigram for {wood}, for example, is called 'thunder' (also described as 'thunder emanating from earth'), and in the Germanic tradition the volcano corresponds to the Indian ⟨agni⟩, 'damp fire': the fire below, which emanates from earth (red fire, black lava), whereas the Indian ⟨fire⟩ corresponds to 'fire above' (rays of the sun and lightning), see Kratky (2000c, Ch. 1.3). We shall come back to this in Ch. 14.3.

Now we come to a noteworthy idea put forward by Müller (2000, Ch. 3). He believes that certain therapies match certain dispositions, in multiple respects: the disposition of the inventor or discoverer of a new therapy method, for example, is related to its nature. This therapy, then, is especially beneficial for individuals of the same disposition. This allows the conclusion that therapies are also particularly beneficial to their discoverers, should they fall ill (or already were). Not only artistic but also therapeutic activity as self-therapy? From a homoeopathic perspective, this is not very remarkable, since there should be a resonance in any case. The same is true for finding the best match for therapist and patient, incidentally. You have probably heard again and again that patients select 'their' therapists.

A study by Schwarz (1998) revealed a comparable truth: Doctors are especially success-ful with their patients when they have the same concept of health and illness (Schwarz speaks of healing equivalency and lists ten concepts). This means it is more important to find the best match (P3) rather than, objectively, the best therapy. Freud and Jung, who subscribed to different concepts, were both successful, and their patients often confirmed their respective concepts. It appears there are patients of Freud and patients and Jung who found their respec-tive best match. This constitutes a problem for the evaluation of therapies. The psychotherapy scene in particular offers myriad therapies with varying theoretical backgrounds (see Feder-spiel & Lackinger Karger 1996). An exaggerated version might be where everyone invents his own self-therapy and markets it. If there are enough individuals of a similar type, this therapy, whatever it may be, can be beneficial in many cases. But how is it to be evaluated? A dispute about this topic including an evaluation of the evaluation can be found in Grawe et al. (1998) and Tschuschke et al. (2001).

In conclusion, let us look at some concrete information put forward by Müller regarding the primary and polar dispositions. Orthodox Western medicine is well suited to the disharmonious and the movement type (i.e. pitta) while homoeopathy, on the other hand, is better suited to the harmonious and sensitive type (i.e. vata). For the nutritional type, Müller especially recom-mends Kneipp and Priessnitz cures. These statements are also interesting for us in connection with the perspectives; see Ch. 7.2 and Kratky (2000c, Ch. 1.4):

a) {Wood} as representative of pitta stands for P1, i.e. Orthodox Western medicine, to which, according to Müller, the 'coarser types' are especially responsive. Further-more, according to Anthroposophical medicine, pitta corresponds to low homoeo-pathic potencies (see Table 10.1), where appreciable chemical effects occur. Here again we find a 'fractal logic'. Homoeopathy is suited to *vata*. If one applies homoe-opathy, however, to *pitta*, then should only use low potencies!

b) {Water} in the centre of kapha stands for P2, which suggests feedback therapies but also (auto-)regulative therapies. The cures that have been mentioned also have a direct relationship to actual water.

c) {Metal} as vata representative stands for P3, which also includes homoeopathy. This concerns the symbolic-analogous level ('simile': matching remedy and clinical pic-ture like the right and left hand). The motto of P3 is: 'on the one hand − on the other hand' (cf. Table 2.1). Moreover, healing prayers belong to this symbolic level, which Müller also recommends for the sensitive type.

An interesting comparison with these considerations is afforded by Gienow (2000), concerning the discrimination of therapeutic methods as well as the span of application of homoeopathy. We shall come back to that in Ch. 12.2-4.

10.3. Cybernetics: Types of Feedback Control

In our account of Western type assignments, we begin with cybernetics. It seems to have little to do with medicine but does allow a comparison to Ayurveda. Cybernetics, developed about 1940 by Norbert Wiener, deals with controlling and regulating organisms and machines. The two terms are not used consistently in literature. For our purposes, regulation is to be accompanied by feedback in order to distinguish it from control. Thus, *control* aims at P1, *regulation* (feedback control) at P2. Today there is also much talk about control technology or engineering. It is a relatively 'old' Western technology, in which P2 plays a role. Regulation shows a connection to the doshas, the Ayurvedic regulatory principles, with respect to name as well as to approach. Within the scope of cybernetics or control engineering, we find the most diverse applications. In the following we shall concern ourselves only with simple questions regarding this subject and look at steering a boat with its steering wheel. There are basically three approaches: the so-called integral, proportional and differential steering or control (I, P, D). This sounds complicated but can be easily explained, see the next paragraph. For those interested in mathematics, we recommend Busch (2002), among others.

The example I shall use to illustrate this comes from personal experience. I was holidaying in Corfu and joined a group excursion in a small boat, which was operated by one man. On the return trip, a strong wind sprang up, and the captain was hard pressed to fasten some items on the boat and instruct his passengers. I was standing by his side, when the wind grew much stronger, and he asked me to take over the wheel. To my dumbfounded question of how I needed to proceed, he instructed me to look back, keep an eye on the wake of the boat, and continue in the same direction. This 'reversed steering' turned out to be very effective. The wake wound around a straight line in the middle, which was the guiding line for me. It was, of course, only a straight line due to the previous expert manoeuvring by the captain.

The technique I was instructed to use was an integral control, which is robust, i.e. a layperson cannot do too much harm with it. The fluctuations of the past are summed up (integrated) to a target value, and the corresponding deviation is adjusted. This is a rather gentle process. If I had instead kept my eyes ahead and had aimed at the distant goal (a certain port), I would have probably ended up using proportional control: I would have steered against the boat, proportionally to its tangential deviation, which could have gone awry easily. The waves kept throwing the boat to and fro and I would have kept steering against this motion … With the aid of integral control I let the wind turn the boat this way and that and only reacted to more abiding deviations.

A differential control is even more sensitive: not the deviation from the direction but the actual change of direction counts in this case. That is to say, if the boat points in the right direction but turns to the side, the wheel is turned depending on the rotational velocity. Considering the angle of deviation from the desired direction as the main variable, we get: For I-control past angles are added up, for P-control the current angle is used, for D-control a reaction to future deviations, calculated (unconsciously) on the basis of current changes in angle, is implemented now.

I -control: taking the past into consideration: slow;   rough but robust.   (10.5a)

P-control: moment-to-moment reactions: medium; medium.   (10.5b)

D-control: anticipating the future: fast;   fine but unstable.   (10.5c)

PI-, PD-, ID- and PID-control systems, which combine the advantages of the various control techniques, are also available. Due to the characteristics concerning speed and stability, one suspects a strong similarity of I, P and D to *kapha*, *pitta* and *vata* (in that order). The mixed controls, then, correspond to the two-dosha types and the three-dosha type, respectively.

This will be substantiated by further observations. In terms of the path of life, a child (assigned to kapha) primarily abides by I-control. As has already been mentioned, this is also suitable for "laymen", and a child is, of course, still in training. Should it get into any danger due to lack of foresight (future aspect!) or react too slowly, then it is the task of adults to intervene and protect it from harm. At the onset of adulthood, a person has gained enough experience to make the transition to P-control. With growing experience, more and more foresight is possible, which then leads to D-control in older age. Without this anticipation, this type of control would be overly sensitive. However, due to the life spiral moving inward (Figure 8.5) only I-control is represented in a (virtually) pure form. P-control also incorporates I-components, D-control also I- and P-components. In the case of the Corfu example, I was not obliged to look ahead (in either sense) while steering since we were in the open sea and all I had to do was keep on course.

The types of control considered so far are linear, which is directly expressed in the name 'proportional controller' (for P-controller). I- and D-controllers are also linear or proportional but not to the deviation (e.g. of the angle of the boat) itself but to the integral over time or the change in deviation over time (differential quotient – see (4.1a-c)). More realistic than linear controllers are threshold value controllers, which do not react until a certain deviation (or its integral or differential quotient) has been reached. Vata reacts in this case as soon as its partner's behaviour changes rapidly beyond a certain degree. Pitta reacts to taunts and humiliation only once they have crossed a certain threshold. The 'cold-blooded' kapha, usually composed (or placid or stubborn as the case may be), swallows taunts and indignities for a long time until the sum of past insolent behaviour has crossed the critical threshold and one last straw breaks the camel's back. Kapha is a 'good' candidate for a person running amok who, before going berserk, was an unobtrusive, even exemplary and 'charming' person.

All this has brought us to the topic of processing stimuli, nutrients, etc. The three types of feedback control also differ in terms of input (intake), throughput (processing, transformation) and output (reaction, elimination). Input, throughput and output are always present, but the type of feedback control decides which of the three variables can be regulated. If we take eating as an example: An I-controller will eat something and only know after a while – by the reaction of the digestive tract – whether it is digestible. He 'listens to his body'. If the fare is inedible, it will be taken care of via a rigorous elimination process. A P-controller reacts immediately to the direct stimulus (e.g. the taste of the food) and adjusts digestion accordingly. He orients himself externally. A D-controller will spit out immediately what is inedible or, better yet, act with foresight and not put such food into his mouth. Once it has entered his system, it is virtually too late. Here experience and precaution are needed. A super-cautious person will only eat in good restaurants, food cooked by people he trusts or – as used to be customary for kings and important men – only after a taster has survived eating the food. Another possibility is that he eats that which he knows or suspects to be healthy.

There is an interesting psychological study by Pudel & Westenhöfer (2003) concerning eating behaviour, compare Mittwede (1998, Ch.10.3) as to Ayurveda. It shows that the importance of internal signals is highest in childhood (kapha) and then continuously decreases and that (pseudo) rational ideas become more and more important during the course of one's life and are dominant in old age (vata). External stimuli take on a role of medium importance and are maximal in midlife (pitta). Overall, we have the following sequences by analogy, with which we shall conclude our excursion into cybernetics:

D-controller: input-controller: vata,   anticipating or rationalising.   (10.6a)

P-controller: throughput-controller: pitta, reacting to external stimuli.   (10.6b)

I- controller: output-controller: kapha, reacting to internal stimuli.   (10.6c)

10.4. Psychology: Basic Feelings and Characters

Now we come to another subject area. In Western psychology and psychotherapy, there are many classifications of emotions, human types, etc. We shall select a few and begin with the *basic feelings* or emotions (Machleidt et al. 1989, Machleidt 1995). In his research, he discovered five basic feelings, which can be distinguished by EEG. Typical patterns of behaviour are also linked to these emotions. A brief characterisation is as follows:

a) curious / longing | cf. TCM: {Metal}: grief   (10.7a)

b) fearful / aloof | {Water}: fear   (10.7b)

c) belligerent / aggressive | {Wood}: anger   (10.7c)

d) sad / self-sacrificing | {Earth}: worry   (10.7d)

e) joyful / enthusiastic / manic | {Fire}: joy / mania   (10.7e)

A closer look at Machleidt's statements also reveals a close connection to the emotions in TCM linked to the five elements. Only {metal} and {earth} – again – require additional deliberations. Curiosity/ longing is not represented in this form in TCM; however in Ayurveda greed is attributed to vata, i.e. {metal}. We shall discuss this in more detail in Ch.14.1. Furthermore, the supplementary characterisation 'self-sacrificing' points to *earth*, which has to do with restoring and sacrifice. Longing on the other hand is more closely connected to potentiality. This is related to the polarity of the trigrams 'heaven' and 'earth' and also to Jewish and Germanic traditions, which we shall address in Ch. 14.2-3.

The first three basic feelings correspond to the dosha *centres*, the other two to the dosha *transitions*. At first glance {flora}, is not represented here. In Machleidt (1995, p.55), however, a remark can be found regarding a special form of fear reduction: not, as usual, by distancing but by merging – seemingly giving up distance and identity. This manner of speaking, however, belongs to P4 and we brought the symbiotic P4 in connection with {flora}, see (7.4). The psychological approach, where merging is a special form of fear reduction, is equivalent to the Tibetan view of {flora} belonging to [water]. Finally, there is also an advanced form of joy/ mania: liberation, being free (Machleidt 1995, p.89). This last step of development can easily be brought into connection with the three-dosha region in the centre of the health disc (Ch. 8.4) and/or the Tibetan type 'stillness' (Ch. 10.2) such that the seven Tibetan types are ultimately represented in the basic feelings.

Wilhelm Reich presents a typology of five *character structures*, which was extended by Lowen and then by Kurtz (Bäurle 1988, p.218). A sophisticated system of so-called body types came about, which get their names from related body-centred psychotherapy forms. Neither the term 'body type' nor the names of the types should confuse us; we shall again look behind the curtain. In the final analysis, it must (also) serve as a classification of 'normal' human beings. The five characters are – supplemented by a brief description (see Bäurle 1988, p.10):

1) Schizoid:	timid		cf. TCM:	SJ / {Flora}	(10.8a)
2) Oral:	powerless			*PC* / {Flora}	(10.8b)
3) Psychopath:	preten-	i) tyrannical / dominant		GB / {Wood}	(10.8c)
	tious	ii) seductive / manipulative		LR / {Wood}	(10.8d)
4) Masochist:	dis-	i) killer masochist		{Water}	(10.8e)
	couraged	ii) trapped masochist		{Earth}	(10.8f)
5) Rigid:	restless	i) phallic: achievement-oriented		{Fire}	(10.8g)
		ii) hysterical: noise-producing		{Metal}	(10.8h)

For a more precise discussion, we refer the reader to pp.25-125 of the afore-mentioned book. In the following, we shall present further statements from this book in quotes. Let us now look at the relationship to the circle representation (cf. Figure 8.1):

With reference to point 1)

"These are special individuals, whose favourite topic is death and who distinguish themselves by their spirituality." This immediately brings to mind {flora} (more *SJ* than *PC* because of the death theme).

With reference to point 2)

"The oral character wants to suck out energy – which was kept from him as a child". Since the natural oral phase is the first after birth, PC is a good match here. If this need was not satisfied at that time, a shift toward PC in the life spiral takes place and continues until this issue has been dealt with successfully.

With reference to point 3)

The description of the psychopath already shows signs of {wood}/pitta and forms, according to Bäurle, the *opposite pole to the oral character*. Indeed, {flora} and {wood} are located at opposite positions in the circle representation. In this respect the *tyrannical* version of the psychopath offers itself as the direct opposite pole to the oral character (poles: *dominant – powerless*) and thus is located at *GB*. The remaining pair, *timid – seductive,* is also a good match, which assigns *LR* to the *seductive* psychopath as the opposite pole to *SJ*.

With reference to point 4)

The characteristics of the masochist imply that he is to be found in the region {water} and {earth}. Furthermore, the corpulence described by Bäurle hints at kapha. The classification 'stubborn and phlegmatic' for the killer masochist points to the centre of kapha and thus to {water}, the melancholia of the 'trapped masochist' to {earth}.

With reference to point 5)

The restlessness of the rigid character already points to vata, more precisely to the Chinese elements that are still available, {metal} and {fire}. 'Spontaneity and the dazzling manner' of the hysteric then, point to {metal}, the 'energy and action' of the phallic type to {fire}.

In summary it can be said that the original five-fold scheme by Reich knew two separate types for {flora}, one for {wood} and one each for the combinations {water} and {earth}, as well as {fire} and {metal}. This also corresponds to the close relationship of the elements in the two pairs (Figure 8.4).

Chapter 11

Chronobiology and Chronomedicine

11.1. Daily and Annual Fluctuations from an Eastern Point of View

In the previous chapters, we have often talked about dynamic processes. We shall now address this in detail. The functions and processes of the organism are not always equal but are subject to a myriad changes and fluctuations: for example during the course of a day, year or life. Whenever it concerns the healthy organism, we speak of chronobiological processes. In addition, there are also reactions to stress and processes of falling ill and convalescence. Here, we need chronomedicine; time and dynamics need to be heeded. In practice, chrono-biology and chronomedicine are often used synonymously. In the West, this is a recent and often underestimated field. In the sense of Ch.2.2 (Table 2.1a&b) it belongs to perspective P2 (dynamic-systemic thinking), while orthodox Western medicine is at home in P1 (logical-systematic thinking). In the East, on the other hand, heeding cyclic processes in healthy and ill individuals has been a steady tradition for quite some time. In Ch.7.3, we have already met the Chinese *meridian clock*, which corresponds to the major energy cycle. This yields the following rhythm of the three circuits, six elements and twelve meridians (starting at 03:00 hours on the 24-hour clock):

Circuit	1		2		3		
Elements	**Metal – Earth**	–	**Fire – Water**	–	**Flora – Wood**		(11.1b)
Meridians	LU LI – ST SP	–	HT SI – BL KI	–	PC SJ – GB LR		(11.1c)
Time of day	03-07 07-11		11-15 15-19		19-23 23-03		(11.1d)
Doshas	*V V P K*		*V P K K*		*K V P P*		(11.1e)

At the indicated time, the energy flow in the corresponding meridian is at its maximum, and conversely, twelve hours later (time shift of half a day), it is at its minimum. In principle, this can be determined by pulse diagnosis. What is striking from the point of view of rhythms is that the physical-astronomical day from midnight to midnight is shifted by one eighth of a day (three hours) from 3 am to 3 am. Incidentally, this arrangement is supported by Western chronobiological research: according to Hildebrandt et al. (1998, pp.72ff) the day can be separated into two half days: a performance-oriented (ergotropic) period from 3 am to 3 pm (03:00 to 15:00) and a relaxing (trophotropic) period from 3 pm to 3 am (15:00 to 03:00). We shall come back to this in more detail in Ch. 11.2. One additional point is the introduction of *daylight saving time*. If an individual requires eight hours' sleep, he typically sleeps from 10 pm to 6 am or from 11 pm to 7 am. This means that the middle of the night is two or three hours *after* midnight for him. In many countries, daylight saving time partly counter-balances the resultant uneven distribution of daylight and thus tricks the individual's natural need.

In TCM, apart from a *daily* rhythm there is also a *seasonal* rhythm, which corresponds to the so-called *creation cycle* of the elements. There are, however, just as in Tibetan medicine, various versions depending on their origin (Kratky 2000b, Ch.1). There are four *core* seasons (elements starting with spring: wood, fire, metal, water) with a varying number of *transition* periods ('doyo'), which are often assigned to earth. As to the expression 'doyo', see Haas (1992, p.549), Kobau (1993, p.443) and Wenzel (1999, p.425). The progression of the seasons is also reflected in pulse diagnosis. The representation in Paik & Yoo (1979, Chs.XIII-XV), in particular, establishes a link to various severe diseases, which can be diagnosed from the deviations in normal seasonal pulses (significance of transition pulses). This is what has brought me in the end to assign the various seemingly contradictory versions of the TCM creation cycles and seasonal sequences to disease states of varying degrees of severity.

Wood,	Doyo,	**Fire,**	Doyo,	**Metal,**	Doyo,	**Water,**	Doyo	–	ideal, healthy;	(11.2a)
Wood,		Fire,	Doyo,	**Metal,**		**Water,**	Doyo	–	slightly ill;	(11.2b)
Wood,		Fire,	Doyo,	**Metal,**		**Water**		–	seriously ill;	(11.2c)
Wood,		Fire,		**Metal,**		**Water**		–	critically ill.	(11.2d)

(11.2a) is the oldest version of TCM, (b) an older version, which I, personally, prefer, (c) a version that is usually worked with today (five-element cycle); (d) does not appear, presumably because therapy at this stage is no longer possible. Due to the sequence of these versions, one could presume that people used to be healthier than they are today. Another interpretation consists of seeing the old TCM as more theoretical and oriented in ideals and the newer version as more practical and realistic. A more fitting interpretation is probably that by its self-conception TCM used to treat the healthy individual (prevention) and today tends to treat the ill person (therapy).

Let us now turn to the pulse of the six seasons as described by Paik & Yoo (1979, Ch. XV). This process takes place not according to the six elements (inner/ outer pairs of the meridians) but according to the bottom/ top pairs (see Table 7.2a-c). Since Paik & Yoo do not speak about pathogenic pulses, we must proceed on the assumption that they are describing a healthy person. A sequence results where three yang pairs are followed by three yin pairs, which correspond to the six divisions of the year of 60 days each. This can be seen in (11.3a-f), where the central month of the respective season is also specified (see Bialas 1998, p.53). The question is, which of the 12 meridians are meant here? For comparison: in TCM, an element is often equated with its yin meridian but other times both meridians are taken into consideration. In this case, it follows from the given information that the meridians in parentheses in (11.3a-c&f) will not come into play. This results in the following assignment of core seasons (in bold) and doyos:

1) March:	*Shaoyang*	*(Yang)*:	(SJ) **GB**		**Wood**	(11.3a)
2) May:	*Yangming*	*(Yang)*:	ST (LI)	Doyo: Earth		(11.3b)
3) July:	*Taiyang*	*(Yang)*:	**SI** (BL)		**Fire**	(11.3c)
4) Sept.:	*Taiyin*	*(Yin)*:	SP **LU**	Doyo: Earth	**Metal**	(11.3d)
5) Nov.:	*Shaoyin*	*(Yin)*:	HT **KI**	Doyo: Fire	**Water**	(11.3e)
6) January:	*Jueyin*	*(Yin)*:	PC (LR)	Doyo: Flora		(11.3f)

Earth represents the transition twice (ST, then SP) and *fire* (HT) and *flora* (PC) once each. All four transition meridians are, incidentally, transition elements in the sense of the circle representation (dosha transitions). For less severe diseases (11.2b), a six-element cycle with *earth* in late summer and *flora* in late winter remains, for more severe diseases (11.2c), only a five-element cycle with *earth* in late summer. As was the case for times of the day, the seasons are also shifted with respect to ours: the traditional Chinese year begins with spring, which means about mid-February there. This moves the four core seasons up by one half season compared to ours, but the year itself begins half a season *later* than ours one eighth of a year – compare the shift of one eighth of a day in the meridian clock). This is probably due to the fact that the physiological rhythms lag behind the physical-astronomical rhythms by an eighth of a period. This merits further investigation.

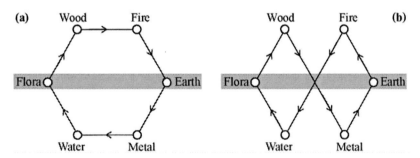

Figure 11.1. a) Succession of seasons of the six elements;
b) Daily progression: Chinese meridian clock.

Now we come to the comparison of yearly and daily progressions of the elements, Figure 11.1. For the purposes of immediate comparability, the six-element version of the yearly cycle was used (with *earth* in late summer and *flora* in late winter). The elements are arranged clockwise in their yearly progression (i.e. *differently* from the circle representation). This representation results automatically in an internal connection between earth and flora (cf. Granet 1993, p.236: sixth element as 'doubling of earth') : The grey strip in Figure 11.1a represents the earth's surface, wood and fire (yang) lie *above* it, metal and water (yin) *below*; metal is interpreted here as hard earth. Moving from water to wood corresponds to moving from the earth's surface *upwards*, from fire to metal *downwards*. Wood emanates from earth, which turns to ash through being burned by fire and falls back to earth. Kubiena (1995, p.51) alludes to both aspects of the earth's surface but does not differentiate by elements: *"The phase of earth lies in between, from which development in both directions is possible: transition to* yin *in the case of dissolution in the earth, or transition to* yang, *when new life is created by new germination!"* Flora could not be described more beautifully than in the last half sentence. The section of the year, 'late winter', which ends about mid-February, also fits in well: nature wakes up from 'hibernation', the first plants emerge from the snow.

For the meridian clock, Figure 11.1b, the same *arrangement* of elements was chosen as in Figure 11.1a; the difference in *succession* is denoted by the links with arrows. This results in an interesting connection between yearly and daily cycles, see (11.1d): the progression *water – flora – wood* is the same in both cases. Then the meridian clock flips to *metal* at 3 am (03:00) and proceeds in the opposite direction: *metal – earth – fire*, where at 3 am (15:00) the system flips back and everything begins anew.

What about the daily and yearly progressions in Ayurveda and Tibetan medicine? We shall limit our discussion to the 'dosha clock' for daily rhythms, since the literature is inconsistent with regard to yearly rhythms and, at times, explicitly points out that this depends on the climatic conditions (e.g. rainy seasons) of the respective region. So we return to the 'dosha clock'. In Ayurveda, the day is divided into six four-hour periods comparable to the elements in the Chinese meridian clock. The periods, however, are shifted forward by one hour. For example, the period assigned to pitta is 10 pm to 2 am (22:00 to 02:00) and not 11 pm to 3 am (23:00 to 03:00). Compare (11.1f), where the assignment of Chinese elements to the doshas is depicted for purpose of comparison. This shift, however, does not prevent a comparison. First, India as well as China are rather large countries and cover several time zones, and secondly these times were determined centuries or millennia ago (problem of local time). Furthermore, in temperate regions there are additional seasonal shifts of one hour in local times due to daylight saving time.

Time of day:	03-07	07-11	11-15	15-19	19-23	23-03	(11.4a)
Types according to TCM:	**V**	**P/K**	**V/P**	**K**	**K/V**	**P**	(11.4b)
Tibetan Medicine:	**V**	**K**	**P**	**K**	**V**	**P**	(11.4c)
Ayurveda:	**V**	**K**	**P**	**V**	**K**	**P**	(11.4d)

In the following, we stick to the Chinese partitioning of daytime, compare (11.1). The results of (11.1e) are summarised in (11.4b). For comparison, the statements of Tibetan medicine and of Ayurveda are shown in (11.4c) and (11.4d), respectively. Let us look at Tibetan medicine first (compare Qusar & Sergent 1997, pp. 65 & 228). The times where the dosha was clear from the perspective of TCM are now confirmed. At the transitions, the respective dosha, in bold type in (11.4b), is confirmed. Where it does not (seemingly) agree, the corresponding meridians (*ST, HT, PC*) are located at the boundaries of the 'correct' doshas. Now let us turn to Ayurveda, (11.4d), see Chopra (1993, pp. 244ff) and Schrott (1994, pp. 146ff). The doshas agree in four segments, in the other two vata and kapha are interchanged. This is an indication that the assignment in Ayurveda is probably not quite correct. This merits its own investigation. In Ayurveda, the daily progression in the circle representation corresponds, incidentally, to a constant counter – clockwise movement (V–K–

P–V–K–P). In Tibetan medicine, this is only true for the period from 3 am to 3 pm, after which it flips into a clockwise movement (K–V–P), which resembles, in one way, the daily change in TCM at 3 am and 3 pm (Figure 11.1a&b). This concludes our journey into Asia and we return to Europe.

11.2. Western Chronomedicine

The intertwined rhythms in the human organism are also observed and examined with growing interest in Western medicine. In this section, we will primarily refer to the compendium by Hildebrandt et al. (1998). In Chapters 1-2 of this book, the ultradian, circadian and infradian rhythms are distinguished (see Table 11.1). Temporal and spatial regions are connected here: the faster the rhythm, the more localised it is. Infradian rhythms often go beyond the individual (fertility and population rhythms). Another criterion for distinction is the autonomy of rhythms. Exogenous rhythms are produced by time indicators such as the sun or moon. They tend to be slow, whereas endogenous rhythms arise spontaneously ('the internal clock') and tend to be fast. A shift toward endogenous rhythms has developed during the course of evolution, i.e. autonomy has become more pronounced. Sometimes there is an interlinking of exogenous and endogenous control, for example in the rhythm of sleeping and waking. The interplay of various rhythms is also important. In this respect, simple number relationships are seen as beneficial (see further ahead regarding the pulse-respiration quotient). Rhythms arising as a reaction to stress stimuli are often also in whole-number relationships to the spontaneous rhythms. The internal coordination of the latter decreases, incidentally, with stress and increases again during periods of rest.

We shall now take a closer look at ultradian rhythms. These are primarily endogenous and concern functional units of the organism. They resemble the Indian regulatory principles in terms of their functions. In fact, Hildebrandt divides the ultradian rhythms into three groups: the information system, the metabolic system and the distribution system of respiration and circulation (see Table 11.2). Hildebrandt's classification is apparently oriented in Anthroposophy – a very similar three-fold grouping can be found there, see Ch.10.1 and Kratky (2002). The dosha assignment comes from there as well. Vata is represented again in all characteristics as a mixed and transitional form.

**Table 11.1. Fundamental division of biological rhythms
by Hildebrandt et al. (1998, pp.3-14)**

Rhythms	Ultradian	Circadian	Infradian
Period length Control	less than a day primarily endogenous	roughly one day endo- & exogenous	more than a day primarily exogenous
Region Examples	cells, organs circulation, secretion	organisms sleeping/waking rhythm	population population rhythms

In orthodox Western medicine, ultradian rhythms are also observed and utilised for diagnosis (electroencephalogram, electrocardiogram), but this is not usually considered to be a part of chronobiology or chronomedicine. Inclusion in these categories is only the case when the interconnections between rhythms and integration into slower rhythms are taken into consideration. A connection with the chaos approach can also be made (see Ch. 4.3 in particular). Glass & Mackey (1988) wrote a pioneering work regarding the connection between chaos research and biological rhythms. The authors talk, among other things, about dynamic diseases (i.e. disturbances in rhythms). This means that even though a relevant measured value is within the normal range, a severe illness cannot be ruled out as long as the dynamics of the measured value are not in order. A too regular (rigid) heartbeat, for example, is just as problematic as one which is too irregular (Morfill & Scheingraber 1991, Ch. II.4). Presumably, it depends on the right 'degree of chaos'. This naturally raises the question as to whether this is chaos in the mathematical sense. There is an on-going intensive discussion about if, and to what extent, coincidental processes play a role in brain function and the facets of the electroencephalogram; see Arhem et al. (2000) and Lehnertz et al. (2000). Of course, we always run the risk of attributing something we do not understand to coincidence. As a rule, one can distinguish deterministic chaos from stochastics, but the quality of physiological tests is in general not sufficient for this distinction. In conclusion, we shall mention a few books with this topic: West (1990), Herbert (1996), Aniscenko & Neiman (1998a&b) and Barbi & Chillemi (1999).

Now we come to a *chronobiological* perspective in a narrower sense. The ultradian rhythms also underlie circadian fluctuations, which in turn are influenced and 'distorted' by sleep, eating and work rhythms. Chronobiological examinations minimise these influences through regular (bed) rest and evenly distributed intake of food and fluids, for example (Hildebrandt et al. 1998, p.49). The upcoming page numbers refer to this book. There, the results of many different daily fluctuations refer in general to the period 3 am / 3 pm instead of midnight / noon. The reason for this is that many minima and maxima occur around 3 am and 3 pm. This shift of about three hours resembles the Chinese meridian clock, see above. The seasonal shifts mentioned there surface again in Hildebrandt's work, (p.63). These ubiquitous fluctuations further lead to the suggestion that we should replace the term *homoeostasis* with the term *homoeodynamics* (p.70).

Table 11.2. Ultradian rhythms in the human being: division into three groups (Hildebrandt et al. 1998, pp. 4 & 11) and assignment to the three systems (Anthroposophy) and doshas

Rhythms	Information System	Metabolic System	Distribution System – Respiration, Circulation*
Form	relaxation oscillation (spikes)	pendulum oscillation (sinus)	transitional form
Time behaviour	fast (0.001 s to 0.1 s)	slow (1 min to 24 h)	medium (0.1 s to 1 min)
Frequency	variable	stable	variable
Amplitudes	stable	variable	variable
Anthroposophy	nervous-sensory system	metabolic-locomotor system	rhythmic system
Doshas	kapha	pitta	vata

* Additional terminology: rhythmic systems of transport and distribution.

Table 11.3. Examples for physiological extrema at 3 am and 3 pm

Minimum/Maximum ca 3 am / 3 pm	Minimum/Maximum ca 3 pm / 3 am	Hildebrandt et al. (1998)
Body temperature: Head; torso (rectal)	Body temperature: Foot, hand	p.68f
Respiratory and pulse rates, systolic blood pressure	–	p.74-76
Muscle power	Capacity for continuous work; response time	p.88 & 94

Some concrete examples (see also Table 11.3) include respiratory and pulse rates as well as systolic blood pressure, which reach a minimum around 3 am and a maximum at 3 pm. The same is true for the temperature of the torso and head (as well as that taken rectally), in reverse time sequence for hands and feet. Analogously, muscle power and capacity for continuous work also run in opposite directions. The former reaches a maximum at 3 pm, the latter at 3 am. The time-of-day fluctuations are especially wide for temperature. The temperature measured at the feet (p.69) is even split into several extreme values: Instead of a maximum at 3 am there are two maxima at about 1 am and 6 am and the minimum at 3 pm is replaced by two minima at about 1 pm and 6 pm. From p.23, we can conclude that this can lead back to a difference in temperature progression for 'morning' and 'evening' people (for whom separate statistics should be produced). In 'morning people', the rectal temperature is lowest at about 1 am, in 'evening people' at about 6 am. Correspondingly, a morning type is unsuited to working night shifts (p.43) and an evening type has difficulty getting up early.

A related problem is 'jet lag', which occurs after one has flown over several time zones. As a rule of thumb, one requires one day of recuperation per hour of time difference, where a westward flight (subjectively staying up later) is easier to handle than an eastward flight. This presumably has something to do with the fact that our diurnal rhythm (measured in a bunker with steady lighting, see p.22) is about twenty-five hours, and thus our regulative capability is already adjusted to around one hour a day. In a westward flight, the shifts *subtract* (easement) while in an eastward flight they *add* (additional strain for regulation). TCM now offers utilisation of the meridian clock. According to Julia Tsuei (personal communication), massaging that meridian which is supposed to have its maximum at the new local time is especially helpful. This results in the meridian clock setting itself to the new time. As far as I know this 'obvious' possibility has not been officially tested but it would be a simple solution to a growing problem.

Our previous considerations inspire further comparisons of Western and Eastern chronobiology (see Table 11.4). The agreements (in part) cannot be overlooked. The last row clearly reveals possible falsifications through eating and sleeping habits: only when one insists that individuals do not eat and sleep at predetermined times, does the time of maximal urine elimination become apparent. Incidentally, we shall deal with the pulse-respiration quotient in some detail in Ch.11.3.

Now we shall look at the reaction to *external* stimuli. According to Hildebrandt this, too, fluctuates depending on the time of day. An individual is especially sensitive to cold stimuli in the morning and heat stimuli in the afternoon and evening (pp. 36f, 70f, 92-94). Maxima/ minima occur around 9 am and 9 pm and vice versa. Sensitivity to pain also varies but is a little more complex. Two protocols must be distinguished: the epicritic and protopathic (p. 57f). In the former, a stimulus is increased until a sensation of pain arises while in the latter, a defined continuous stimulus is set, and the time that elapses before the onset of pain is measured. The characteristics work in opposite directions: epicritic algesia (pain sensitivity) reaches its maximum around or after midday and its minimum around or after midnight, while in the protopathic case it is the other way around (pp. 92-5). At first, this seems paradoxical, but it also can be seen in the analogy of power and endurance, which run in opposite directions in their diurnal progressions (see Table 11.3).

Table 11.4. Comparison of meridian timetable according to the Chinese meridian clock with Western chronobiology (page references refer to Hildebrandt et al. 1998)

Meridian	Time	Occurring at the indicated time
Gallbladder	1 am – 3 am	p. 81: Minimal contraction of gallbladder after stimulation
Lung	3 am – 5 am	p. 77: Optimal pulse-respiration quotient PRQ
Large Intestine	5 am – 7 am	p. 81: Afterwards: maximal frequency of bowel movement
Stomach	7 am – 9 am	p. 81: Maximal basal pH value in the stomach
Heart	1 pm – 3 pm	p. 74: Maximal pulse rate and systolic blood pressure
Kidney / Bladder	3 pm – 7 pm	p. 83: Maximal urine elimination

Not only sensitivity to pain but also the reaction to pain medication fluctuates according to the time of day. The effect of such medications as well as general and local anaesthesia reaches its maximum at 3 pm (p. 36f). The duration of effect of a defined local anaesthesia around the jaw depends heavily on the time of injection: four and a half hours for an injection around 2 pm or two hours at 6 pm (p. 95). Even the placebo effect fluctuates with the diurnal rhythm and reaches a maximum in the afternoon. At that time, the placebo component of a common pain medication is also the highest (pp. 93 & 95). Overall, there is a wealth of good evidence regarding chronomedical facts (see also Geyer & Stacher 1992). Unfortunately, these discoveries are not much heeded, especially with regard to optimising the effect of medications by administering them at the appropriate time. This is the field of chronopharmacology; see Redfern & Lemmer (1998), Lemmer (1996 & 2004) and Touitou (1998). For medications that are taken only once in a 24-hour period, a simple way of ensuring that the lowest possible dosage is taken would be to administer them at the time when their effect is greatest. Naturally, the diurnal progression of side effects and the placebo effect should also be taken into consideration.

This leads us briefly to the altered dynamics of the organism when subjected to strain or during illness (more on this in Ch. 11.4). Diseases often exhibit a rhythm as well, but this differs from the spontaneous rhythms. These internal dynamics correspond to natural healing progressions in diseases. We can deduce from this that recovery often takes its time, and for this reason, periods of rest and convalescence should not be curtailed. Strong medications can be used to circumvent this need for time in the short run, but the question is how does this affect the organism in the long run? In this context it is worth mentioning that in the typical 'modern' chronic diseases (cancer, diabetes), the time structure is only weakly pronounced. There is no definite beginning and no tendency toward self-healing (p. 33 in Hildebrandt). Personally, I believe that it would be worth trying to implement strong external time indicators in cases of chronic diseases in order to aid the organism to regain a natural chronobiological order.

11.3. The Breath and the Pulse

An especially interesting parameter is the pulse-respiration quotient PRQ, the number of heartbeats per breath. The PRQ shows strong inter-individual diversification during the day (from ca 2.5 up to 7), while between 3 am and 6 am it is generally close to its optimal functional-economic value of 4 (pp. 5, 42, 76f). According to the Chinese meridian clock, *metal* is especially active during this time and, in particular, the *Lung* meridian LU from 3 am to 5 am; see (11.1b-d). Hildebrandt investigated the diurnal progression of the PRQ in a trial combining test subjects into five groups (see our Figure 11.2). These groups brought the following median values for the period from 9 am to 9 pm (in the waking state):

Five PRQ groups: PRQ $\approx$ 2.8, $\approx$ 3.3; $\approx$ 4.3; $\approx$ 5.3, $\approx$ 6.3.   (11.5)

A comparison with Ayurveda and Tibetan medicine is interesting here (see Ch. 8.1). In Sachs (1997, p. 37), the PRQ was stated for the three doshas, see Ch. 8.7, where the typical Chinese elements (in parentheses) for the respective dosha can also be found:

Kapha (water):	PRQ below 4,
Pitta (wood):	PRQ approaching 7,
Vata (metal):	PRQ from 5 to 6. (11.6)

On average we expect a PRQ of 5-6; see Qusar & Sergent (1997, p. 182). In Kratky (2000b, Table 6), a formula giving the PRQ as a function of the position on the circle can be found. On the disc, the following simplified formula results:

$$PRQ = 5.25 + 3.2\ r\ \cos(\alpha - \alpha_{SI}),\ \alpha_{SI} = 105°.$$ (11.7)

r denotes the distance from the centre (boundary: r=1) and α the angle (starting from earth, counter-clockwise); see Figure 9.1b. The Small Intestine meridian has $\alpha = 105°$. Referencing the angle to this meridian results in the highest agreement with the information given in the literature. The PRQ estimates resulting from the localisation of the meridians (Figure 8.4) are given in Table 11. 5.

PRQ

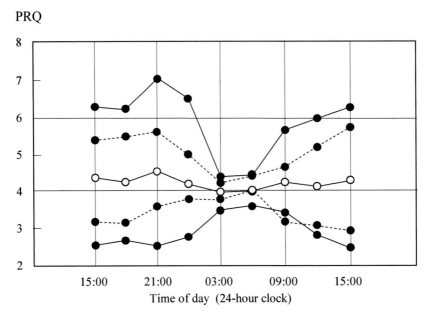

Figure 11.2. Pulse-respiration quotient (PRQ) of a total of 89 healthy test subjects, divided into five groups based on the 24-hour median value of the quotient. Modelled after Hildebrandt et al. (1998, Figure 46).

**Table 11.5. The pulse-respiration quotient (PRQ)
for meridians according to (11.7) and Figure 8.4**

Dosha	KAPHA				PITTA				VATA			
Meridian	PC	KI	BL	SP	ST	LR	GB	SI	HT	LI	LU	SJ
PRQ	3.0	2.7	3.3	4.0	5.3	6.4	6.7	6.7	6.4	5.7	5.3	4.9

Due to the reference value of α_{SI} the meridian axes, $KI - SI$ and the axis $ST - LU$ perpendicular to it enjoy an exceptional position. In the latter the PRQ value of 5.25 results automatically for both meridians, cf. (11.7). To the right of the axis $ST - LU$ the PRQ is *greater* than, to the left less than 5.25. The PRQ minimum of 2.7 occurs at KI, the maximum of 6.7 at GB and SI. Whole numbers or nearly whole numbers occur for PC (3.0), ST (4.0) and SJ (4.9) – twice for flora and once for earth. The especially beneficial PRQ of 4.0 (Hildebrandt et al. 1998, pp.25, 42 & 76) occurs at *earth* (SP, again 'in the middle' in a certain sense); at *flora* the median value of the two meridians is also 4.0. Comparing this with Figure 11.2 or (11.5), we get the following results for the grouping there:

PRQ $\approx 2.8, 3.3$: *PC, KI, BL;* ≈ 4.3: *SP, SJ;*

           ≈ 5.3: *ST, LU, LI;* ≈ 6.3: *LR, GB, SI, HT.*   (11.8)

The relationship between respiration and pulse not only demonstrates itself in the PRQ but also in a remarkable linking (p.110f in Hildebrandt), showing a preference to inhalation during certain phases of the heartbeat. This linking is easily disturbed and more noticeable during phases of recuperation. People in a state of relaxed introspection also demonstrate processes of synchronisation between electroencephalogram and heartbeat (see Song et al. 1998). This kind of linking could present a way to investigate more closely those phenomena, which are sometimes reported by meditating groups: the participants allegedly are linked to each other with regard to respiration, heartbeat and even brainwaves. Presumably, collective breathing is the starting point that leads to the linked heartbeat and electroencephalogram. Returning to Hildebrandt, another interesting phenomenon is the rhythmic alternation of sides in breathing through the nose. While lying on your side or with rhinitis you have probably been aware at times of only breathing through one nostril. In healthy individuals, too, there is one 'dominating' nostril and it alternates about every four hours. This can be tested by placing a piece of plexiglass horizontally under one's nose: the dominating nostril leaves a longer trace of moisture. There are big differences between individuals, but the diurnal rhythm in a single person remains unchanged over more than a week (pp.98-100). The discussion includes the possibility of this spontaneous breathing through alternating nostrils being connected to the side-specific changes of cerebral activity (pp.92). Compare this to the discussion of right and left brain activity.

Here we find a connection to the Indian tradition. In yoga as well as in Ayurveda, pranayama, directing energy with breathing techniques, plays an important role (Maheshwarananda 2000, pp.16-31; Chopra 1993, pp.346-350). Chopra describes the exercise of alternating nostril breathing, where with the aid of the thumb pressed on the ala of the nose the individual alternates inhalation and exhalation on the left and then right side. The goal of this exercise is to interlink the right and left sides of the brain. The relative duration of inhalation and exhalation as well as the two pauses in between are also important (Tatzky et al. 1995, pp.79ff). There are three rhythms: the calming, the stimulating and the stabilising, which recall the sedating, tonifying and neutral (creating eutony, harmonising) setting of acupuncture needles, respectively (see Ch.9.4 toward the end). The quoted site from the book by Tatzky et al. is also reminiscent of TCM in other ways, such as the pauses between breaths in repletion (when the lungs are full after inhalation) and in vacuity (when they are empty after exhalation). The examples given there reveal the following pattern:

$$\text{Rep:Vac} = 1{:}1 \text{ calming, } 4{:}1 \text{ stimulating, } 2{:}1 \text{ stabilising,} \qquad (11.9)$$

where Rep and Vac denote the pauses in repletion and vacuity, respectively. Here, again, we see simple number relationships.

In conclusion, we should mention one generalisation of the PRQ, the so-called *autonomous* or *autochronic* image (Moser et al. 1999&2008, von Bonin et al. 2001). In this process the heart rate is analysed in the region of 0-0.5 Hz (heartbeat: ca 1 Hz); correlations of heartbeat and respiration at ca 0.25 Hz and fluctuations in blood pressure (ca 0.10 Hz) appear in the image as maxima. The higher frequency components are dominated by the parasympathetic, the lower by the sympathetic nervous system. In healthy individuals, the average maximum during sleep is about 0.25 Hz. The autonomous image offers the possibility of a progression control after therapeutic interventions, e.g. with cancer patients; see Moser et al. (1999). Furthermore, the positive effect of therapeutic speech (rhythmic speech) on the variability of heart rate can be tested (von Bonin et al. 2001). This has opened a way for testing Anthroposophical approaches (as, for example, in curative eurhythmy).

11.4. Cross-Cultural Dynamics of Illness

Apart from the given human types and the long-term additional changes during the course of a lifetime (Ch. 8.4), there are also diurnal and seasonal fluctuations (see Ch. 11.1-2). Moreover, there are processes that result as reactions to internal or external stimuli and serve to maintain a state of health or accompany illness progression. We have mentioned this in passing many times and now we shall delve into it. Health as balance is mirrored in the suitable change of location on the health disc. If flexibility is impaired for whatever reason, it can serve as a trigger for illness. Within the frame of the circle representation, in Kratky (2000b, Ch. 3) the assumption was stated and also justified that crossing the boundary vata/ kapha (at flora) is in general not possible or only with great difficulty. In certain situations, however, this might be necessary in order to maintain health. A thick line denotes this presumed difficult transition in the *disc* representation (Figure 8.4). It corresponds to a divergence of the spiral, a region characterised as 'abyss' and 'beyond' in Ch. 8.4.

If one assumes falling ill to be a typical journey along the spiral moving out towards flora, then, according to Hering's Law, recovery would mean a reversal, i.e. moving inward from kapha to vata. The longer the duration of the illness, the longer is the process of convalescence. Crossing the boundary directly at flora, however, would open a shorter path of healing. Indeed, exceptional cases of spontaneous or miraculous healing have been reported, where a patient suffering from a life-threatening illness, instead of dying, has rapidly recovered. References to this can be found in ethnomedicine, where reports are made of special forms of healing in trance or altered states of consciousness; see Kratky (2000b, Ch. 3). The (symbolic) death and rebirth phenomena described in this field could refer to crossing this special boundary, especially since flora is, in any case, connected to birth and death. The decisive electroencephalogram rhythms here are presumably the δ-waves, see (10.1a).

Table 11.6. The six stages of illness in TCM and Ayurveda

Stage	TCM			Ayurveda	
	F/H Pair [a]	Meridian [a]	Characteristic	Morrison [b]	Chopra [c]
1	*Taiyang*	SI	hot, outer	Accumulation	Accumulation
2	*Yangming*	LI	hot, outer	Start	Aggravation
3	*Shaoyang*	GB	mixed	Overflow	Dispersion
4	*Taiyin*	SP	cold, inner	Establishing	Localisation
5	*Shaoyin*	KI	cold, inner	Onset	Manifestation
6	*Jueyin*	LR	mixed	Developments	Onset

[a] Foot/ hand pair of meridians.
[b] Morrison (1995, pp.68-72), see Table 7.2a-b & Figure 7.5.
[c] Chopra (1993, pp.115-118).

Now let us look at a typical illness progression as described in detail in TCM (Table 11.6). Originally it referred to diseases induced by cold and was later generalised to include all external causes (Focks & Hillenbrand 1997, p.431). It involves six *stages* or *layers*, which are described in terms of *bottom/ top pairs* instead of elements (Kaptchuk 1996, pp.292ff). The idea here again is that illness progresses from the outside in. For this reason, the three pairs of *outer* meridians (yang) are listed first, followed by the three pairs of *inner* meridians (yin), see Table 7.2a-c and (11.3a-f). Now, the meridians of a bottom/ top pair are practically on opposite sides in the circle representation (Figure 11.3). Proceeding from this and with the aid of information from the literature, *that* meridian which plays the larger role was determined for the respective pair, (Table 11.6). Since, according to Kaptchuk, stages 1 and 2 are connected to *heat* (fever) and stages 3 and 4 to cold, these stages are assigned to those meridians of bottom/ top pairs located on the respective sides of the horizontal temperature axis (Figure 8.1). So, for example, for the 1st stage, *taiyang*, *SI* and not BL was chosen and for the 5th stage, shaoyin, *KI* and not HT. This fits in with the type associations given by Terrades (1996, pp.48-52) of taiyang being *fire-* and shaoyin being *water*-dominated (i.e. SI and KI, respectively). Kaptchuk (1996, p.294) describes the 4th stage as deficient spleen yang (*SP*), the 5th as deficient yang, especially kidney (*KI*). Two meridians lying in kapha are then ascribed to yang deficiency, which is consistent with kapha as yang deficiency (Figure 7.4). In this context, *SP* is confirmed for the 4th stage and *KI* for the 5th.

Such concrete evidence is not available for stages 2, 3 and 6. Because of the assumption that an illness first stays in the region of vata (supported by Ayurveda and homoeopathy), the second stage is assigned to *LI* and not ST (Table 11.6). The remaining stages 3 and 6 are special cases. According to Kaptchuk, they are neither clearly outer nor inner but *mixed*. In the 3rd stage, heat and cold alternate in *time*, in the 6th stage in *location* (depending on the body part). For this information, apart from the references which have already been mentioned, Maciocia (1994, p.391f) was also consulted. This 'mix' in stage 3 is logical, since the 2nd and 4th stages are a transition from outer to inner and from hot to cold. That the 6th stage is a mixed stage as well points to the fact that the cycle can be closed after this succession (and begin again with the first stage). Indeed, both cases are mentioned in TCM:

a) An illness getting more and more severe finally gets stuck in stage 6
    (usual viewpoint).   (11.10a)

b) Where the illness progresses further, the cycle repeats itself
    (Kaptchuk 1996, pp.298).   (11.10b)

In Kratky (2000b), both meridians were left in stages 3 and 6. Now we want to go a step further and choose one meridian from the corresponding pair. The fact that they are located *half outside* and *half inside* in both stages speaks against the flora meridians: according to the life spiral, *SJ* is the innermost and *PC* the outermost meridian (Figure 8.4); for this reason the choice of GB and LR. In the 6th stage the mixed temperature also speaks clearly against the meridian PC, which according to the disc representation is always cold. Furthermore, Focks & Hillenbrand (1997, p.437) suggest that there is a need to 'regulate the liver' in the 6th stage. All in all, this confirms the choice for LR for this stage. However, one thing is still unresolved: why are GB (3rd stage) and LR (6th) not obviously hot? We shall come back to this in

Ch. 13. At this point, we merely want to mention that the indicated succession of stages is the one usually referred to and that deviations from this do occur (Kaptchuk 1996, p. 292).

Let us look at the succession of meridians *graphically*; see the 6-cycle ('illness dynamics I') of Figure 11.3. Falling ill starts at *SI (fire*, pitta at the boundary to vata) and progresses toward *LI* (metal, vata), see the direction of the arrows. Then it moves to *GB* (wood, pitta), continues to *SP* (earth, kapha at the boundary to pitta), *KI* (water, kapha) and finally to *LR* (wood, pitta). There, the succession is either completed or the whole cycle starts again (dashed line from stage 6 to stage 1). This, however, is a simplified representation with the assumption that the locations of the meridians remain the same. Due to the increase of the severity of the illness, one must rather assume that these locations keep moving closer and closer to the boundary. However, since there is no quantitative model for this available at this time, the cycle was drawn as *closed* in itself.

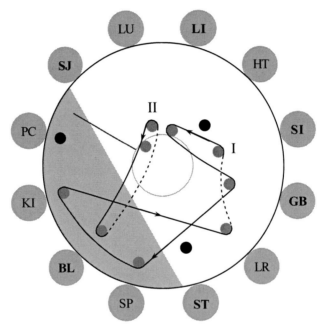

Figure 11.3. Health disc with illness dynamics I and II depicting the integration of the TCM meridians into the dynamics of falling ill and recovering (in the direction of the arrows and in the opposite direction, respectively). Dynamics I and II of falling ill start at SI and LU, respectively (marked I and II), then move in the direction of the arrows. Meridians not involved in any dynamics are marked in black (PC, ST, HT). The dashed curves indicate the closure of the cycle. The vagotonic grey region was taken from Figure 9.4.

In Ayurveda, too, there is a six-stage model of illness – in two variants, which deviate slightly from one another (Table 11.6). This, again, is about a *typical* illness progression; the terms used are characteristics of the doshas or the illness. The approaches of these two medicine systems are now identified on a trial basis. The 1st Ayurvedic stage, 'accumulation' (of the dosha), points to the condition moving towards the illness, one must assume that these locations keep moving closer and closer to the boundary of the disc and thus triggering the subsequent dynamics ('aggravation' as the 2nd stage). This moving outward was not depicted in Figure 11.3 – as has already been mentioned. The 3rd stage, 'overflow' or 'dispersion', fits in well with toppling from vata to pitta. Stages 4 and 5 correspond to localisation and manifestation in kapha. The expression 'developments' mirrors the jump to pitta, where the illness really breaks out, according to Chopra (for Morrison this is already the case in the 5th stage).

There are similarities, then, between Ayurveda and TCM. A crucial difference, however, stands out: in TCM, the first stage is already connected with fever, and therefore the illness has already emerged. This discrepancy can be reconciled by the assumption that there is *indeed* more than one illness cycle in dynamics I. The six stages of Ayurveda refer to the *origin* of illness, TCM to the subsequent cycle of illness *progression*. From this perspective, Ayurveda would be 'finer' and more geared towards prevention than TCM. This might correspond to the difference concerning the site of pulse diagnosis; see Chs.7.3 and 8.1, after (8.4a-c). Furthermore, the meridians and acupuncture points are measurable in a certain sense, according to Ch.7.4, but the Indian counterparts (nadis or channels of Ayurveda, and chakras in yoga traditions) are not.

The six-stage progressions of TCM and Ayurveda can thus be reconciled, if they are true cycles, see (11.10b). This opens up another possibility, which is emphasised again and again in TCM and Ayurveda: the progressions described there are *typical* progressions but are not the only ones. In the case of cycles, the illness can 'spring up' at certain sites in the cycle (onset of illness). It then continues in the direction of the arrows while it continues to increase in severity. In this case, too, Figure 11.3 offers a good guideline to the dynamics to be expected. It should be noted that, according to Kaptchuk (1996, p.298), every stage lasts one day. The connection between the six stages and the bottom/ top pairs by the same name was not established until about 1100 A.D.

As a final point, a comparison with the seasonal progression is interesting (11.3a-f). In the stages 1-3, the two cycles move in opposite sequence, whereas stages 4-6 correspond to each other (taiyin – shaoyin – jueyin, cf. Table 11.6). This resembles an analogous phenomenon regarding the inner/ outer pairs (elements) in comparison to the progression of seasons and the meridian clock (Figure 11.1); there, the *second* half of the elements moves in the opposite direction.

Hildebrandt et al. (1998) also emphasise the interplay of various rhythms and mention the fact that in reactive dynamics (processes of falling ill and recovering) a rhythm emerges which is not found in healthy physiological rhythms: the circaseptan periodicity, i.e. a weekly rhythm (p.32f, pp.113ff). This circaseptan reaction periodicity often appears in self-healing processes, even when accompanied by therapeutic measures. Fever progressions in scarlet fever, for example, show a slow normalisation, which is accompanied by smaller and smaller but noticeable fever spikes on the 7th, 14th and 21st, ... day after the initial outbreak. A similar situation holds for rejection reactions after a kidney transplant and for progressions during a stay in a sanatorium over several weeks. At the days mentioned above (after beginning of treatment), critical extreme digressions occur, which slowly wane until the patient is healthy again. This is especially apparent in sleep disorders and acute tooth abscesses. Circaseptan aggravations are, incidentally, an indication of a good cure progression – despite the fact that they are troublesome.

These statements can be easily interpreted within the frame of the TCM cycle of the *six* stages (during recovery in the *opposite* direction of the arrows). In traversing the complete cycle, one keeps returning to the 'same' point. It even fits in well with the *week*: if, according to Kaptchuk, every stage lasts one day, then after six days a full cycle has been traversed. If we assume that the step that starts the next cycle is a particular healing crisis and requires an extra day, this just totals one week. This leads one to contemplate why we have a seven-day week and if we indeed need a day off on Sunday. In the creation story of the Old Testament God worked for six days and rested on the seventh. No matter what we think about this statement, the conclusion that we, too, should always rest on the same day, is, in the light of Hildebrandt's work, decisive for our state of health. We then (after a longer settling time) shift our 'critical' days to a fixed day, for example Sunday, where they can pass without harm due to the period of rest.

Now let us return to Figure 11.3. Apart from illness dynamics I (with six stages), which we have discussed, it also lists a dynamics II (with three stages). I discovered this, not via TCM, but via the dynamics of miasms and through the *enneagram*. As far as homoeopathy is concerned, Gienow (2000, p.76) describes two such successions, which he, however, does not see as closed cycles. We shall come back to miasms and their relationships to Chinese elements in Ch.12.4. Here is just the result: The first succession corresponds basically to dynamics I, which has already been described. The second encompasses three stages and reads, in terms of Chinese elements and meridians:

Dynamics II: Metal – Flora – Water (LU – SJ – BL or LU – PC – BL)   (11.11)

From the Chinese elements, we get the meridians, based on the assumption that every meridian already involved in dynamics I is no longer available. Since both meridians of flora are still available, the following two versions of (11.11) result: Figure 11.3 shows the first variant, and dynamics II is completed to form a cycle modelled after dynamics I. The cycle starts at *LU* (marked by II), moves to *SJ* and then along the inside passing by the 'forbidden flora zone' (line in the figure) to *BL*. In the second version it would go from *LU* on the outside, passing *PC* and then back to *BL*. The entire cycle would then bypass the forbidden zone altogether and not – as in the first version – pass it on the inside.

It should be mentioned that dynamic processes and transitions do not only occur during the progression of falling ill and convalescence, but also in healthy life. These processes can also be interpreted in terms of the life spiral; see Kratky (2005b; 2006a&b).

Now to the enneagram, see Rohr & Ebert (1991), which will be treated in more detail in Ch.14.4. This consists of nine (psychological or spiritual) types, which are all equipollent and have their own advantages and disadvantages. They are distributed over three 'fundamental energies', HEAD, GUT and HEART, which have close connections to the doshas. None of those three types, however, represents any of the three fundamental energies in pure form. They are divided into one group of six and one of three types, each with separate cyclic dynamics. Each type is represented in a disintegrated, a normal and an integrated form. Integration and disintegration, however, often do not occur within the type but within the corresponding 6- or 3-cycle. *Disintegration* increases in one direction, *integration* in the opposite direction. If we look at the two directions as analogous to falling ill and recovering, these statements can be applied to the health disc. This was done in Figure 11.3. The characterisation of the enneagram types suggests that *SJ* and not PC is part of the 3-cycle.

This leads us back to TCM. First we notice that flora is not involved in the 6-cycle of the *cold-induced, heat-related diseases* (dynamics I), which is linked to 'overlooking' this element in TCM. In Ch. 8.3 we talked about this possibly being a result of the flora type (blood type AB) not being in existence until 1000 years ago. Taking a closer look at the books on TCM does reveal other illness progressions, which, however, are not elaborated. These include the four-layer concept and the sanjiao/ triple-heater concept (Maciocia 1994, pp. 190 & 493-5), which is partly brought into connection with it. It would be interesting to investigate a possible connection of these concepts with dynamics II. At any rate, they are from a later period (ca 1700 or 1800 A.D.) and belong to the few more recent discoveries in TCM. Thus, they were developed during a period when blood type AB was already in existence (see Ch. 8.3).

11.5.* Stability of the Meridians

The above considerations confirm Figure 11.3, i.e. the meridians *HT, ST* and *PC* are not involved in dynamics I or II. They are marked in black in the illustration. As can be seen, all are located at dosha transitions and form an equilateral triangle on the circle. In the sense of chaos and systems research (Ch. 3-4), the results we have discussed suggest that the twelve meridians can be divided into three groups: into one group of six and one of three with cyclic dynamics (periodic movement) and three fixed points. Interestingly we have denoted just these three meridians as fixed points from an Anthroposophical point of view (Ch. 10.1, see also Kratky 2002): *PC as* 'body's body', *ST* as 'soul's soul', *HT* as 'mind's mind'. Since these do not appear as types in the enneagram, it stands to reason that they are not attractors ('stable') but repellors ('unstable'); see 3.2. Accordingly, it is quite unlikely that one would meet one of these in real life. They appear to be those types that would represent the three fundamental energies of the enneagram in a pure form: *PC* for HEAD, *ST* for GUT and *HT* for HEART.

Furthermore, according to (11.3b, d-f) these three meridians belong to the group of four which constitute the seasonal transitions. The fourth is *SP*. This opens up a completely new perspective on the various creation cycles and successions of seasons, see (11.2a-d) and (11.3a-f). Therefore, the transitions are characterised by instability and must be stabilised by the organism (Ch. 4.3). A healthy organism succeeds in doing so fully; see (11.2a). In a progressive illness this happens less and less, namely in the order of steadily decreasing instability. ST and HT are the most unstable, because these meridians are already eliminated as transition meridians in less severe diseases. Overall, we have:

Unstable Meridians:	1st (coequal): ST & HT,	3rd: PC,	4th: SP.	(11.12a)
Stable Meridians:	SI,	LU,	KI, GB.	(11.12b)

SP is the least unstable according to (11.2c) & (11.3d) and also appears in the enneagram. The meridians representing the four seasons are apparently stable. They are listed in (11.12b).

The remaining four meridians do not appear explicitly in the four seasons, i.e. they are not as stable as the four mentioned in (11.12b). Nothing more can be said about them for the time being. Each dosha now contains one stable and one unstable meridian. In addition, there is a second unstable meridian in kapha and a second stable meridian in pitta. The two meridians (*SP, ST*) located at the positive x-axis (yin) are both unstable; the two (*GB, SI*) at the positive y-axis (yang), on the other hand, are stable.

The three unstable fixed points (repellors) have an interesting impact on the path of life (the inward spiral from flora to flora counter-clockwise, see Ch.8.4). This path can be described by a single variable, namely the angle, α (Figure 9.1b). Due to a constant change in parameter, which represents increasing age, α attempts to grow continuously (counter-clockwise movement). Right after the dosha boundaries, the repellors stand in the way like mountains and stop movement at these boundaries. Thus, in order to cross them, the parameter must continue to grow for a while until it can then leap across, which happens fairly quickly. Thus, the path of life is not even but pauses for a while at the transitions and then overcomes them in spurts. *PC* is responsible for the 'holding back' of birth and then (after one revolution) for death, *ST* for the transition to adulthood, *HT* for the midlife crisis and shock of retirement. Before every step (of integration), there is a pause. Incidentally, in most cultures transition rituals support and ease the transition into the next stage. In our society, such rituals are still present to some extent – for example, baptism. Since both *ST* and its neighbouring meridian *SP* are unstable, this means that the transition from puberty to adulthood is especially crucial.

Unlike the life spiral, illness dynamics I and II cannot be described by one single variable. They run their course in the plane, and finally even in space – the seeming crossing of the trajectories comes about by projection onto the plane from the point of view of complexity research. Figure 11.3 shows that dynamics I passes quite near the repellors, *ST* and *HT*, but dynamics II stays far away from all repellors.

Chapter 12

Recent Developments around Homoeopathy

12.1. Homotoxicology

We shall now address a form of illness dynamics that was developed by the homoeopath Reckeweg in the middle of the 20th century. After lengthy studies, Reckeweg formed the opinion that, in the final analysis, illness can be traced back to external or self-produced poisons, which are harmful to the individual (for this reason, the term homotoxins). Ayurveda uses the term *ama* for toxic or waste products of digestion, which also play a crucial role in health problems.

The organism attempts to excrete these homotoxins or to render them harmless. The symptoms that arise during this process are usually interpreted as illness. Six stages (or phases) can be distinguished which correspond to six strategies of the organism (see Table 12.1). First, the organism attempts to excrete the toxins, which, for example, may manifest in increased perspiration (physiological stage 1). If this attempt is unsuccessful or insufficient, the reaction is increased and fever occurs (pathological stage 2). If this fails as well, the toxins are stored where they do the least harm (stage 3). The first three stages are of a humoral nature – no harm has yet come to the cells and the prognosis is favourable. Thereafter the so-called biological division takes place, which consists of a changeover to vegetative processes (see Table 12.2). The subsequent stages 4-6 are of a cellular nature; now the cells become increasingly damaged. These are primarily silent stages: the patient appears to be well, but the clinical findings are alarming. In stage 4 precancerous conditions might emerge, in stage 5 degenerative processes occur and finally, in stage 6, tumours.

An overview over these six stages can be found, incidentally, in Doerper Reckeweg & Maschke (1996, pp.49-58) and in Reuter & Oettmeier (2001, pp.54-56). A change in stage in general brings with it a change in the tissue and germ layer. Reckeweg (1978, Ch.4) speaks about vicariation. The crucial point lies in the biological division. These statements bring to mind Ayurveda, especially the change from its 3rd to 4th stage as a transition from dispersion to settling in the new dosha (Table 11.6). Moreover, the six TCM stages also display a changeover between the 3rd and 4th one: from yang to yin, from outer to inner, from heat to cold. Reckeweg (1978, pp. 151-3) also refers to the TCM stages and connects them with his own stages. Accordingly, Table 12.1 specifies the meridian assignment resulting from the previous chapter.

Table 12.1. The six stages of illness from the point of view of homotoxicology (Reckeweg 1978, Chs. 4 & 27)

Stages of illness	Characteristics	TCM [a]
1: Excretion	Secretions	SI
2. Reaction	Fever	LI
3: Deposition	Benign deposits	GB
4: Impregnation	Precancer	SP
5: Degeneration	Degeneration	KI
6: Neoplasm	Tumours, cancer	LR

[a] see Table 11.6 & Figure 11.3.

Table 12.2. The grouped stages of illness of homotoxicology

Stages of illness	Principle	Characteristics	
Humoral stages 1-3	Excretion	Sympathi-cotonic:	acid, warmth, high metabolic rate
Biological division			
Cellular stages 4-6	Conden-sation	Parasympathi-cotonic:	base, coldness, low metabolic rate

This also enables a connection to Anthroposophical medicine. According to Figure 10.1, tumours can be expected in those quarters of the disc encompassing the meridians SP, ST and LR (with the neighbouring meridians, BL and GB), see Figure 9.3. SP, LR and (as a neighbour) GB are involved in the 6-way dynamics. Interestingly, Reckeweg lists benign deposits such as cysts and myomas in stage 3 (GB), in stage 4 (SP) precancerous conditions and in stage 6 (LR) tumours, while in the intermediate stage 5 (KI, further away), they are not mentioned. There, in turn, he specifies degeneration, which fits in with Anthroposophical medicine, as well as sclerosis and auto-aggressive diseases, which he also assigns to stage 5. A connection to homoeopathy can also be made (syphilis or destructive diathesis as 'degeneration', see Table 5.2).

The biological division can also be regarded in the light of our previous considerations. Some of its characteristics are listed in Table 12.2. This *pushing out* (excretion) compared to *drawing together* (condensation) fits in well with the three yang and three yin stages of TCM. According to Reckeweg, the change from yang to yin corresponds to the biological division, the changeover to vegetative processes: a transition from the dominance of the sympathetic system to that of the *parasympathetic* (or vagal) system, which entails many changes. The grey region of Figure 11.3 is now dominated by the parasympathetic nervous system, the white region by the sympathetic (derivation in Ch. 9.2). Thus, the stages 1-3 (*SI, LI, GB*) are automatically located in the sympathicotonic region, and the dynamics turn into the vagotonic region (4-5: *SP*, *KI*). Only the last stage lies again in the sympathicotonic white region. Incidentally, in dynamics II the first two stages (*LU*, *SJ*) and the third stage (*BL*) are located in the white and grey regions, respectively.

Reckeweg was a homoeopath who, at first, attempted to treat all six stages with the aid of classical homoeopathy. He discovered that he was only successful in the early stages of an illness. After this, he had to use combinations of various therapies (including orthodox Western medicine) or complex remedies. This led him to start his own company (Heel), which manufactured complex remedies. We have already encountered some of the problems involved in the use of complex remedies in Ch. 5.2. Another aspect is addressed in a study investigating the complex remedy Traumeel, (Oberbaum et al. 2001): compatibility of complementary medicine and scientific studies.

The starting point of this study was a side effect of chemotherapy in form of stomatitis (inflammation of the mouth), which is practically impossible to get under control with orthodox Western medicine. A possible positive influence of Traumeel, which is recommended for inflammations, was thoroughly investigated. 30 patients were evaluated, 15 of whom received Traumeel and the other 15 a placebo. The result was significantly in favour of the complex remedy. The quality of this work is demonstrated by the fact that it appeared in the orthodox medical journal *Cancer*. As far as I know this was the first article on complementary medicine to be published by this journal.

12.2. The Three Laws of Indication

With these considerations, Gienow (2000) allows a good comparison regarding the difference of therapy forms as well as the field of application of homoeopathy. First, we shall look at the so-called laws of indication. In Ch. 2.1, Gienow (2000) begins his discussion with the two laws of indication by Hippocrates, which show that the simile principle is indeed very old:

1st Law of indication: *Law of opposites*: Opposite is cured by opposite. Application whenever the cause of illness is known.

Comment: This principle relates to orthodox Western medicine ('allopathy'), called 'antipathy' by Gienow, which describes the principle quite adequately but is an unfortunate choice given the underlying meaning of 'antipathy'.

2nd Law of indication: *Law of similarity*: Like is cured by like. Application whenever the cause of illness is unknown.

Comment: This law of similarity is pivotal to the homoeopathy developed by Hahnemann.

Now a few thoughts about 'cause' (see also Ch. 2.1): The success story of the *natural* sciences of modern times is based on the fact that it has focused on relatively simple, easily comprehensible parts of the problem. What these sciences do *not* do is get involved with nature itself (otherwise, they would not be sciences); rather they only look at a very limited model of nature. For these simplified processes, which lend themselves to many experiments, the successions and correlations over time are researchable. One speaks of causal-analytical thinking, although this has nothing to do with the more 'profound' or 'true' causes, which philosophers and theologians have batted around for millennia. On the contrary, modern sciences have started to turn from the 'why?' to the 'how?'. We find this limitation of nature repeatedly in our everyday lives, the keyword being 'technology'. For example, human beings are able to hike up a mountain and down a valley, but for our cars we must build roads that are as level as possible, and this requires a great deal of space. The advantage of this approach is that within this limited scope it is possible to achieve a great deal.

This brings us to the field in which the 1st law of indication can be applied, according to Gienow. Many infectious diseases exhibit a clear pathogen, against which one can take action in a concrete fashion. This is the success story of orthodox Western medicine, which regards itself as scientific. Nonetheless, there is a problem: the complexity of a human being. Either medicine addresses the *whole* person, but this then is not science, or the human being is reduced, for example, to 'the stomach in bed 18'. Since nobody consists of only a stomach, this brings about – in the *long* run – unexpected effects ('side effects'). This narrow view of science also expresses itself over *time*. Long-term predictions are practically never possible. Orthodox Western medicine is first and foremost an *acute* and *emergency* medicine. After initial success, the consequences of interplays that are not understood become prevalent. However, every therapy has a typical behaviour over time. In homoeopathy we often find an initial worsening of the condition (homoeopathic aggravation), but after a few days it brings about the desired improvement (see Ch. 5.1). Whereas in orthodox Western medicine a rapid improvement is often the case but there is the risk of getting worse (chronification) in the long run. However, this worsening does not occur after days but after months of therapy – far beyond our usual horizon of time.

This short-term thinking of ours also makes orthodox Western medicine unreliable just where it is most successful. For example, antibiotics have been prescribed not only when necessary but also 'just to be sure' on all kinds of occasions with the result that their success is already toppling. Because of the excessive use of antibiotics, bacterial resistance has advanced to such a degree (feedback!) that it has become a growing problem. In addition, many diseases whose incidence had dropped dramatically – at least in the West – have re-emerged. For example, the incidence of TB is growing at an alarming rate in the USA. The 2nd Hippocratic law of indication can, however, be interpreted to say that the opposite of what is expected will take place, whenever the situation is not fully under control.

The problem of a reversal (in the long run) occurs again and again in more general contexts. In our short-term thinking, we base our interventions on the current situation and do not take into consideration – or not sufficiently – the reactions of others involved. Just as the classical approach of solving, the ever-growing problem of too much traffic is to build more roads. This is only helpful, as long as humanity quits reacting to more roads by driving even more. Furthermore, after every accident in a tunnel, a call for the construction of a second tunnel can be heard. On the other hand, one could argue that this would not save lives in the long run, because many people would drive faster, whenever safety is increased and thus take more risks driving in a tunnel and cause more catastrophes. Another example is development aid. The drought in the Sahel zone, for example, was partly caused by an international well project. 'Surprisingly', the natives accumulated more animals, which then overtaxed the improved situation. This fits in with the expression: the road to hell is paved with good intentions.

A thought experiment on the subject of reversal might be as follows. Someone gets the idea in the summertime to use his refrigerator as an 'air conditioner'. He opens the refrigerator door and leaves it open for a while. In order to avoid side effects, first the contents of the refrigerator are eaten. What happens in the first few minutes and what after one hour? In the short run, the kitchen cools off, but after only one minute, the condenser turns on and keeps running. This generates more heat on the outside than coolness on the inside so the kitchen starts to warm up. The consequence of opening the refrigerator door in the longer run could be called a 'side effect', or better counter effect. Side effects in general pose a serious problem in orthodox Western medicine. We have already looked into this in Ch.1.3.

In classical Antiquity, there was already a dispute about opposites and similarity, which is still current today. In Greek drama, gruesome murders were depicted not for the purpose of enticing the audience to imitate these atrocities but for the cleansing effect (catharsis) of these dramas as a deterrent. A Chinese saying on this subject says "Once yang gets too strong, it topples into yin." The philosophers, especially Plato, as opposed to the poets, believed this to be erroneous. They in turn believed in contrariness therapy, the counter effect. Aristotle was one of the first believers in catharsis. Today there are still discussions about whether violent movies pose a risk of imitation or conversely have a positive effect because of the audience being able to let off steam.

Gienow moves beyond these two laws of indication in Ch.2.2. First, he looks at the polar effect of remedies that emphasise one or the other pole. Digitalis, for example, can raise or lower a patient's heartbeat, independent of the dosage. In addition, this phenomenon might depend on the original condition of the patient. However, harmonising the polarity of symptoms in a suitable manner constitutes a third way of healing:

3rd Law of indication: *Healing by harmonising*. This is directly linked to 'vital force'. In most cases this is not possible, however, and a detour via the first or second law of indication is necessary.

Comment: Gienow is somewhat unclear here. In any case, he also uses the word *love* for vital force. Furthermore, Gienow describes the ideal regulative therapy: a remedy with a polar effect is administered which triggers a regulation toward the mean value in every case. For example, if you know what is important, digitalis can be used to normalise heartbeat, no matter whether the patient's heart is beating too slowly or too fast. In Chs.3 & 4 complex systems and their control are discussed. In complex systems, the relationship between stimulus and response, dose and effect is not quite as rigid as in simple systems, which are those usually studied. The term 'self-organisation' already suggests that structures and processes are not coerced by external forces but at most activated – perhaps by changing one of the parameters.

Complex systems are not easily understood due to their non-linearity and feedback loops and are not controllable by the usual means (Kratky 1989, 1990). This effect of digitalis independent of dosage – according to Gienow – is an example of unusual behaviour. Words such as love and longing can be interpreted in the present context in the sense of parameters. An aphorism says that, in order to make someone build a boat, it is better to stimulate his yearning for the sea rather than explain to him – which seems obvious – how such a boat should be built. As long as the general framework is set, he will figure out on his own how to accomplish this task. Similarly, orders are only useful if one is sure that they will be followed. It is said that if you want to get something done, you should either do it yourself or else forbid your adolescent child to do it (which opens up a new aspect of Adam and Eve's 'sin'). The child revolts in his attempt to gain independence but remains just as dependent as before, just the wrong way round. One more step is necessary for his release into independence: no (more) rules, which only serve to polarise the situation further, but accompanying the child with love into adulthood. Then he will find his own way, one his parents might not even have imagined! This would be an example of regulative 'therapy'.

12.3. The Starting Point and the Direction of Effect

Now we shall go one step further. According to the generalised simile principle, (see Table 5.1d) the direction of the effect of therapy can also depend on the patient's state of health or the starting point of therapy. Interesting but little known research by Pavlov can be found regarding this subject. He not only investigated conditioned reflexes but also alertness (activation, tonus of the cerebral cortex) and its inhibition. He discovered that the expected relationship between stimulus and response only takes place during waking consciousness (high tonus) but that, with growing inhibition or deactivation of the cerebral cortex, the behaviour changes in a stepwise manner:

1) Normal phase: weak stimulus   – weak response
                         strong stimulus – strong response   (12.1a)
2) Equivalent phase: (strong) response – independent of stimulus intensity   (12.1b)
3) Paradoxical phase: weak stimulus   – strong response and vice versa   (12.1c)
4) Ultra-paradoxical phase: response in the opposite direction.   (12.1d)

An example of the ultra-paradoxical phase is when aromas that are usually experienced as pleasant become repulsive and vice versa. Incidentally, usually only the three phases which deviate from the norm are considered, but here we shall talk about phases 1-4. Pavlov's results can be found in several sources including Sargant (1958, pp.33ff) and Sponsel (1995, pp.564ff). It is essential not to confuse Pavlov's phases with Reckeweg's stages of illness.

How does one get into these various states of activity or phases? It is not internal controls (such as in falling asleep and waking up) or conscious relaxation which play a role here but external influences such as suppression of stimuli (in soundproof spaces, dark caves, lying in a tank of tepid water) or the opposite, a flood of stimuli (e.g. loud and fast drumming). Pavlov originally worked with dogs, which he subjected to more and more stressful situations.

This path via external influences introduces a complication inasmuch as stimuli lead to a certain tonus, which in turn determines the stimulus-response scheme (double role of stimuli).

Stimulus deprivation as well as inundation will, if they are profound enough, lead to strong inhibitions and thus to the ultra-paradoxical phase 4. This is also true for particular threats and stressors, where in phase 4 what was originally experienced as unpleasant is now experienced as pleasant and vice versa. This makes comprehensible how victims can develop a positive view of perpetrators in extreme situations (e.g. a bank robbery with hostage-taking). Since in these ultra-paradoxical phases reprogramming is possible, which apparently still holds in later normal states, this is where conditions for brainwashing are optimal (Sargant 1958). However, positive applications are also possible – just bear in mind healings in ethnomedicine, conveyed in a trance. With the proper music, for example, a state is induced in the patient, in which pathological processes apparently can be reprogrammed into healing processes. The schooling of shamans is also characterised by exposure to extreme conditions (stimulus deprivation and inundation with strong stressors, states of fear and the threat of death) (Gruber & Kratky 2002).

The four phases can be interpreted as tonus- or inhibition-dependent reversal effects of stimuli, which is a supplementation to the dose- and time-dependent reverse effects discussed in Ch.5.1. The effect of a stimulus varies depending on the tonus of the brain. In normal waking consciousness, stimuli have the usual effect; with growing inhibition, a sequence of differing stimulus-response relationships takes place. Just as we illustrated in Figure 5.1.a&b the reverse effects discussed in Ch.5, we shall do the same here. Figure 12.1 shows a simple trigonometric function as a response curve that is in accordance with the four phases by Pavlov (the thick sine curve in the middle). The formula for a circle with radius r with the same centre as the disc (with radius R=1) is given by

$$\text{Response} = r\sin(60°-\alpha); \quad \alpha_{wood}=60°, \quad \text{circle representation: } r=r_c=0.7; \tag{12.2}$$

cf. (9.11) & Figure 9.1b. First, let us look at the normal waking state (high tonus). In this case, the reference value for the disappearing stimulus is right over to the left, at the vertical line, where the value of the trigonometric function is zero. This means: no stimulus, no response. Let us take a blood-pressure lowering drug as an example. An increasing dosage means movement from the origin to the right. First, the blood pressure rises and in higher doses (in the middle of the illustration), a dose-dependent reverse effect occurs. The part of the curve to the right we shall address later.

Following these preparatory remarks, we shall assume that realistically high doses will not exceed a certain window, which has the width of a (grey or white) stripe in Figure 12.1. The normal waking state (high tonus), then, refers to the part of the curve in the left grey stripe. Response is normal; it grows along with the stimulus, and is almost linear (phase 1). The maximal dose is indicated by the vertical dashed line. The other regions of the curve remain hidden for now. They are not accessible until the tonus changes. Increasing inhibition or declining tonus causes the zero point of this window to be shifted to the right in this model; the width does not change. Once the shift has reached exactly the width of one stripe, the window is congruent with the white stripe to the left (phase 2). This part of the sine function shows that the organism now responds strongly and almost independently of the dose. If inhibition continues to grow, we shall wind up in the grey stripe in the middle (phase 3). Now the dose-effect relationship is reversed: small doses have a large effect, large doses a small effect. For strong inhibition (the white stripe in the middle, phase 4), the effect is again approximately proportional to the dose but now in the reverse direction (i.e. blood pressure *lowering* in our example).

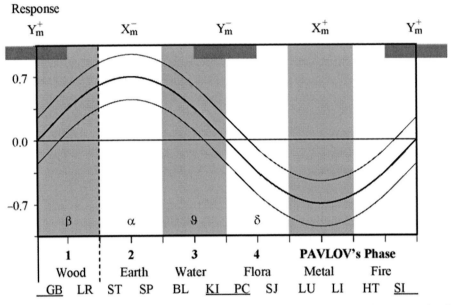

Figure 12.1. Reverse effect dependent on inhibition (Pavlov's phases: 1-4). Assignment to the circle representation. For explanations of the band around the curve and other explanations, see text.

These statements can now be linked to facts that we have already developed. The starting point is the claim by Sargant (1958, p.33) that phase 2 can also occur in overly fatigued individuals. Different states of activity (sleeping, waking) and their connection to the EEG and the Chinese elements were discussed in Ch.10.1, see (10.1a-d) & (10.2). In our geometric model (circle representation), increasing deactivation or inhibition corresponds to a clockwise path beginning with wood, continuing in to earth and water and ending in flora. In this process, the four phases are traversed in order. In Figure 12.1 the brainwaves, phases and Chinese elements are listed accordingly.

Of course, Pavlov's phases only cover two thirds of the Chinese elements, which means that the response curve in *metal* and *fire* is still open for now. However, due to the circle representation of the elements one can proceed with the assumption that the curve will have the same value at the right edge as it did at the left edge (the same point on the circle). The periodic sine function is the simplest curve that satisfies this condition and also reflects the four phases correctly; it was chosen for this reason. The modes of behaviour in the region of metal and fire can now be developed. First *metal*: just as was the case with *earth*, located on the opposite side, the effect is practically independent of the dose, only the direction is reversed (lowering the blood pressure instead of raising it). In an analogous manner we find a practically linear dose-effect relationship for *fire* – and its opposite, *water* – (where small doses have a large effect and vice versa) but in the opposite direction.

All in all the elements located at the lower half of the circle, *wood, earth* and *water*, exhibit an effect in the expected direction, and the elements located on the top, *fire, metal* and *flora* an effect in the opposite direction. With regard to this subchapter, the lower half of the circle is connected to the *first*, the upper half to the *second* law of indication. However, we encounter a language problem here: Since from our Western perspective contrariness (contrariness principle) is 'normal', the effect of the elements of the upper half of the circle, which is opposed to it, becomes 'contrary to contrariness' and thus indirectly becomes the same or similar (simile principle). The upper half of the circle thus has a close connection to homoeopathy, which will be elaborated on later. Now where does the *third* law of indication come into play? Candidates on the circle are the transitions between top and bottom, i.e. a region around the points Y_m^- (on the left edge of the circle) and Y_m^+ (on the right edge), cf. Figure 9.1a. On the disc, this results in a horizontal zone around the horizontal yang axis, which encompasses the three-dosha region near the centre of the disc (the point of origin). For the moment, however, we shall stay with the circle representation.

For clarification, we shall refer to Figure 12.1 again. Since Y_m^- and Y_m^+ are located exactly between two elements, their windows are shifted by half a window with respect to the stripes of the six elements. The two windows are now marked in dark grey at the upper edge of the illustration. At Y_m^+ the circle closes; for this reason the respective window appears twice (at the right and left edges of the figure). If we look at the middle sine curve again in the respective regions, a dose-dependent reverse effect is apparent in both cases. At Y_m^- the response is allopathic in small doses (above the zero line); in high doses, the effect is in the opposite direction (homoeopathic, below the zero line). At Y_m^+ the reverse is the case. In both cases, the curve goes through zero for medium doses. Exactly at this point regulation towards the mean value is addressed (3rd law of indication); especially at this point, the nonspecific effects of a stimulus come to bear (see Ch.9.4). Analogous to Figure 9.5, Figure 2.1 also specifies a band around the middle sine curve, which represents the harmonising nonspecific effect. For the sake of simplicity, we shall not consider a threshold S, but rather set it to zero.

Now let us think about which meridians near Y_m^- or Y_m^+ the 3rd law of indication applies to. This is probably the case for the meridians underlined in Figure 12.1; that is for *PC, KI* (right at Y_m^-) and *SI, GB* (right at Y_m^+) – in their respective windows, the middle sine curve goes through zero. As far as the subsequent meridians are concerned, e.g. *HT*, the answer depends on the width of the band. In the assumed width of the band in Figure 12.1, not the middle sine curve but a part of the band around the window region of *HT* crosses the zero line. An analogous situation results for *LR, BL* and *SJ*. For *ST* and *SP* on the other hand the contrariness principle applies, for *LU* and *LI* the simile principle. This is what the circle representation shows us.

For the *disc* representation, however, we must make a small change (Figure 12.2). In the dark grey ('bow-tie' shaped) region the 3rd law of indication (regulation, harmonisation) applies as the sine curve goes through zero here (Figure 12.1). The subsequent light grey region follows from the width of the band around this curve. The width of the band was assumed equal on the disc and chosen according to the following conditions for consistency:

the region of harmonisation in the sense of the 3rd law of indication should encompass the three-dosha region ($r=1/4$) of Ayurveda. Accordingly, no part of the inner disc is white. It is a minimal condition. The band could be made wider; the light grey region in Figure 12.2 would then spread upward and downward, the four additional 'rectangles' of the region having width B:

$$-B \le [\text{response} - r\sin(60°-\alpha)] \le B; \text{minimum: } B = (\sin 75°)/4 = 0.2415 . \qquad (12.3)$$

The locations of the meridians in the circle representation are the points of intersection of the radial lines with the dashed circle (Figure 12.2). Because of the life spiral, the meridians are shifted for the disc representation (black, grey and white dots). Relevant changes with respect to the circle representation result for the meridians, *LU* and *LI*, which move toward the boundary of the region of harmonisation. *BL* and *LR*, on the other hand, move outwards and also come to rest at the boundary. All other meridians remain in their respective positions on the circle representation. Thus, *SP* and *ST* clearly remain in the contrariness region; even if the light grey region is expanded by choosing a greater value for B, see (12.3).

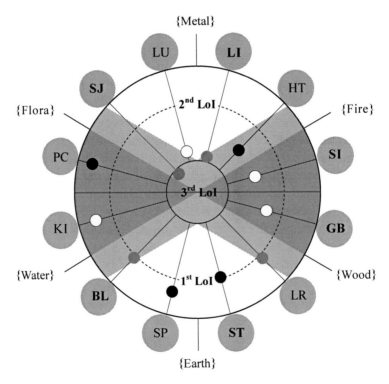

Figure 12.2. Assignment of the meridians to the three laws of indication (LoI); white zones: region of oppositeness (1st LoI, bottom), region of similarity (2nd LoI, top); in between (grey): region of harmonisation (3rd LoI).

The meridians of (11.12a) are marked in black (unstable), those of (11.12b) in white (stable), and the rest (four meridians) are grey. Three of the four white meridians are located in the inner, dark grey region of harmonisation, where *SI* is especially close to the horizontal yang axis and thus is in the best position for harmonisation. In addition, it is the only meridian, according to Figure 9.4, with a neutral total energy. For this reason, it can be surmised that it is the usual reference meridian in a healthy person and/or has a standby function. Illness arises only when harmonising no longer works for whatever reason. In this sense, it is not surprising that in dynamics I (which is frequently seen) illness begins at *SI* (Table 11.6, Figure 11.3). Of the other five meridians of this dynamics *GB* and *KI* are also located in this region of harmonisation. *SP* lies in the contrariness region; *LI* and *LR* – as already mentioned – are borderline cases. This is also true for two of the three meridians of dynamics II, *LU* and *BL*, while *SJ* clearly lies in the region of harmonisation.

The regions of the laws of indication are not strictly divided. The first law of indication dominates the entire lower half of the disc, the second the upper half. Both aspects are still represented in the grey region in between, and for this reason harmonisation or regulation is still possible there (3rd law of indication), but not over the entire range of doses (cf. Figure 12.1). With growing distance from the (horizontal) y-axis, regulation becomes more and more difficult; the first or second law of indication (bottom or top) dominates more and more. Near the boundary of the bar, we are still formally in the zone of harmonisation, but regulation there has only limited possibilities.

Now to those meridians which are outside or only just within the zone of harmonisation. *SP* and *ST* are clearly outside (in the contrariness region), but *BL* and *LR* are positioned right at the border. Incidentally, both of these are the last illness stage in both, dynamics I and II, as long as it does not continue in a cyclic fashion. *LU* and *LI*, the two meridians of *metal*, are located on the border with the simile region. They only come this close to the region of harmonisation because the life spiral is already approaching the point of origin there – contrary to *ST* and *SP*, which are on the opposite side. The restlessness in vata might originate in the effort of trying to achieve harmonisation there.

Vata, especially *metal* in its centre, is then the natural region for homoeopathy. This corresponds to Müller's statement quoted in Ch. 10.2 that homoeopathy is an especially good match for the sensitive type – for it corresponds to *metal* according to Table 10.2a, the central element of vata (psora). According to Figure 12.1, *metal* is largely independent of the effect of the dose. This can be interpreted to mean that information plays the major role here. If you read a book, ten times you have not gained *more* in principle than by reading it only once. Indeed, the information aspect of homoeopathy is emphasised repeatedly. Accordingly, the dose in terms of the quantity of sugar globules or fluid to be ingested is of secondary importance. With regard to the dose in another sense, the potency, opinions are inconsistent, but here too it appears that the right dose is not as important as the choice of the correct homoeopathic remedy. In any case, vata has a very deep connection to homoeopathy. It corresponds to the miasm psora, which is pivotal to homoeopathy. We have discussed this on several occasions, especially in Ch. 5.4, where we also introduced the miasms. The next subchapter will serve to deepen this connection further.

12.4. The Extended Miasms

At first, Hahnemann only looked at a patient's individual and current symptomatology for the purposes of diagnosis and the simile principle for therapy. With growing success, more and more difficult cases (and chronic diseases) were presented to him, and this method no longer sufficed. A thorough anamnesis was called for, as was the determination of the patient's underlying constitution and illness type (Ch. 5.4). This in turn let him to the discovery of the concept of the miasms psora, sycosis and syphilis, with psora being pivotal. Instead of only using the simile principle, Hahnemann now spoke of anti-miasmatic remedies, an expression more suited to allopathy than homoeopathy. From the perspective of illness dynamics and the laws of indication discussed in Ch. 12.3, this can be interpreted in the following way: more serious diseases, and chronic diseases in particular, have in general already left the region of psora and are therefore no longer responsive to the simile principle alone. Compare also Table 12.3, which is based on Table 5.2 and the laws of indication. The table should remind us that psora, sycosis and syphilis correspond to vata, pitta and kapha, respectively.

It should be noted that Hahnemann only described a very few anti-miasmatic remedies; the individual no longer seemed to be central but rather what was typical. This might also be connected to the observation that there are more individual differences at the onset of an illness than after it has become chronic. We shall come back to this in Ch. 13. In any case, not all homoeopaths went along with Hahnemann's idea of miasms and those who work with miasms (or rather diatheses), have a different understanding of this concept; see Pschyrembel (2000), keywords miasms and theory of miasms.

The number of miasms considered also varies. Often a fourth, tubercular miasm, is recognised, but the literature is not consistent. It can be found between psora and sycosis or between sycosis and syphilis. Other systems offer five or more miasms. Masi-Elizalde on the other hand speaks of only one miasm (psora), which expresses itself in inappropriate attitudes and distorted perceptions. The primary psora corresponds to good health, which can turn via the secondary (= customary) psora into the tertiary psora (sycosis or syphilis). This presumably refers to dynamics I and II – the more so because Masi-Elizalde also speaks of a masked sycosis that becomes manifest in somatic changes despite apparent good health. It resembles the description of stages 4-6 in homotoxicology (Ch. 12.1), where the latter, in turn, is located in sycosis.

Table 12.3. The three diatheses of homoeopathy – comparison with the miasms, the doshas of Ayurveda and the laws of indication (LoI, cf. Figure 12.2)

Nomenclature	Lymphatic	Lithemic	Destructive
Dorcsi Ortega Miasms	Fearful Deficiency Psora	Loud Overabundance Sycosis	Rigid Degeneration Syphilis
Ayurveda LoI *	Vata 2, 3	Pitta 1, 3 (2)	Kapha 1, 3 (2)

* Laws of opposites (1), similarity (2), harmonisation (3).

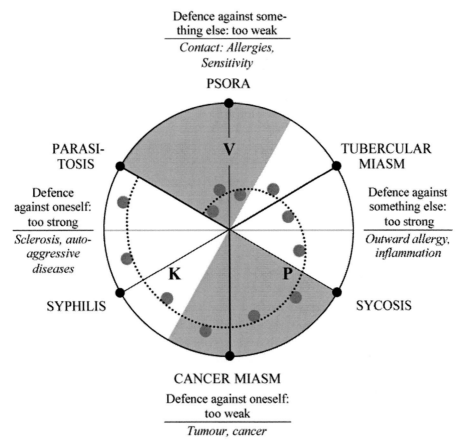

Defence against some-
thing else: too weak

Contact: Allergies,
Sensitivity

PSORA

PARASI-
TOSIS

Defence
against oneself:
too strong

Sclerosis, auto-
aggressive
diseases

SYPHILIS

TUBERCULAR
MIASM

Defence against
something else:
too strong

Outward allergy,
inflammation

SYCOSIS

CANCER MIASM

Defence against oneself:
too weak

Tumour, cancer

Figure 12.3. Comparison of the extended miasms by Gienow (2000) to Ayurveda (**V**: vata, **P**: pitta,
K: kapha) and Anthroposophical medicine. The illustration is based on Figure 10.1.

The controversial discussion concerning miasms also shows itself in the main topics of
two issues of homoeopathic journals (see Weisshuhn 1997 and Weinschenk 2002). In van der
Zee (2001), the process of birth is connected to a specific sequence of miasms. A comparison
of several systems of miasms can be found in Payrhuber (1997, Ch. X); he also refers to
Ortega and Masi-Elizalde. Original literature concerning these two can be found in Ortega
(2000) and Faust (1993). Sankaran, who ascribes to yet another system of miasms, is also
often quoted in this context. The tubercular miasm is located between sycosis and syphilis in
his system, a version that cannot be reconciled with my understanding of the subject matter.
A synopsis of his system can be found in Sankaran (1997, App. 1; 1999, Ch. 24).

Now let us move on to the extended miasms as described by Gienow (2000); the following page numbers refer to this book. Of the three usual miasms, psora, sycosis and syphilis,
Gienow considers psora as the most important and calls it the primary miasm. Sycosis and
syphilis are secondary miasms (p. 105) in his system and all three constitute the main miasms.
Apart from these, he also refers to three other miasms as transitional: tubercular miasm,
cancer miasm and parasitosis (intermediary miasms). He regards the tubercular miasm as a
transition between psora and sycosis, where psoric immune deficiency is combined with

sycotic over-reaction (p. 42). According to Gienow, it lacks internal substance and is comparable to a bladder or vesicle. Translated to TCM, this corresponds to yang excess and yin deficiency. According to Figure 7.4, this is exactly the location of {fire}, which indeed corresponds to the psora/ sycosis boundary. There are so many agreements between Gienow's approach and mine that I shall refer to his version of miasms.

Gienow assigns the 'primary colours' blue, yellow and red to psora, sycosis and syphilis, and the 'mixed colours' to the transitions. On the back cover of his book, he represents the miasms with their colours arranged in a circle. Because of the relative location of the (extended) miasms to one another, links to other typologies are also possible. Their connection to the dispositions can be seen in Table 10.2a&b. This, in turn, leads to a connection to Ayurveda (see Figure 12.3), which also depicts the four fundamental illness types as described in Anthroposophical medicine (Fintelmann 2000). The exact region of the four illness types is given by the white and grey quarter-circle sections (cf. Figure 10.1). All in all, a four- and a six-way system contrast each other:

Top:	sensitivity, contact: allergies	– psora	(12.4a)
Bottom:	swelling, cancer	– cancer miasm	(12.4b)
Left:	sclerosis, auto-aggressive diseases	– parasitosis & syphilis	(12.4c)
Right:	inflammation, outward allergies	– tubercular miasm & sycosis	(12.4d)

In (12.4a&b) the connection is obvious, as is that in (12.4c&d) after some contemplation. A few points (which have already been dealt with immediately before Figure 10.1 when discussing Anthroposophy) can be made here: Allergy usually corresponds to an over-reaction during contact (psora, dynamics in the direction of sycosis). However, the reaction can also be insufficient (psora, dynamics in the direction of syphilis) – for example, allowing parasites to enter the organism. The former case corresponds to the tubercular miasm, which Gienow also connects with allergies on p. 42. The second case, however, refers to parasitosis. The exact characterisation of the primary miasm, psora (Ch. 5.4 in Gienow), incidentally, reads just like the Indian description of vata and is in many aspects reminiscent of *metal*. A short characterisation would be:

Psora: *Changeability* (vulnerable equilibrium), instability; occurrence of opposite symptoms (e.g. heat and cold); worry, dryness; deficiency (feelings of emptiness), frailty, sensitivity (to stress, inappropriate reactions).   (12.5)

The statements by Gienow (on pp. 51, 61, 74-79, 104-107) can be summarised as follows: in addition to the latent psora, there is also an *exhausted* and a (*hyper*) *active* form. The exhausted form is fixated via parasitosis in *syphilis*, the activated form via the tubercular miasm in *sycosis*. For this reason, Gienow considers psora to be bipolar. It has two faces: one corresponding more to *sycosis*, the other more to *syphilis*. This, in turn, resembles the statement in Tibetan medicine about vata being temperature neutral per se but having a tendency to topple over into cold or heat (Qusar & Sergent 1997, pp. 82, 184 & 205). According to Gienow, the entire spectrum of types is already contained in *psora*, but individual expression is more accentuated in the other miasms. This allows the following interpretation (cf. Figure 8.4): in vata (psora), V-K (*SJ, LU*) represents the left half of the health disc and thus also refers to kapha, whereas V-P (*LI, HT*) represents the *right* half and also refers to *pitta*. The entire disc (twelve meridians) is represented in vata (four meridians) in a self-similar fashion. This fractal-like behaviour can be taken one step further as everything is again represented in *SJ.* From an Ayurvedic perspective, it is the only meridian that lies in the three-dosha region. From the perspective of TCM, it forms a connection to all areas of the organism.

Gienow also offers evidence for this. For, indeed, behind the six miasms there is a primordial psora, Tsora-at (pp.28, 38, 209), which apparently is identical or closely related to the latent psora (pp.106 & 172). It is characterised by deficiency. All diseases begin and also end here. SJ fits into this picture rather well. It is located in the three-dosha region containing everything but, alas, is in V-K, a 'region of deficiency'. Illness arises whenever a connection of all three regions cannot be established. In this case, the outward spiral appears to be a possible path of illness. This has led us to the most interesting point, the dynamics of miasms, first mentioned in detail by Gienow in Chs.4-5.

After many examples, the following scheme becomes apparent (for easier reading the Far Eastern terminology and the health disc will be used): Any stress first shows itself in vata, because of its instability and sensitivity. In the region of vata, which at first sight corresponds to equilibrium (with a latent weakness), fluctuations in the state of health arise on the disc. These fluctuations grow with increasing stress. At first, everything remains in the functional region; somatisations are not expected due to the changeability of vata. The pendulum-like movement typically begins at the vertical axis, an over-reaction carries it to the right (LI), where exhaustion soon takes its toll (left, LU), with a (short-term) movement back to the starting position and so on; that is, an ellipsoidal movement results. Once the stress proves too much for the organism, movement breaks away to the *right* (via fire to wood) or to the *left* (via flora to water). This also brings about somatic fixations.

On p.76, Gienow describes the resulting two forms of illness dynamics (as a reversal of the forms of healing dynamics):

A) Activated psora (*metal*) – tubercular miasm (*fire*) –
   – sycosis (*wood*) – syphilis (*water*);   (12.6a)

B) Exhausted psora (*metal*) – parasitosis (*flora*) –
   – syphilis (*water*).   (12.6b)

The Chinese elements are included in this case. In the sense of the circle representation, A moves clockwise, B counter-clockwise; they are two opposite movements from psora to syphilis. Dynamics A is similar to dynamics I of Figure 11.3 (TCM), dynamics B is entirely consistent with dynamics II. Interestingly, according to Gienow, both successions have the same origin: oscillations around the vata centre. On p.99, Gienow describes dynamics A as the main path after suppression of psora. The first discrepancy with dynamics I is that it begins with the succession metal – fire instead of fire – metal. However, since Gienow describes larger and larger fluctuations in psora before the onset of illness, until the movement overshoots the tubercular miasm and lands in sycosis, this can easily be interpreted as an initial fluctuation between metal and fire, where Gienow settles for the succession metal – fire and TCM for the reverse. Movement continues via *wood* (corresponding to Figure

11.3) to *water*, where Gienow fails to mention earth (cancer miasm), which lies between them. Either it was overlooked or the cycle only remains at earth (*SP*) for such a short period that it can be counted as part of the cycle or disregarded. The latter confirms that *SP* is the fourth unstable meridian; (11.12a), the other three do not participate in any dynamics.

The succession of miasms ends in syphilis (water) for Gienow. He presents the example of infection with scabies on p.42, where the step toward parasitosis (flora) also takes place, but in his opinion, this is an exception. He does not mention a return to sycosis (stage 6: *LR*). As a whole, the dynamics of miasms corresponds to an outward spiral (clockwise movement) and thus to my original understanding of illness processes. On the other hand, dynamics I breaks away from a clockwise direction of movement by returning to *LR* in closing the cycle. Nonetheless, one must assume that dynamics A and I are one and the same and that the outward spiral is merely a first approximation of the actual relationships of illness dynamics. An additional comment on dynamics II may be made: It comprises the three stages *metal – flora – water*. The meridians that come into question, *LU – SJ – BL*, are shown in Figure 11.3. There, however, this dynamics also has been completed to become a cycle (which is not mentioned by Gienow).

Healing occurs in the reverse direction according to Hering's Law. While the severity of the illness is increasing, the subsequent miasm is the pathological miasm, the one in the opposite direction the healing miasm. The latter must be activated (facilitation of miasms) in order to push the illness one step back. This continues until the level of the latent psora or tsora-at has been reached. Only there is true healing possible with administration of the correct simile (pp.106 & 172). That is, according to Gienow, there is a 'division of labour' within homoeopathy: first (anti-)miasmatic treatment; the decisive last step is given by application of the simile principle.

Several times, we have heard about possible connections between the doshas and the type as well as the severity of illness. Accordingly, illness progression – simply stated – moves from vata via pitta to kapha, where the situation shifts from functional via acute to chronic illness. This also means that diagnosis from vata to kapha becomes easier but the possibility of therapy, on the other hand, more and more difficult. Orthodox Western medicine occupies a 'position in the middle': it is strong in acute diseases, less strong in functional and chronic diseases. Early recognition (functional disorders and feelings of malaise, including prevention) on the other hand is the strength of many complementary medicine systems. This requires, however, subtle methods of diagnosis, such as pulse diagnosis. In return, therapy is gentle in general; here, diagnosis is the shortcoming of orthodox Western medicine.

Orthodox Western medicine comes into play one step later, for the treatment of acute diseases (typically in pitta or for the movement type, for which orthodox Western medicine is especially beneficial, according to Müller). It has powerful therapies available, but these no longer suffice for chronic diseases. In this situation, in turn, it is the therapy and not the diagnosis that hinders success. The question is: which method is better suited to chronic diseases. In the ideal case, they should not even come about, so that this problem of therapy should not even arise. It is Gienow himself who gives a hint about what to do: miasmatic treatment. In my terminology, this means: the problem is shifted on the health disc until it is located at a site (in vata) where complementary medicine (in this case homoeopathy) can be applied successfully. This site can be different for different methods (see also Kratky

2002). Thus, there is no reason why orthodox Western medicine should not be able to treat a case like this successfully. In a difficult case it makes an exact diagnosis, allows another medicine system to 'shift the illness to pitta', and then tackles the problem at pitta. This would be one possibility of integrating various healing methods.

The above-mentioned book of Gienow is focused on psora. There is another book concentrating on sycosis (Gienow 2003). Incidentally, the characterisation of miasms by Gienow makes possible a cross reference to the four primal complexes by C.G. Jung (Eschenbach 1996, Ch. 7):

Primal sin:	separation from unity:	unsuccessful aspect of P4;
		SJ in {flora};	(12.7a)
Primal talent:	creativity, potentiality:	ambivalent aspect of P3;
		{metal} & vata;	(12.7b)
Primal rivalry:	ambition, hate, power:	unsuccessful aspect of P1;
		{wood} & pitta;	(12.7c)
Primal fear:	depression, destruction:	unsuccessful aspect of P2;
		{water} & kapha.	(12.7d)

The right hand sections of rows (12.7a-d) represent my interpretation (the sequence of rows corresponds to a clockwise movement). P1-P4 refer to the perspectives or approaches to reality introduced in Table 2.1a&b. It is not surprising that ambivalence is associated with P3. Moreover, talent and creativity have two sides is explicitly discussed by Eschenbach on p. 173f (for example the impostor and the swindler). Fintelmann (2000, p. 84) makes a fitting remark regarding the ambivalence of allergies (in vata as well, cf. Table 10.1 and Figure 10.1): "hysteria (overly sensitive, fleeting symptoms) … also hypochondria. Phantom pregnancy, creative imagination … theatrical talent." According to Eschenbach, being creative is a central theme of life, which has a connection to the other three complexes. About the negative side of talent and potentiality: *"I won't make it!"*– premature giving up (vata!). In addition: *"True creative potential often is very unpleasant, for the creative person as well as those around him."*

A few other points made by Gienow will now be mentioned briefly. First of all the duration of the healing process is a tenth of that of falling ill in the best case (p. 206). Furthermore, considerations of 'mirror' miasms play an important role in therapy and impediments of therapy (pp. 15, 73-88). These are miasms on opposite sides, e.g. tubercular miasm – syphilis. Compare the bottom/top pairs of meridians, Table 7.2a-c, which also play a certain role in TCM. Finally, the term breakpoint should be mentioned (pp. 17, 62, 104). This refers to the 'miasmatic scope' of a homoeopathic remedy. Making use of the simile principle, for example, by administering a purely psoric remedy to a patient in a sycotic region of illness, might alleviate the patient's symptoms, but the underlying process will not be stopped and death cannot be prevented.

In conclusion, we shall take a closer look at a disease and healing progression described by Gienow (pp. 76 & 153f) as being less frequent. This progression, which has nothing to do with the spiral, is based on the exhaustion phase of psora. The progression is tsora-at – psora – parasitosis – syphilis; the healing progression takes place in reverse order. The affected person slaves away in exhaustion unsuccessfully, he turns into a parasite, becoming a burden on others but he can also be infected by parasites (P1). This statement referring to parasitosis is interesting inasmuch as flora (which is located at this same site) stands for P1/P4, for the exaggerated P1, which in its exaggeration turns into P4. Now symbiosis is a successful P4-relationship (see Table 2.1a&b). Thus, parasitosis corresponds to a failed symbiosis. There is a pronounced tendency to move in a particular direction, mainly because of lack of energy. This concludes the discussion of the extended miasms. The following subchapter will be devoted to another facet of homoeopathy.

12.5. Homoeopathy of the Elements

Investigating the homoeopathic characteristics of the chemical elements is a new field, which originated with Scholten (1997). Disregarding high potencies, homoeopathic remedies consist of molecules or mixtures of molecules in addition to the solvent. About 3500 are known in principle, about 2000 of these have undergone some remedy proving, only 200 being well-tested. They are called single homoeopathic remedies, even though they are mixtures, since they have been proved and manufactured as such. With the aid of the computer, the above-mentioned number of 200-2000 homoeopathic remedies can easily be managed. On the other hand, an arbitrarily large number of combinations or mixtures of such homoeopathic remedies is possible, which leads to the so-called complex remedies and thus goes beyond classical homoeopathy. Nonetheless, intuition and power of deduction limit the possibilities here as well, as remedies are usually only combined when they have a comparable effect on the main symptoms to be treated. However, the problem of non-linearity and thus non-additivity remains; there is no guarantee that the mixture will have the effect one might expect from the individual components; see (3.1a&b).

Proceeding from the homoeopathic remedies we can, however, also go in the other direction: namely from the molecules to the chemical elements from which they are made up. There are a number of calcium compounds in homoeopathy: for example, Calcium carbonicum (calcium and carbon), Calcium sulphuricum (calcium and sulphur) and Calcium phosphoricum (calcium and phosphorus); oxygen, too, can be found in some of the calcium compounds. One can attempt to attribute similarities in the respective rows to the common element (in our example calcium), and the differences to the respective different element. The advantage would lie in the fact that there are only about 100 elements, which makes the situation relatively manageable. However, the same applies here as for the complex remedies: (homoeopathic) characteristics of the elements can only be extrapolated from the molecules if we assume linearity. Thus, further provings of the elements and of many molecules have still do be done in order to get more insight into how the effects of the elements combine in the molecules built up by these elements.

It is possible, of course, to compare the presumed characteristics of elements with direct results from the remedy provings of elements. Admittedly, up until recently only relatively few elements had been tested or used as homoeopathic remedies. These include Argentum metallicum (silver), Sulphur and Cuprum (copper). For this reason, Scholten initiated remedy provings for those elements that had not undergone such tests, but a number of provings remain to be conducted. The result will be exciting, since there will be at least a partial answer to the question of linearity of effects. Investigating chemical elements is also interesting for a different reason: they are not merely listed side-by-side but are embedded in the row and column structure of the periodic table of elements. With the aid of this structure, blank spaces were recognised as such by physics and chemistry, and this recognition led to the discovery of elements that, until then, had been unknown. Scholten proceeds from the hypothesis that this structure is reflected in the homoeopathic effect. This then results in further predictability of 'blank spaces' in the homoeopathic effect of elements, if the row and column neighbour of an element is known, for example. This, too, can of course be tested via remedy proving.

The periodic table of elements will be discussed briefly because of the connection between physics/chemistry and homoeopathy. An element is characterised by the number of protons, i.e. the positive charge on its nucleus. This charge is counter-balanced by an equally large negative charge of the electron cloud surrounding it. This electron cloud has a shell structure and in general is filled from the inside out, where more and more (2, 8, 18, 32, ...) electrons can occupy the outer shells. The chemical characteristics are primarily determined by the outer shell. A constellation with 8 electrons is particularly stable (the exception being where there are 2 electrons in the case of the 1st shell). The corresponding element, then, is a noble gas, which does not readily take part in chemical reactions. If an atom with one lone outer electron (e.g. sodium) encounters another atom that just needs one more electron to fill its outer shell (e.g. chlorine), this electron is transferred to the other atom and a strong ionic bond is formed (in our example, sodium chloride, i.e. table salt). According to Scholten, the varying degree of willingness to form bonds is reflected in human characteristics, which are assigned to certain elements (give and take).

The elements from hydrogen (atomic number $Z=1$) to uranium ($Z=92$) can all be found in nature. Most isotopes of the elements up to and including $Z=83$ are stable – with the exception of $Z=43$ & 61. Starting with $Z=84$, on the other hand, all elements are unstable, i.e. radioactive. This includes uranium, although it has a half-life of millions of years. The artificially produced transuranic elements follow, starting at $Z=93$ (and currently going up to $Z=111$), some of which decay very quickly (minutes to fractions of seconds). For homoeopathy, only those elements can be considered potentially useful which are stable or have a relatively long half-life. There are about 100 in total. It should be noted that the atomic nucleus also contains *neutrons* as well as *protons*, but these have no influence on the atomic number. As a result, in general there is not only *one* atom for every Z but several isotopes with varying degrees of stability. The previous statements about stability refer to the *most stable* isotope in each case.

Each row in the periodic table begins with an element with a single electron in its outer shell and ends with an element whose outer shell is filled (noble gas). Because of the growing number of electrons needed to fill the shells, the number of elements also increases from row to row. Scholten (1997, pp.22-8) calls the rows *series* and names them after the typical element featured there. Each series is assigned to one theme and one age (see Table 12.4). The elements of a series correspond, in sequence, to a succession of *stages*, which denote the rise, highpoint and decline of the respective theme. At the end, a noble gas represents a time-out period, where the old *no longer* applies and the new is *not yet* born. This period could just as well be placed at the beginning of the new series. Our time-out period of the week, Sunday, represents an analogous situation. Sometimes we find it placed at the beginning, sometimes at the end of the week.

Table 12.4. Characterisation of the elements series by Scholten (1997, pp.29-67)

Series	No. of elements	Name	Theme	Age
1	2 (Z= 1 to 2)	Hydrogen	Being, symbiosis	Unborn
2	8 (Z= 3 to 10)	Carbon	Individuality	Child
3	8 (Z=11 to 18)	Silicon	Relationships	Juvenile
4	18 (Z=19 to 36)	Iron	Purpose, work	Young adult
5	18 (Z=37 to 54)	Silver	Ideas, arts	Adult
6	32 (Z=55 to 86)	Gold	Power, leadership	Old
7	(incomplete)	Uranium	Magic	Very old

The *stages* (succession of rise and decline) correspond to the *columns* of the periodic table. The number of stages is not constant but increases with the series (see the number of elements of a series, Table 12.4). Scholten (1997, pp.29-67) elaborates on the succession of stages in the case of 18 stages. The rise takes place from stage 1-9, the highpoint is at stage 10, then the decline follows from 11-17 (18 is the time-out period). Thus, the climb is a little longer than the fall.

The elements of one row of the periodic table thus – from a homoeopathic perspective – have the same theme, those of one column belong (approximately) to the same stage. In this respect, the elements of one row or column can be compared. An interesting aspect is the assignment of elements to stages of life (age) (last column in Table 12.4). If one takes life per se as one large episode of rise, highpoint and decline, the series can be interpreted as a kind of series of stages, this time referring to life as a whole. The curve of rise and decline then is still more asymmetrical than for the 'true' stages. The highpoint (power, leadership) does not appear until series 6 (golden series), i.e. in advanced age. Overall, a self-similar structure of the course of life is revealed. Accordingly, there are a few special elements where series and stage match perfectly, regarding their level of rise or decline.

The 1st series (elements: hydrogen, helium) takes place in the mother's womb. It is a question of yes or no (being born or not). The subsequent series can be combined into the pairs: childhood – youth, middle age – advanced age. This reminds us of an analogous representation in Ayurveda (life spiral, Figure 8.4). It suggests a comparison of the series 2-7 with the six Indo-Tibetan ⟨elements⟩ and the three doshas:

Series:	2	3	4	5	6	7		(12.8a)
⟨Elements⟩:	⟨Water⟩	⟨Earth⟩	⟨Agni⟩	⟨Fire⟩	⟨Air⟩	⟨Ether⟩		(12.8b)
Dosha:	Kapha	Kapha	Pitta	Pitta	Vata	Vata		(12.8c)

The angle brackets are used again in order to avoid confusion with the elements in the sense of Scholten. Incidentally, with one exception, all radioactive elements are located in the 6th and 7th series, i.e. in *vata*. Each series corresponds to two of the 12 main meridians. The 1st series is 'beyond' normal life and thus finds its place on the line segment of flora (between death and birth) which closes the life spiral. The characterisation of the 1st series as 'symbiosis' fits in as well. Furthermore, two meridians belonging to the so-called extraordinary meridians can also be assigned to this region: namely the governing and conception vessel, also called sea of the yang and yin meridians (Kratky 2000c, Ch. 3). They play a primary role and are probably the first meridians formed in the embryo (David Dapra and Kuo-Gen Chen, personal communication).

According to Scholten, each element, starting with birth, is assigned to about one year. This then results in a typical lifespan of around 90 years, where the end of puberty is placed at ca 16 years, the end of the middle adult age at 52 years. The formal structure of the periodic table, in which the rows (series) get longer and longer, has a biological parallel: First, a child develops very quickly. Thereafter, the older a person gets the less he changes and in return, the processes surrounding him appear to take place faster and faster. Seen from outside with time measured objectively, a series which goes through all stages takes longer and longer with growing age. This seems more realistic than a fixed number of seven years per developmental jump as in Anthroposophy.

Scholten was not the only one to consider the connection between homoeopathy and the chemical elements. De Schepper (2003) came to very similar conclusions although he started from a more classical homoeopathic viewpoint. The concept of considering remedies as members of groups that share common characteristics (kingdoms and families), which was introduced by Farrington in the latter part of the 19th century (new editions: Farrington 2002a&b), has recently been advanced by Rosenthal and Sankaran; see Rosenthal (2000) and Sankaran (2005). Rosenthal distinguishes between the mineral, plant, animal and human kingdoms. He considers the basic properties of homoeopathic remedies coming from the different kingdoms. Sankaran follows similar lines and distinguishes three kingdoms: mineral, plant, and animal. In an effort to find a common theme in remedies belonging to a given plant family he has studied the various plant families in depth, which has resulted in a detailed description of the plant kingdom, comparable to the description of the inanimate kingdom by the rows and columns of the periodic table. Sankaran has also studied the relation between the botanical families and the miasms, which has yielded a periodic table of miasms and remedies. It is not surprising that Scholten wrote the foreword to Sankaran's *An Insight Into Plants* (see Sankaran 2002).

Finally, it should also be mentioned that Scholten went one step further considering the elements in minerals and plants (Scholten 2000, 2001 & 2002). Thus, the work of Scholten, Rosenthal and Sankaran has birthed new facets of homoeopathy.

Chapter 13

A Deeper Understanding of
Falling Ill and Recovering

13.1. Description of a Landscape Model

In Chs.7-10, we looked at various approaches, which have led us to the health disc or rather could be reconciled with it. In Chs.11-12, this was augmented by an analysis of illness dynamics, to which TCM and homoeopathy made the primary contributions. These considerations can now be illustrated with the aid of a simple landscape model, which varies according to the location of a point on the health disc. To demonstrate this we shall look at a landscape of potentials in which a ball is in motion. Just as in a real landscape, the ball has a tendency to seek the lowest point. If we take friction into consideration, the ball will come to rest at a minimum (bottom of the valley). The point (measured horizontally) at which the ball comes to rest determines a stable state of the system described by the landscape. For the sake of simplicity, we shall work with one single variable s, which we shall interpret presently. The landscape, the potential $E_{pot}(s)$ as a function of s, which is to describe the most important characteristics of the doshas and/or elements, will be chosen to be as simple as possible, i.e. as power functions of s.

The following functions will be used: s^6, $-s^4$, s^2 (parabola) and $-s$ (straight line, linearity). Figure 13.1a shows the behaviour of these functions near the origin, which is to be our reference point. Right around s=0 the straight line makes the greatest contribution, then, in decreasing order, the parabola, the function of degree 4 and finally the function of degree 6. For values of s far away from s=0, the reverse order applies. The exact locations of the transitions depend on the coefficients. If the magnitude of the coefficient is 1, the transition is exactly at s=±1, most easily seen in the left upper corner of the light grey square in Figure 13.1a. $E_{pot}(s=0)=0$ holds for all potentials considered. As the starting potential we shall choose $E_{pot}(s) = 2s^6 - 3s^4$. It is to hold for V_m^+, i.e. the topmost point of the circle representation (x=-0.7, y=0). Accordingly, this symmetrical potential can be found in the topmost graph of Figure 13.2. The coefficients 2 and 3 do not curtail generalisation. They were chosen for simplicity, so that the minima would be at s=±1 and the value for E_{pot} would be exactly –1. In this way, the other cases can be easily compared. The landscape at V_m^+ exhibits three positions of equilibrium (see top of Figure 13.2 again): one unstable at s=0 and one stable each at s=±1. Farther away, the landscape becomes increasingly steep and in every case drives back the ball, whose value of s represents the state of the system. That is, it ultimately comes to rest at s=±1.

However, we may imagine a noise produced by the organism or external disturbances as additional jiggling of the landscape. In a steep landscape, the ball will then jump around near the bottom of the valley, in a shallow landscape it can also jump over the hill into the next valley. Overall, the effect of a gentle jiggling can be compared to a slight levelling of the landscape. The probability that the ball will be able to surmount larger differences in height is less. Let us suppose that the above-mentioned noise typically aids the ball to surmount differences in height of up to 0.5. For differences in height of 1, however, it would take a very long time before the ball could jump over the mountain. In this situation, a ball at V_m^+ in general can no longer surmount the hill and jump into another valley. The *left-hand* valley (*l*) represents *kapha*-like states, the *right-hand* one (*r*) *pitta*-like states. Both have a stable equilibrium at V_m^+ (the bottom of the valley). *Vata* – in the *centre or middle* (*m*) – is characterised by an unstable equilibrium at s=0. One can imagine the variable s as temperature increasing to the right, where the order left (kapha) – middle (vata) – right (pitta) results automatically. The statement from Tibetan medicine mentioned in Ch.8.1 (Qusar & Sergent 1997, pp.82, 184 & 205) that vata (Tibetan: *lung*) is temperature neutral per se but tends to topple over to cold or hot is reflected in the chosen potential (the neutral middle temperature is unstable).

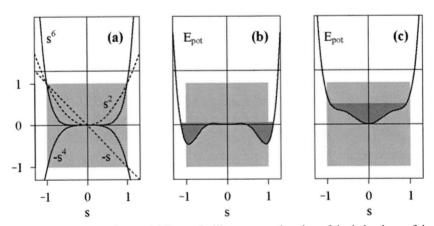

Figure 13.1. Landscape of potential E_{pot} to facilitate comprehension of the behaviour of doshas and elements. **a)** According to (13.1), the following power functions of s contribute to E_{pot}: s^6, $-s^4$, s^2 (parabola) and –s (straight line, linearity); **b)** E_{pot} for x=–0.35 and y=0; **c)** E_{pot} for x=0.35 and y=0.

Some further remarks need to be made regarding Figure 13.1-2: each depicts the interval –1.3≤s≤1.3. In Figure 13.2 the same holds for the *potential*, while in Figure 13.1 the double positive range of values (i.e. up to E_{pot}=2.6) is illustrated. Figure 13.1 illustrates that the power curves grow very quickly and that leaving out this range in Figure 13.2 does not result in the loss of important information. In any case, the small square frames of the 'window structure' in Figure 13.1-2 are 1.3 units high and wide. Furthermore, the combined region $-1 \leq s \leq 1$ and $-1 \leq E_{pot} \leq 1$ is specified as a light grey square. In the other graphs in Figure 13.1-2 the potential of the absolute (i.e. deepest) minimum up to a value of 0.5 units higher are marked in dark grey. This is to illustrate which ranges of potentials are made accessible by the jiggling.

The control of complex systems mentioned in Ch.4.3 now expresses itself as a balancing at the maximum; it is now an instability control. This means that the organism is able – with a great effort of balancing – to keep the ball (i.e. its own state or condition) in V_m^+ at s=0, which, however, is made even more difficult by the jiggling of the landscape. For this reason, the ball will keep rolling around near the maximum under constant risk of falling, which corresponds to the instability (going to and fro between V-P and V-K) of vata (psora) described in Ayurveda and homoeopathy. Should the ball fall, it would be almost impossible (at least in V_m^+) to land at s=0 again without help. In rare cases, jiggling can here have a positive effect. The discussed potential function is completely symmetrical. On average, the ball lands – also during mishaps – in the left or right minimum with equal probability. Nonetheless, in every single case where balancing fails the symmetry is broken in the act of rolling down (the result being either left or right) – compare this with the air coils turning clockwise and counter-clockwise discussed in Ch.4.2. The potential landscape in V_m^+ is unmistakably vata. Nonetheless, a loss of balance mimics a toppling to kapha or pitta (the *landscape* did not change but the *condition* assumed in it did). This corresponds to the opinion that all possibilities are already represented in psora (vata).

Now we come to the landscape of potentials on the disc (x, y) with the *yin* axis (or x-axis) as *vertical* axis (*downward*) and the *yang axis* (or y-axis) as *horizontal* axis (positive axis towards the *right*), cf. Figure 9.1b. Here the parabola and the straight line, whose contribution and influence on the disc vary, come into play:

$$E_{pot}(s) = 2s^6 - 3s^4 + (9/8)*[1+(x/r_c)]\,s^2 - (y/r_c)\,s\,;\ r_c = 0.7;$$

$$-1 \leq x \leq 1,\ -1 \leq y \leq 1,\ x^2+y^2 \leq 1. \tag{13.1}$$

The coefficients will be explained shortly. For a given x and y, a landscape of potentials develops as a function of the abstract variable s. For selected values of x and y, the corresponding curve of potentials is given in Figure 13.1&2. Figure 13.2 shows the landscape of potentials $E_{pot}(s)$ for the seven characteristic points of the disc: for the centre as well as the points $V_m^+, K_m^-, P_m^+, V_m^-, K_m^+, P_m^-$ of the circle representation; cf. Figure 9.4 for integration of the circle representation (r=r_c=0.7) into the health disc (r=R=1). This integration is, incidentally, the reason for the appearance of the parameter r_c in (13.1). Along the temperature-neutral *yin* axis (y=0; from x=-1 to x=1) the linear term $- (y/r_c)s$ in (13.1) drops out and only the *even* powers remain ($s^6, -s^4, s^2$). Thus, E_{pot} remains left/right symmetrical, where with increasing x the parabola opening upward (cf. Figure 13.1a) makes an ever-greater contribution.

In Figure 13.1b another condition in vata can be recognised (x=-0.35, y=0) whose locale corresponds to point 'b' in Figure 13.2. It already shows a stabilisation of the equilibrium which was still unstable in V_m^+ at s=0. In addition, the other two valleys come a little closer to s=0. They are also not quite as deep, which enables the ball to return with the aid of a slight jiggling in case it jumps out of the central valley. The difference in height between the left (or right) maximum and the left (or right) minimum is barely 0.5; the flat minimum at s=0 is just below the maxima.

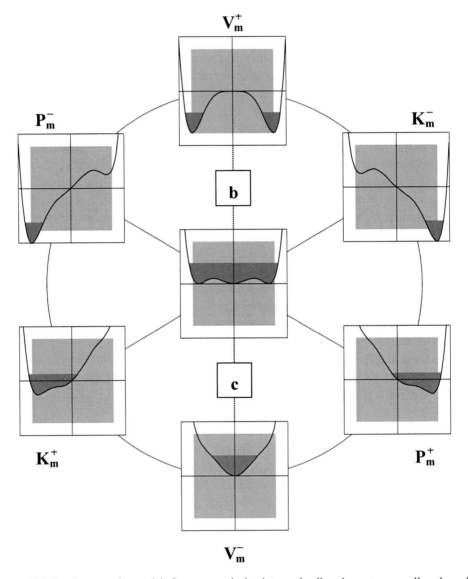

Figure 13.2. Landscapes of potentials for seven typical points on the disc: the centre as well as the points V_m^-, K_m^-, P_m^+, V_m^-, K_m^+, P_m^- (cf. Figure 9.4). Two additional positions (**b**, **c**) specify the sites, whose E_{pot} is given by Figure 13.1a&b.

As x grows, the central valley becomes larger (see Figure 13.2, graphs in the middle from top to bottom, and Figure 13.1c). In the centre of the disc (x=0) the three valleys are of equal depth, which corresponds to an equipoise of V, P and K. This condition, incidentally, forced the coefficient in equation (13.1) to be (9/8). As x increases, we move along the border of V/P and finally arrive at V_m^-, {earth}. Already at x=0.35 (Figure 13.1c, locale of point 'c' in

Figure 13.2) we see that the central valley has absorbed the other two. Nothing of kapha or pitta remains at V_m^- (x=0.70, bottommost graph in Figure 13.2). No balancing is required here and jiggling no longer plays a role. This automatically results in the stable vata principle being actualised not in {metal} or in vata itself but at the opposite site, in {earth}. This is a different wording for the confusion of {metal} and {earth} and/or perspective P3 (a modified version is: *"One stands for the other"*).

The parabola thus plays a role in the variability of the potential on the yin axis (or x-axis). In (13.1) there is an additional term, representing a straight line whose slope is $-(y/r_c)$. This term breaks the previous left/right symmetry of the potential curve. Because of the negative sign of the additional term, the potential is lower on the *left* than on the right for y<0, and for y>0 it is lower on the *right* than on the left (cf. the two outer graphs in Figure 13.2, on the right and left side). One more comment needs to be made to simplify the comparison of the seven positions on the disc depicted in this Figure: note how the two graphs on the right result from reflecting the graphs on the left about the vertical axis (and vice versa). If we look just at the two graphs on the right, we can see that in the upper curve the valley on the left is only expressed very weakly while the one on the right is particularly deep and dominating. In the lower curve, only the right-hand valley is stable (however, it reaches all the way into the vata region).

Here a wide range of conditions comes about with their focus in pitta, which corresponds to the location P_m^+ /{wood} of the chosen point, while in the upper picture, K_m^- /{fire}, kapha-like conditions are (weakly) represented, too. This is interesting inasmuch as {fire} is located exactly *opposite* to kapha (an analogous situation applies to {flora} opposite to pitta). A similarity in the respective axes is obvious here. In conclusion, it should be pointed out that the landscape in the centre of the disc is particularly wide and more and more accentuated toward the edge. In parallel, the organism is increasingly compelled to fight against possible disadvantages of the landscape, which promotes a tendency to falling ill. Admittedly, this also depends on the direction. In the upper half of the disc the landscape is more accentuated and thus 'more critical' than in the lower half. This, however, is counter-balanced by the fact that the life spiral comes closer to the centre there.

Now we turn to the comparison between V_m^+, K_m^- and P_m^- (see the upper three landscapes in Figure 13.2). Vata-like conditions (the region around s=0) are *unstable* in all three cases. An organism derailed to the right at V_m^+ (after pitta-like conditions) might behave in a similar manner as in K_m^-, for the valleys to the right of each look very similar. However, there is one crucial difference: In the first case the organism COULD behave differently, the landscape itself is symmetrical. In the second case, the symmetry is no longer innately present. Gienow talks about *functional* disturbances in the first case, which are *fixated* (somatised) in the second case, and in Ayurveda the argument is similar. In our present interpretation, not only the *behaviour* (position of the ball) but also the *landscape* itself has changed. The fact that the respective right-hand valleys of psora and the tubercular miasm are so similar is probably the reason why the latter is often called *pseudo-psora*. In an analogous manner, *parasitosis* should also be seen as (the other side of) pseudo-psora (see the left upper graph of Figure 13.2 at P_m^-). Indeed, Gienow (2000, p.86) speaks of parasitosis being the 'other pseudo-psora'. On p.105 a comparison between the tubercular miasm and parasitosis shows that the first erupts in the direction of *activity* and the second in the direction of *exhaustion* (for us here this means to the *right* and *left*, respectively).

13.2. The Health Disc:
Division into Zones, Dynamics

Before we take another step, let us divide the disc into zones to indicate the respective valleys specified by the landscape of potentials. We have already discovered that in K_m^- / {fire}, for example, there are two valleys, namely the right (r), pitta-like and the left (l), kapha-like, where the latter is only accentuated weakly. In Figure 13.3, the solid curves mark the borders of the zones; the resulting seven zones are characterised by the indication of the number and location of the valleys (m stands for the *middle* vata-like valley). K_m^- (in Figure 13.2 top, right in direction of K_e^- but on the dashed circle), for example, is located in zone **2** (l,r). That is, there are two valleys, $l\&r$, in K_m^-. Due to its proximity to zone **1** (r) with only one valley, (r), the right valley of K_m^- is considerably deeper than that on the left. In P_m^+, only the right valley is well-formed. However, the border between the two-valley region **2** (m,r) is in close proximity, which is expressed in the levelling mentioned in Figure 13.2, bottom right.

Around the centre (in the region of the *three-dosha* and the *metal* types) we find a trapezoidal region **3** (l,m,r) with three valleys. Further down (at V_m^-), zone **1** (m), which has already been mentioned, appears where only the central valley is stable. The other zones result by symmetry of reflection about the vertical x-axis, where l and r must be exchanged in the representation of the respective valleys; m remains unchanged. In all cases, a comparison with Figure 13.1-3 is helpful. The borders of the zones, incidentally, arise wherever flex points and extrema (maxima, minima) of the landscape merge. This requires solving equations of degree two. Only the solution where y_{border} represents the y-value at a zone's border will be presented here:

$$y_{border} = \pm (r_c/50) * [(Q+6)/5]^{1/2} * [6Q-9-45(x/r_c)],$$
$$\text{with: } Q = \pm [21-15(x/r_c)]^{1/2}, \; r_c = 0.7. \tag{13.2}$$

Thus, there are four solutions in all for y_{border} as a function of x (see Figure 13.3). The four boundaries can be recognised easily. They form two pairs, each pair a result of reflection about the x-axis. The twelve meridians are distributed over the seven zones in such a manner that each zone contains at least one meridian, three zones contain two, and the zone characterised by three valleys even contains three meridians. It is striking that the largest zone, **2** (l,r), does not contain a single meridian on the left-hand side (where the kapha-like valley is deepest) – and this is just close to the vata/ kapha border, which stands for birth and death. In the context of Ch.9.5, we came across a similar question. There, we argued that at this border the superordinate meridians, governing and conception vessel, find their place. However, they are not part of the 'usual' meridians considered here. If we include them in Figure 13.3, then there will be four meridians in the large zone **2** (l,r), two on the left (governing vessel, conception vessel) and two on the right (HT, SI).

Here we need to make one more remark about the linear term in (13.1), $-(y/r_c)s$ or rather more general $-F(y/r_c)s$ (F: positive constant). The minus sign simplifies interpretation. A ball in the potential landscape on the right, $s>0$, typically corresponds to the behaviour in locations on the right of the disc; in other words, you do not have to think backwards. Now to the factor F: it can neither be chosen arbitrarily like the coefficients of s^6 and $-s^4$, nor does it result automatically like the coefficient of $[1+(x/r_c)]$ s^2. As expected – as in the case of the other terms in (13.1) – it has a magnitude of around 1. An aid in determining the choice of F is the fact that the zone (borders) are more and more compressed toward the yin axis with increasing F and are stretched more and more with decreasing F (the extension is proportional to the respective $|y|$, and the behaviour on the yin axis remains unchanged). For $F>2$ the two **1**-zones (on the right or left respectively) dominate the disc; for $F<1/2$, on the other hand, these two zones are pushed off the disc. But the health disc represents the whole spectrum of human behaviour and for this reason should be as comprehensive as possible. A reasonable distribution of the zones results at or near $F=1$. For this reason we shall just consider the case $F=1$; see (13.1).

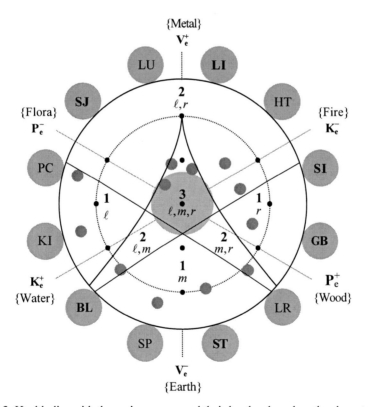

Figure 13.3. Health disc with the various zones and their borders based on the characteristics of the landscape model, E_{pot}. **1**, **2** or **3** refer to the number of valleys of the potential function E_{pot} in the respective zones. The letters refer to the location of the valleys: left (l), middle (m) or right (r). The position of the twelve meridians (●) is the same as in Figure 8.4. The small black dots are sites playing a particular role in this chapter. Note especially V_m^+, K_m^-, P_m^+, V_m^-, K_m^+ & P_m^-, which lie in direction of V_e^+, K_e^-, P_e^+, V_e^-, K_e^+ & P_e^-, namely on the dashed circle in the circle representation ($r_c=0.7$).

The zone borders have something to do with transitions and dynamics. For this reason, comparison with the dynamics of falling ill in Ch.11 is interesting; see Figure 11.3 for the 6-cycle (dynamics I) and the 3-cycle (dynamics II). Furthermore, we can compare the zone borders with the division of the disc discussed in Ch.12 (see Table 12.2). In Ch.11, we saw that *SI, LI, GB, SP, KI* and *LR* participate in Dynamics I (the order of sequence being according to TCM interpretation). *GB* and *LR* are located in zone **2** (m,r) and the remaining four meridians in different zones. In four steps of the 6-cycle *two* zone borders are crossed, in the step from *KI* to *LR three*, but from *SI* to *LI* only *one*. Since a change in zones is connected with a change in landscape and a possible jump of the ball into another valley, it stands to reason that the change is more improbable and more lengthy the more the landscape changes. Going back and forth between *SI* and *LI* is easy, since only one border needs to be crossed.

In Ch.12.4, incidentally, another argument led to the conclusion that the differing order of succession SI – LI or LI – SI, according to Gienow and TCM respectively, can be explained by the rapid movement to and fro. From *KI* to *LR* it is the other way round: here the ball must cross three borders. Gienow does not even mention the resulting jump from kapha to pitta. This could be because the cycle – if it occurs at all – gets stuck in stage 5 (*shaoyin, KI*, Table 11.6) and not, as assumed in Ch.11.4, in stage 6 (a *delay* instead of getting stuck symbolically means a day off on *Saturday* instead of Sunday). Indeed, TCM often regards stage 5 as the critical state (Kaptchuk 1996, p.294).

Now let us look at the other meridians and, first, the ones involved in dynamics II (*LU, SJ* and *BL*). The first two stages of falling ill are in zone **3** (l,m,r), the third stage (*BL*) in the adjacent zone **2** (l,m), which was the last zone remaining open but has now been filled. In order to reach it and close the cycle, the same zone border must be crossed. Since all stages are adjacent here, a rapid to and fro is to be expected. Perhaps this is why this form of dynamics is not explicitly accounted for in TCM. Finally, we get to the three meridians not involved in any cycle, *HT, ST* and *PC*. All three have yet another meridian in their zone. A closer look at Figure 13.3 reveals another interesting point: the last meridians of the two cycles, *LR* (dynamics I) and *BL* (dynamics II), lie almost as mirror images with respect to the x-axis, and are the only ones that exhibit this behaviour. Thus, their landscapes are also reflected in a close approximation about the vertical axis.

Another question from Ch.11 arose with regard to the assignment of *GB* (at shaoyang, 3rd stage) and *LR* (at jueyin, 6th stage) in dynamics I. In both cases, according to TCM, there is confusion regarding temperature. This mostly concerns the question of which stages are *hot* or *cold* (although, since the central valley corresponds to neutral temperatures, we shall now interpret the issue as *hot* versus *not hot*). At first sight it looks as though *GB* and *LR* must be excluded, because they are clearly *hot* (both to the *right* in the circle representation corresponding to a *positive* y-value). However, the y-value in our present perspective only contributes to the shape of the landscape and does not yet tell us the actual condition of the system. The landscape of P_m^+ (Figure 13.3) applies approximately to both meridians. Accordingly, the landscape there is very wide and flat (Figure 13.2) and medium to high temperatures are possible. This implies wide fluctuations in temperature in both cases, which is also described in TCM (see the comments on Table 11.6). On the other hand, *PC* is located near P_m^-, which clearly corresponds to a low temperature (Figure 13.2-3). For this reason, *PC* will not be considered as a candidate for the last illness stage of dynamics I, as opposed to *LR*. It should be noted that *BL* exhibits a wide range of lower to medium temperatures as 3rd stage of cycle II due to the mirror symmetry to *LR*.

After a cycle of falling ill, the organism ends up at *SI* (dynamics I) again or at *LU* (dynamics II), but now both are located closer to the boundary of the disc. As has already been mentioned in Ch.11.4, *falling ill* can be interpreted as the meridians moving towards the boundary of the disc. This process also causes the respective landscape to become more accentuated, which thus makes 'breaking away' even more difficult. In the case of *recovery*, then, the meridians move *inwards* (the cycle moving in the reverse direction). This brings with it a levelling of the landscape and the respective valley is easier to leave. Falling ill and convalescence can also be described by way of a change in *noise level*. A more vigorous jiggling of the landscape aids the ball to surmount the hills – as if the landscape were levelled. This heightens the system's flexibility. Now we imagine a very high noise level that overcomes, for example, all unevenness near s=0 for all sites on the disc (x, y). This corresponds to a total potential in which practically only the leading power proportional to s^6 remains (Figure 13.1a). This, in turn, becomes so steep away from s=0 that even the strongest noise cannot overcome it. Overall one potential remains, which is symmetrical around s=0 and similar to the usual potential of V_m^-, or {earth}; cf. Figure 13.2 (bottom).

13.3. Valleys, Lakes and Stochastic Resonance

In dividing the zones, the respective number of valleys of the potential function E_{pot} was important, more precisely the minima, which define a valley. In the sense of the pure landscape model (with friction and without noise), the ball can always be found in one of the lowest points of the valleys (locations: s_{min}). Furthermore, in the description of our model in Ch.13.1 we also spoke of the contribution made by noise, which is able to move the ball away from the minima. The noise level can be seen as the water level in the potential landscape. The landscape is filled with water up to a certain level H; only the parts of the landscape hidden by the water are accessible to the ball within a reasonable time frame. As a mental exercise supported by Figure 13.1-2, we can imagine that a spring emerges from the floor of the valley (the minimum of the respective valley), which allows the water to rise from zero to a certain level. This 'lake' in the valley will initially be rather small and its centre $s^{\#}$ at the surface will be close to the minimum s_{min}. The centre will be displaced upwards and, parallel to it, the parameter $\delta^{\#}$ representing the length of the lake, will grow. It spans from $[s^{\#}-(\delta^{\#}/2)]$ to $[s^{\#}+(\delta^{\#}/2)]$. At a critical height, the water will reach an adjacent maximum (the 'top of the dam'). As a result a waterfall will flow into a neighbouring valley, which then creates a second lake until the maximum of this valley is reached and the two lakes merge into one (H then represents the height measured from the lowest minimum). An example of this (with three valleys) is given in Figure 13.1b, where first the small valley is filled proceeding from the low minimum, $s_{min}=0$, and then the water spills over into both adjacent valleys. Finally, shortly before reaching the final height of H=0.5 in Ch.13.1, the two hills are flooded from the outside and one continuous lake results.

The zone borders given in Figure 13.3 apply to the absence of noise (water level zero). As the water level rises, they are being displaced in the direction of a zone with a higher number. Once a noise level of H=0.5, for example in Ch.13.1, is reached, only the structures in the upper region of the circle representation will still be visible. The part of the disc below about x=-0.35 (Figure 13.1b) will soon form a large 1-zone. The effect of the noise (water level H) can be characterised in two ways, the 'upper' and the 'lower'. The *upper* method measures the *surface* of the lake (centre $s^\#$, length $\delta^\#$) and the *lower* method estimates these values by way of (s_{min}, δ). In this process the landscape 'below' (near the bottom of the valley, s_{min}) is replaced by a parabola, whose minimum lies at s_{min} and whose curvature at s_{min} is the same as that of the potential function. For example, the *minimum* of the parabola, as^2, is at s_{min}=0, the *curvature* is 2a, the length of the lake at height H=0.5 is δ=(2/a$^{1/2}$). Expressed more generally:

Parabola a(s–s$_o$)^2: s$_{min}$= s$_o$, length of the lake at height H: δ_H=2[2H/a]$^{1/2}$.   (13.3)

The upper method yields *exact* values for $s^\#$ and $\delta^\#$, but these must be determined numerically and individually for each height. The lower method only gives *estimated* values for s_{min} and δ_H (which are exact for small values of H), but one single analytical Formula δ_H can be used for all H, see (13.3). This results in two complementary statements regarding the landscape around a minimum. The difference between the results of the two methods is a measure for the deviation of the landscape from the shape of a parabola up to height, H. In Figure 13.1 the results for eleven sites on the disc are given. They include the (2+7) locations of Figures 13.1b-c & 13.2, cf. Figure 9.1, supplemented by the points Y_m^- (x=0, y=-0.7) and Y_m^+ (x=0, y=0.7). Incidentally, all 11 sites are marked as black dots in Figure 13.3. Returning to Table 13.1, we see that (for H=0.5) $s^\#$ and s_{min} as well as $\delta^\#$ and δ are given for the lowest minima, supplemented by s=0 where we have a minimum but not the lowest minimum, i.e. for (x=-0.35, y=0), Figure 13.1b. In this case – just as at the centre – there are three minima. For this reason, there are also two specifications of sites and lengths (for lakes that originate from the central and right minimum, left and right are symmetrical). Due to the overflow into the neighbouring valley, the upper method is only useful for comparison to a limited extent and is therefore shown in parentheses.

Table 13.1 shows pairs of rows, where the results for the *upper* method are given in the top row and the results from the *lower* method underneath. Because of the symmetry of re-flection, only the lengths of the lakes are given on the left and only their centres on the right. The reader can easily fill in the rest. As to the centres and sites: it should be noted that $s^\#$ and s_{min} (on the right) deviate notably from one another, which implies a deviation from the parabola shape near the minima. The decisive factor, however, is the general trend, which is the same for both methods if one compares the results from one of the two methods for the eleven positions on the disc. From top to bottom (whether vertically or at an angle), the *locations* $s^\#$ and s_{min} approach the value 0 or land exactly on this value (cf. Figure 13.1-2). In the end only the middle valley is stable ($s^\#$ =s_{min}=0). For the *lengths* $\delta^\#$ and δ, the behaviour is more interesting: If one ignores the middle valley, the length keeps increasing from top to bottom (vertically or at an angle). If, on the other hand, *only* the middle valley is considered, the reverse is the case! In Ch.13.4, we shall come back to this and draw conclusions regarding the mode of action of yin and yang. For now, we shall just point out one thing: the centre as well as the length of the lakes in the kapha-like left valley of V_m^+ (*metal*) closely agrees with the result for *flora* (the best match by comparisons within the same method). The same goes for the pitta-like right valley of V_m^+ and *fire*. This means that *flora* and *fire* can mirror or rather simulate a partial aspect of *metal*. The same is true for parasitosis and the tubercular miasm as partial aspects of psora ('pseudo-psora'). We had already discovered this by looking at the shapes of the landscapes in Figure 13.2. This is now demonstrated in the characteristic parameters of the location and the width of the landscape near a minimum.

Table 13.1. Characterisation of the potential landscape by centre ($s^{\#}$, $s_{\min}$) and length ($\delta^{\#}$, δ) of a lake of height H=0.5 above the minimum. Eleven sites (pairs x, y) on the disc are considered (cf. Figure 13.1-3). The locations (centres) are given to the right of the vertical midline, the lengths on the left. The reflected values on the other side would need a minus sign at these locations, but the lengths would not change. In each pair of row, the upper row shows the results ($\delta^{\#}|s^{\#}$) of the 'upper' method and the lower row the results ($\delta|s_{\min}$) of the 'lower' method

x ↓	$\delta^{\#}$ / δ				$s^{\#}$ / $s_{\min}$			
−0.70				0.46	0.92			
-"-				0.41	1.00			
−0.35		0.46	(2.27)	2.27	0	(0)	0.92	
-"-		0.43	0.50	1.89	0	0.94	0.98	
0	0.69		(2.18)	2.18	0	(0)		0.78
-"-	0.51		0.67	1.33	0	0.87		0.93
0.35		1.21		1.82	0		0.47	
-"-		0.71		1.09	0		0.84	
0.70				1.14	0			
-"-				0.94	0			
y →	−0.70	$-0.35*3^{1/2}$	0	0	0	0	$0.35*3^{1/2}$	0.70

The model of potentials contains only one fixed component and one varying as a function of the location on the disc. The latter encompasses the *parabola* and *straight line*, cf. (13.1). The organism keeps healthy by suitable movement on the disc (x, y) and thus indirectly by changing the potential landscape (straight line and parabola component). This location also offers a starting point for therapeutic measures (see below). Furthermore, we discussed noise in general and *instability control* near V_m^+ in particular. One might assume that the noise level can be varied by the organism to a certain degree – in other words, that there is a possibility of an external influence serving as a therapeutic measure. These questions will also be addressed in Ch. 13.4.

Now we shall compare the division into zones, which has been discussed, with the regions displayed in Figure 12.2, which illustrates the laws of indication. Above all, it becomes apparent that the organism cannot accomplish regulation at the bottom or top of the disc.

There are similarities between Figure 12.2 and Figure 13.3, but also differences. The latter refers to the ball being trapped in the left and the right valley at P_m^- and K_m^-, respectively (cf. Figure 13.2), whereas both points lie in the region of harmonisation of Figure 12.2. However, there is agreement concerning V_m^- – the ball being trapped in the middle valley, where the meridians SP and ST are located. According to Figure 12.2, these are the only meridians that unambiguously lie outside the region of harmonisation. Even more interesting are the meridians that lie on borders of this region: BL and LR lie in both figures at the lower border; LU and LI lie in both figures at the analogous upper border. Variants of both models may be compared, too: in Figure 12.2, width B of the 'rectangles' may be varied according to (12.3), and the same is possible for height H of the 'water level' or noise. This is, however, beyond the scope of our present considerations.

Let us go back to another research field of complex systems that has a close connection to our model here: stochastic resonance (Ch.4.3). This concerns the paradoxical phenomenon that helps weak information to get through with the aid of noise. To illustrate this let us look at the potential function in V_m^+ (Figure 13.2, top). Here we have two valleys of equal depth; the ball cannot get from one to the other unaided. One remedy is to add noise, i.e. jiggle the landscape. If the jiggling is very weak, this will not help the situation. With strong jiggling, the ball will jump around from valley to valley. There is a medium noise level, however, which elicits an occasional change of valleys but at irregular intervals. The funny thing about stochastic resonance lies in the fact that the landscape, too, is 'rocked' in a rhythmic manner (at one time the left minimum is a little lower than the right, at another the reverse is the case). This rocking frequency also expresses in the frequency with which the ball jumps around. Simply stated, the ball will jump into the lower minimum in phase with the rocking motion. The information on the rocking frequency is not suppressed by the noise but augmented.

In stochastic resonance, there is usually one signal for which an optimal noise level must be determined. Similarly, one could optimise the rocking of the landscape for a given noise level. On the disc, the rocking corresponds to a going to and fro between two sites (x, y). This, then, brings us back to vata / {metal} / psora and the fluctuations always reported there with regard to heat and cold as well as humidity and dryness (see Ch.7.2 and Heise 1996, p.11). We must not get confused by the fact that in medicine systems often only *one* side is emphasised (TCM: dryness of {metal}, Ayurveda: coldness of vata, homoeopathy: the 'too little' of psora). Now the two valleys in vata along the vertical axis have equal depth; going back and forth from right to left has exactly the effect of rocking the landscape mentioned in stochastic resonance. By the way, there is one additional concern in vata: instability control. The ball needs to be stabilised on top of the hill (maximum). We shall have to take a closer look at this.

That vata is easily brought out of balance and just as easily gets back into balance can be accounted for by taking noise into consideration. On the one hand, jiggling the landscape endangers stabilising the ball at the maximum at s=0; the ball rolls off the summit whenever control fails. On the other hand, it is this jiggling that brings the ball back to the top where it can be stabilised anew. However, although we assumed that noise could typically counterbalance differences in height of 0.5 units, near V_m^+ the difference is greater. Here stochastic resonance can be of help (with the additional process of instability control). For this process, however, the system must go back and forth between left-skewed and right-skewed potentials (V-K, V-P). In this way, with the aid of noise, the ball has a high probability of being brought over the hill out of one of the two valleys and rolling – hopefully relatively slowly – to the maximum. Now here again the stabilising process comes into effect and captures the ball at the top. This, of course, must happen at the right moment, otherwise the ball will continue to go to and fro. This typical vata behaviour, then, has much to do with keeping healthy. However, it can get out of control through too much movement back and forth, and then one of the two illness progressions that we have already discussed takes over.

One more comment needs to be made concerning the capture of the ball once it is on the top of the hill: the slower the ball passes by, the easier it is. For this process, weak noise is beneficial, but then the ball only gets there relatively infrequently. However, one result of stochastic resonance is helpful here: the ball rolling over the hill in phase with the rocking motion. In our example, this result can be seen in a new light: the organism, by setting the rocking into motion itself, is able to guess when the ball will go over the hill, which makes catching it easier (however, this may happen).

One of the ways in which the two-facedness of vata expresses itself is in the particular characteristics of the main remedy for psora (vata), sulphur. There are two completely different types which both require homoeopathic sulphur: the more mental ('white, cold') sulphur type and the more body-oriented ('red, hot') sulphur type. The fact that the same remedy can be beneficial in such contrary cases can be explained with the aid of the potential at V_m^+. The same person (characterised by the same potential function) can derail into two opposite directions, kapha-like or pitta-like. Thus, because of an unsuccessful balance two 'identical people' can appear completely different but need the same homoeopathic remedy (sulphur). This brings us to the question of how remedies can be effective within the frame of our model and will be addressed in the next section.

13.4. Unipolar and Bipolar Remedies

In our model, the organism is able to change the potential function by varying the component of parabola and straight line and also making use of the noise component for control. Therefore, it seems logical that these three possibilities can also be applied *externally*. In TCM, internal and external heat are distinguished, e.g. for {fire}. Both are connected to the component of straight line of the potential, cf. Figure 13.1a and (13.1) – caused once by *inner* and once by *outer* influences. This makes the potential deeper on the right. Through internal reactions to outer influences, however, the relationships become even more complicated. Let us stay with the example of temperature: according to Ayurveda, hot weather means that the organism switches to cooling, that is to say that external heat in general is connected to internal cold and vice versa. From the point of view of dynamics, the body heats up when external temperature in hot weather suddenly rises, but an internal counter mechanism is quickly put into action, which, by overreacting, first produces an excess of cold and then levels off to the right amount. In other words, periods of worsening and improvement occur in turn.

Regulation mistakes can occur in typical situations, apparently including the 6-cycle of falling ill (dynamics I, Figure 11.3). In TCM, one speaks of 'cold-induced heat disorders', which characterise the first part of the cycle. If the system is hit in *SI* by external cold, this corresponds to a shift to the left (temperature axis) in direction of *LI*. An overshooting counter regulation produces an internal heat, which drives the system back to the right in the direction of *GB* passing *LI* (the motion in a vertical direction is ignored in this simplified consideration). The illness cycle then runs its course.

Chopra (1993, p.109f) talks about 'hundreds of thermostats' in Ayurveda. This refers to the considerable number of variables that interact in a cybernetically interlinked system. For the sake of simplicity, we only consider *one* variable, s, in our model, which consequently stands for many things. Adding one more variable would result in a three-dimensional landscape, but a more realistic version would include higher dimensions. Some of these variables are interlinked to such a degree that a derailing of one variable in general would throw the other variables of that same group out of balance as well. Depending on the susceptibility, there are typical illness pictures for any one person. The classification into types can be made to varying degrees of refinement. We have mentioned during the course of this book the numbers 3, 4, 5, 6, 7 and 12. In homoeopathy, there are well about 200 well-documented remedy pictures. Discovering complex connections and combining them into suitable types would also be a worthwhile endeavour for orthodox Western medicine, but presumably statistics in its current form is still overtaxed by such an endeavour. In Far Eastern medicine, lengthy experience and intuition have solved this problem.

Depending on the individual's predisposition and weakness, balancing a group of variables – represented by the variable s – is particularly difficult in vata. The unproblematic variables can be completely ignored in this situation. On the other hand, during a remedy proving of a certain homoeopathic remedy, the ball can be made to fall (in the ideal case) in a healthy person especially with respect to those variables that are expressed in the remedy picture. But with the aid of the simile principle this same homoeopathic remedy enables an individual who has been derailed with regard to these variables to be healed. You can think of it as follows: A homoeopathic remedy raises the noise level of those variables that make up the remedy picture. The organism, taken by surprise by the remedy proving, will then show a tendency to lose its balance exactly with respect to those variables. Conversely, in a person who has fallen ill with respect to those variables, the ball can be brought back up the hill by jiggling the 'critical' variables. As soon as the ball is on the top and the system attempts to catch it again, the symptoms recede and the homoeopathic remedy should no longer be taken because, from this point on, the jiggling will hamper the balancing process and act counterproductively. Indeed, continued use of a homoeopathic remedy during a substantial improvement in symptoms is considered malpractice.

This is how the simile principle can be explained. Admittedly, only the case of a loss of balance in vata or psora was considered, more precisely near $\alpha=180°$ (the median angle of vata). On the other hand, this goes nicely with the statement of Gienow that the simile principle of homoeopathy can only be applied successfully there, in the region of the latent psora (see also Figure 12.2). Before this, the patient must be met at that place (on the disc) where he is currently situated and the illness must be shifted with the aid of (anti-)miasmatic remedies from there via the healing miasms to psora. Depending on the cycle of recovery, one ends up at *LI* (6-cycle) or *LU* (3-cycle). There, the simile principle can be brought to bear. The discussion among homoeopaths as to whether miasms are important or unimportant finds a suggested solution here in terms of a chronological division of labour.

Now let us go back to the variation of the potential function itself, see (13.1). In (13.4a) a corresponding modification through external influences is built in. The factors, N and L, can be positive or negative; N stands for *non-linear*, L for *linear*. Eq. (13.4b) is equivalent to (13.4a); it shows how to convert an external influence into a corresponding change of position on the health disc from (x, y) to (x', y'):

$$E_{pot}(s) = 2s^6 - 3s^4 + (9/8)*[1+(x/r_c)]\,s^2 - (y/r_c)\,s + Ns^2 - Ls\,; \qquad (13.4a)$$

$$E_{pot}(s) = 2s^6 - 3s^4 + (9/8)*[1+(x'/r_c)]\,s^2 - (y'/r_c)\,s\,,\ \text{with}\ x' = N(8/9)\,r_c,\ y' = B\,r_c\,. \qquad (13.4b)$$

Let us look first at the straight line as a typical case of orthodox Western medicine: If s, for example, stands for blood pressure, then a medication that *raises* blood pressure corresponds to a *positive* coefficient L, which for the sake of simplicity will be proportional to the dosage. No matter what the potential $E_{pot}(s)$ looked like before, the change occurring as a result of the medication shifts the ball in the variable s corresponding to s_{min}-shift to the right, see (13.4a). In (13.4b) the same process is interpreted as a movement on the health disc, where additional internal consequential reactions are ignored. For small doses L, the shift s is proportional to the shift in y (a linear effect). Increasing the dose, however, can change the structure of the landscape (the number of valleys, Figure 13.3). As soon as the border of a zone is crossed, the position of the ball can change suddenly. In any case, all movement is in one direction only (horizontally on the disc as well as with respect to s_{min}): to the right for L positive (medication raising the blood pressure), to the left for L negative (medication lowering the blood pressure). We shall refer to this as a *unipolar* influence. This is the primary field of orthodox Western medicine.

There are also substances with quite a different mode of action. Here we can take digitalis, which we have already mentioned, as an example since it can both lower and raise the heart rate, virtually independent of the dosage. It therefore acts (potentially) in two directions, which we shall from now on call a *bipolar* effect. It can be represented by a change in the *parabola* (factor N). The independence of the dosage cannot be accommodated completely (what happens in case of negligibly small doses?) but nonetheless, for simplicity, we shall assume N to be constant (N can, of course, have different values for different bipolar remedies). N<0 (parabola opening downward) corresponds to destabilising (polarising) substances, N>0 (parabola opening upward) to stabilising substances. Since the parabola has its origin in s=0, these expressions refer to the vata-like state or the middle valley (*m*), and the reverse is true regarding the pitta- and kapha-like states. So stabilising the middle valley automatically means destabilising the other two valleys. The influence of a bipolar medication corresponds to a fixed *vertical* shift of location on the disc – up for N<0, down for N>0, see Figure 13.3 and equation (13.4). N>0 makes the hill in vata flatter in the potential landscape or may even turn it into a *hollow* (in the case of a corresponding zone border being crossed); in any case it facilitates balancing in the vata region.

Thus, it looks as though *stabilising* also means *making healthy*. Furthermore, it appears that the region of earth where the central valley is innately stable is especially healthy. However, these two sentences are only true as long as s=0 is the desired value. Depending on which variable(s) s represents and the varying demands by the individual's surroundings, going away from s=0 can be desirable. In this case, one will not be able to get out of the deep hollow at earth near s=0 and a bipolar polarising (destabilising) remedy is indicated. This, then, allows the organism to regulate in the direction of the desired valley (to the right or left). The following holds overall:

x<0 (upper half of the disc): bipolar-stabilising remedy is beneficial;   (13.5a)

x>0 (lower half of the disc): bipolar-polarising remedy is beneficial.   (13.5b)

In both cases movement is toward x=0 (the horizontal y-axis of the disc), where the organism is self-regulating (see Figure 12.2). Thus, we have found a connection to the 'stratification' of the disc in view of the laws of indication, with the broad horizontal region of harmonisation. In this region, an unspecific or, alternatively, neutral stimulus (zero crossing in Figure 9.5) is sufficient to trigger a process of regulation. Thus, the two approaches have different starting points, but produce similar results.

The fact that digitalis causes the heartbeat to increase or decrease in some people, points to a bipolar remedy. However, this does not tell us whether it is *polarising* or *stabilising*. In the former case it would destabilise a normal heartbeat and – proceeding from a normal heartbeat – lead to a higher or lower rate; in the latter case, it would help to establish a median heart frequency in all individuals, i.e. lowering the rate when it was too high or raising it when it was too low. This kind of therapy belongs to regulative medicine, but perhaps homoeopathic remedies also act in this way. By flattening the landscape at s=0, stabilising remedies make it easier for the organism to return the ball to this location. If a depression is formed, the ball rolls into the minimum by itself. Once the effect of the homoeopathic remedy subsides, the organism must again take over the balancing process; the organism's active cooperation is then required.

Thus, we have been introduced to two possible ways of describing the effect of homoeopathic remedies. At this time, there is no telling whether homoeopathy is best described by the effect of noise or by bipolar stabilising effects. The problems that may occur with prolonged unnecessary therapy with homoeopathic remedies can also be explained with the current approach: after some time, the organism ceases (or limits) its efforts to stabilise 'unnecessarily' the situation; then, as soon as the homoeopathic remedy is discontinued, the ball inevitably falls down. A similar process occurs with the simile principle (remedy proving): the support of the homoeopathic remedy is also answered by a ceasing of the organism's own efforts. In both cases, the negative consequences presumably do not emerge immediately but after the homoeopathic effect has subsided. However, the rules for the use of various potencies of a homoeopathic remedy point to the fact that we are dealing with a *combination* of bipolar effect and noise, in the sense that raising the homoeopathic potency decreases the noise component and increases the stabilising component. The effect of high potencies is usually prolonged, so that longer intervals may be left between doses than with lower potencies. This is only sensible if *quick* stabilising is guaranteed, which cannot be accomplished with noise.

Repeated use of *lower* potencies is, in turn, an indication of *noise*, since several attempts are necessary to ensure success. It is also possible that N increases along with the potency, so that, from a certain potency on, s=0 becomes a stable minimum and from then on one single dose suffices. Thus, the two modes of action of homoeopathic remedies might be distinguished in the following way: In the bipolar-stabilising case. there should be – in principle – one *universally* acting homoeopathic remedy apart from the ones which are acting on an individual level; and this should stabilise all possible variables in s=0 (the so-called polychrests might be a partial solution here). A universal remedy that shakes up all possible variables is, on the other hand, *not* suitable as a homoeopathic remedy, since it would also endanger the many variables already in balance.

There are also substances that display both unipolar and bipolar effects. They might even be in the majority, since the case N≠0 *and* L≠0, see (13.4), is the more general. They can be recognised by the drug descriptions – for example, a laxative which has constipation as a side effect. In this case, we have a combination of *unipolar* and *bipolar-polarising* effects. Should the bipolar effect be virtually independent of the dosage then, especially with small doses where the unipolar effect (L proportional to the dose) is not yet strong, the possibility arises of the polarising effective component letting the system topple in the wrong direction. Perhaps this is the reason why orthodox Western medicine prefers to deal with higher doses.

These thoughts about bipolarity lead us back to the inconsistencies connected with the yin axis regarding which direction is *damp* and *dry*. For the temperature or yang axis, all is clear: *hot* is to the right, *cold* to the left. This axis (variable: y) could be called a unipolar axis, because it is connected with the unipolar effect of the straight line, see the term containing y in (13.1). The moisture or yin axis (variable: x), on the other hand, is connected to the bipolar effect of the parabola and could thus be called a bipolar axis. In this case the question concerning damp and dry has been stated incorrectly so far ("Where is damp, where dry?"). It should be: Where on the axis is moisture *stabilised* and where is it *polarised*? As we shall see shortly, a stable central dampness can be found at the bottom (at {earth}). *At the top* (at {metal}) moisture splits into *wet* and *dry* (polarisation). Depending on whether the aspect of dryness or that of dampness is emphasised, a 'forced unipolar interpretation' results in a top/ bottom assignment of either dry/ damp (Ayurveda, TCM) or the reverse (Greek Antiquity). Which of these aspects is determined to be the primary aspect of this axis? This depends on whether the therapy focuses on the *healthy* or the *derailed* vata.

To understand this we shall return to the landscape. There the temperature is expressed in the position s of the ball: as s increases, the system gets hotter, s=0 corresponds to a neutral temperature. Which characteristic parameter expresses the degree of moisture? If we want to stick to one variable s, then the width of the valley in which the ball is located or rather the curvature (δ or $\delta^{\#}$, 'lower' and 'upper' method) is foremost to be considered for this role. This also makes sense as *yang* has a connection to unipolarity and determines the *direction* (right or left), while *yin* is related to bipolarity and determines *coherence* (narrowness and breadth, narrow or wide hollow). The systematics of δ or $\delta^{\#}$ on the disc discovered with the aid of Table 13.1 can thus be interpreted as a systematics of *moisture*. For clarity, we shall now concentrate on Figure 13.2. The comparison K_m^+ / {water} – K_m^- / {fire} immediately makes apparent the assignment *wet* = large lake, *dry* = small lake, which can also be easily remembered. (Instability control, incidentally, keeps the condition at s=0 in a narrow range and is therefore dry). Because of the left-right symmetry of the landscapes we also have equality of moisture in the comparison of left and right. P_m^- / {flora} is as dry as K_m^- / {fire}, K_m^+ /{water} is as damp as P_m^+ /{wood}. It is well known in Ayurveda that kapha as well as pitta are damp. However, since the only undisputable Indian element of pitta is the dry ⟨fire⟩, problems arise here, which are at times 'solved' by attributing ⟨water⟩ to pitta as well (see Table 8.4). I, on the other hand, suggested adding the element, ⟨agni⟩, the damp fire of digestion (Figure 8.2).

In conclusion, let us look at what happens in the comparison bottom – top. Going up on the right or left starting with damp, things get dryer and dryer. If we climb the vertical central axis, however, we find a different situation: starting at the bottom, moisture increases as we go up (Figures 13.1b-c & 13.2) until at the split into the kapha-like and pitta-like valleys it topples into dryness, which then increases further as we continue to ascend. Thus, the two-faced character of vata is also confirmed with regard to moisture. In the healthy case (the vata region relatively near the centre of the disc) vata is wet (the Greek interpretation of air as damp), in diseased regions (farther out), on the other hand, it is dry (the Ayurvedic interpretation of vata and the usual interpretation of {metal} in TCM). Only after scrutiny of the literature does one realise that the description of this region is not clear at all but ambivalent. More precisely, the horizontal rocking in vata causes steady changes in the landscape but jerky changes in the ball's position (in the left or right valley). Vertical motion also causes constant changes in the landscape but the accessibility to the valleys changes abruptly at x=–0.35, y=0 (Figure 13.1b) due to the given water level.

Thus in vata, apart from the split hot/cold and wet/dry, there is also ambivalence regarding discontinuity (discrete) / continuity (constant); see Chs. 3.2 & 4.2. The ambivalences all come together near the point x=–0.35, y=0 (Figure 13.1b). This location is thus crucial for good health. With small measures of control the organism attempts to keep its condition in the valleys *l*, *m* or *r* as needed. According to Figure 13.3, incidentally, the two meridians of metal, LU and LI, are very close to this point, thus confirming their special role once again.

Chapter 14

Unity in Diversity:
Ethnological and Spiritual Aspects

14.1. Mind and Spirituality:
Indo-Tibetan Approaches

In Ch. 14, we shall make a spiritual journey, beginning in the realm of Hinduism and Buddhism, for doshas (Ayurveda) or nyepas (Tibetan medicine) also have a spiritual meaning. Bauhofer (1997, p. 72f) looks at Ayurveda on two connected levels: the concrete level of life (AYUS) and the abstract level of the mind or consciousness (VEDA). The classification into the physiological doshas – vata, pitta and kapha – corresponds to a division into the consciousness components rishi, devata and chhandas (see Table 14.1). For example, *seeing* refers to the seer (subject), the process of seeing (activity, subject-object relationship) and to being seen (object). Ultimately, they form a unity. However, concentrating too much on the observed object can cause the observer to disappear behind that which he observes. On the physical level, kapha is about building structure, pitta about energy production and vata about rhythmic and balancing processes. The associated gunas ('characteristics', qualities of energy) are also specified in Table 14.1; among other things, they are attributed to different foods. For instance, if a pitta type ingests food that is dominated by rajas, he runs the risk of strengthening pitta too much. For this reason such a diet must be avoided (the allopathic approach). It is noticeable that sattva only embodies the positive side of vata, while the typical characteristics of pitta and kapha are attributed to rajas and tamas. This is also true for the interpretation of the gunas as a kind of mental dosha (Rhyner 2001, p. 56f, p. 99f, p. 138f).

The assignment to the central three channels of the Indian yogic tradition can also be found in Tibetan medicine and is listed here as well. Sushumna, the central, neutral channel, runs along the spine and ends on the crown of the head. To its right is Pingala (hot, sun), to its left Ida (cold, moon); see Meyer (1988, pp. 117ff). The brain is associated with Ida and thus with kapha. This might seem strange at first but it is consistent with statements of various other medicine systems. That Sushumna has a central role is not astounding, however. It also corresponds to the observation in all the literature that vata represents a kind of mixture or integration of kapha and pitta (see the rows 'Digestion' and 'Temperature' in Table 14.1). Anabolism, incidentally, leads to the building up of the texture of the body (seven tissues in Ayurveda), catabolism to the production of energy. The product of the last, finest step of processing foods is called *ojas* (Bauhofer 1997, p. 78 & pp. 194ff). It stands at the transition to the mental level and also at the beginning and end of the digestion process, and it controls the interplay of vata, pitta and kapha, guards their balance and integrates them into a whole.

Table 14.1. Correlation of the three doshas with other classifications

Doshas	Vata	Pitta	Kapha
Consciousness [a]	Rishi	Devata	Chhandas
Assignment [a]	Rhythm	Transmutation	Giving form
Digestion [b]	Metabolic	Catabolic	Anabolic
Gunas [c]	Sattva	Rajas	Tamas
Temperature [d]	Neutral	Hot	Cold
Channels [d]	Sushumna	Pingala	Ida

[a] Bauhofer (1997, p. 51f, p. 73)   [c] Tatzky et al. (1995, p. 31f)
[b] Schwarz & Schweppe (1998, p. 39)   [d] Meyer (1988, pp. 117ff)

The expressions 'transition', 'beginning' and 'end', as well as 'balance' and 'wholeness' point to a localisation at the border of V and K, at the inner end of the spiral – that is, in the region of the TCM meridian *SJ*, which belongs to {flora} or ⟨ether⟩, see (8.12b). This choice is confirmed in Bauhofer's book, where the corresponding mental components – rishi, devata and chhandas – are described and where *soma* represents the connecting element and thus takes on the role of *ojas* at this level. One of his characterisations is 'nectar of immortality', which brings to mind the 'gate of life' *mingmen* and/or flora, cf. Chs. 7.5 & 8.4. In Waterstone (1996, p. 18f) soma is the potion of immortality; it stands for coolness as well as the moon and furthermore is the personification of a hallucinogenic plant (where the trance induced by it again points to *mingmen*). Central to a Vedic sacrifice are *agni* and *soma*, the ritual fire and the ceremonial potion (Bäumer 1996, pp. 204f & 208f). In the first Vedic script, the Rig Veda, they are depicted as gods Agni and Soma and related to one another (masculine / feminine principle). The fact that element ⟨agni⟩ is located opposite ⟨ether⟩ on the circle substantiates the above assumption. More precisely, *soma* corresponding to *SJ* yields an assignment of *agni* to *LR*. Further thoughts on this subject can be found in Ch. 8.2.

In another context, the masculine and feminine principles are at times depicted as two opposing triangles (Aihara 1992, pp. 43ff). As they interpenetrate, the shape of a star emerges (Waterstone 1996, p. 168). The six elements can be represented not only by three polar pairs but also by two triangles, one masculine and one feminine (cf. the Star of David, Figure 14.1). Examples are the Trimurti (Brahma, Vishnu and Shiva) of Hinduism but also the trinity of Christianity. In classical Antiquity Artemis had three shapes and in Europe there are still traces of three related goddesses, the three Beths (Kutter 2003). In the Yoruba religion (in Africa and America) there is a divine couple with three shapes (Früh 1998, p. 200), where Shango is definitely comparable with the deified Agni , and his wife's name, Oya (or Oja), gives pause for thought (in Ayurveda, ojas and soma are equivalent). In the Star of David,

Agni or Shango would occupy the dosha centres, Soma or Oya the transitions. More precisely, Agni (=yang) as {wood}, with the 'wings' {water} and {metal} – and Soma (=yin) as {flora}, with the 'wings' {earth} and {fire}.

Let us now continue with the Rig Veda or the Rk Veda: It contains hymns to 33 gods, although most are addressed to Indra, Agni and Soma (Waterstone 1996, p.17). Agni is the very first word of Rk Veda and thus of all Vedas (Bauhofer 1997, p.148). The sounds (phonemes) of the first two letters, **A** & **G**, are important in the understanding of Ayurveda, as are the sounds of **R** & **K** of the Rk Veda: they correspond to a certain kind of dynamics, the dynamics of stillness. The dynamics of the rolling **R** is stopped by **K**, the limitless motion ends at a fixed point. These two poles now form a unit (Bauhofer 1997, p.48). On p.53 he points out that yoga also stands for absolute stillness, and on p.83 he says the same of **AG** of Agni in place of **RK**. **A** embodies fullness and limitlessness. But wholeness must also contain the point – it must contain emptiness. **G** symbolises the pause, excess (repletion, fullness) is transformed into deficiency (vacuity, emptiness) and then the cycle begins anew. The choice of words (excess – deficiency) again points strongly to the axis {wood} – {flora} or ⟨agni⟩ – ⟨ether⟩.

Bauhofer describes a way in which one can imagine the dynamics of stillness with a different picture on pp.71-79. Vata, pitta and kapha are compared to three blades of a propeller turning with arbitrary velocity. Through this motion, however, the propeller appears to be standing still. The infinite dynamics produces total silence. Nonetheless, one is aware of the dynamics because it produces a pull. That which holds together the propeller is the *ojas*, which we have already mentioned. We find an analogous situation on the abstract level for rishi, devata and chhandas and the coherence through *soma*. In conclusion, Bauhofer mentions an example in physics on p.50: Vacuum, too, is 'nothing', apparently completely still and yet has an inner dynamic. Here the analogy of ⟨ether⟩ and vacuum is apparent. At the beginning of the 20th century ether was replaced by vacuum which, over the course of the decades, received more and more attributes of the earlier ether: from nothing and stillness to ⟨energy⟩ repletion and dynamics.

As far as the structure of the Vedas is concerned, the Rk Veda is the first and fundamental script, which functions like the trunk of a tree. Bauhofer (1997, pp.49-56) makes a division into six branches, each consisting of six aspects. All in all a fractal/self-similar structure results, which is said to reflect the realities in nature and in the microcosm of the human body. This statement can be interpreted as a clue to the six elements. With regard to the branches, it is worth mentioning that the third encompasses yoga and the fourth Ayurveda. Each of the six aspects is characterised by going from stillness to dynamics and back to stillness (three aspects each) or from rishi to chhandas and back.

Now we shall approach the three doshas (nyepas) from the *Tibetan* perspective. These determine the individual's constitution, have their bright and shadowy sides and correspond largely to the miasms of homoeopathy. Dosha and miasm both mean 'ill' – in other words, they emphasise the negative aspect. This is justified whenever the focus is on the origin and dynamics of disease. One can adopt a physical or mental viewpoint again in this matter. In Tibetan medicine, which is strongly influenced by Tibetan Buddhism, there is talk of the *three poisons* of the mind, which lead to related diseases. In terms of the doshas of Ayurveda:

Vata: greed   (lust, affection, attachment, desire)   (14.1a)

Pitta: hatred (anger, antipathy, rejection, aggressiveness, malevolence)   (14.1b)

Kapha: illusion (ego-delusion, indecision, confusion, ignorance)   (14.1c)

See Qusar & Sergent (1997, p. 73), Tatz & Kent (1993, pp. 30-36) and Reichle (1997, p. 166). Some thoughts pertaining to this can be found in Ch. 8.1, where the ambivalence of vata in *not having enough* as well as the tendency of kapha towards self-seclusion are addressed. What is striking is that the terms mentioned have to do with doing and tension rather than allowing and relaxation. There is an interesting reference to existential-analytical psychotherapy. In this therapy 'letting' (letting happen, allowing) is attributed an important therapeutic role, and that in three ways (Kastrinidis 1994, pp. 112-121):

Letting go: desisting, not wanting to hold onto.   (14.2a)

Letting be: being open, letting something be or stand (e.g. a secret),
             neither controlling nor being controlled.   (14.2b)

'Letting':   approaching someone, taking *respons*ibility, trusting,
             getting involved (giving oneself to someone or something),
             willing to confront something.   (14.2c)

According to Kastrinidis, *letting go* is of primary importance. All three modes of letting (initially) have something to do with fear. Enduring and overcoming fear leads to equanimity, high spirits, being open to the secret and thus to transpersonal or spiritual experiences. It is self-evident, therefore, that the three ways of 'letting' correspond to the 'transformed' poisons (same sequence). This is further substantiated by the central role of letting go, which corresponds to the leading role of vata in Ayurveda (Chopra 1993, p. 69). If letting go is not a problem, then the dynamics of falling ill do not come into play (from vata via pitta to kapha). Recovery takes place in reverse order: I must be willing first to get involved in something, then allow whatever comes of it to be and finally let it go.

In the last few paragraphs, we have looked at the psychological aspects more and more. In this context, it is fitting to mention the wheel of life of Buddhism, which concerns the dynamics of life, death and rebirth, where the rebirth – depending on the deeds in the previous life – can take place in one of six realms. The final goal is to attain enlightenment, which gives freedom from rebirth so that one 'gets off the wheel'. The six realms are those of the Devas (gods or divine beings), the Asuras (jealous gods), the animals, the hungry ghosts, the hell beings and the humans. Even though it is possible to be reborn in any of these, it is only from the human realm that it is possible to attain enlightenment and thus get off the wheel.

Aside from a literal interpretation, a figurative one is also possible. Many Buddhist teachers in the West will interpret the wheel of life not just in its traditional way but also in terms of one's everyday life: being happy in the realm of the gods, being angry or jealous in the realm of the Asuras, being greedy and self-centred in the realm of the hungry ghosts or being devoid of insight in the realm of the animals. Tatz & Kent (1993, p. 24 & p. 35f) talk about a geography of states of consciousness, and Epstein (2000, Ch. 1) takes the wheel of life as a model for the neurotic mind. We shall consider this in the same sense here so that the sequence of realms of existence corresponds to the dynamics of (mental) illness and recovery during the course of one's life. In this interpretation, a connection to Ayurveda and Tibetan medicine can also be made.

Now let us look at the wheel of life and its six realms of existence in more detail. There are two illustrations of the wheel of life in Tatz & Kent (1993) and what catches the eye right away is that the two pictures are not consistent: the one on p.25 specifies five sections, the one on the cover six (resembling Figure 8.5 without the life spiral). This already hints at certain speculations concerning our discussion of five versus six elements. But let us continue (in the 6-version): The six realms stand for the six *karmic assignments*, but the arrangement is different from that in our representations. In the upper half of the wheel, the three higher assignments are located – from left to right:

$$\text{Asuras,} \qquad \text{Devas,} \qquad \text{humans.} \tag{14.3a}$$

The Asuras are also referred to as demigods, titans, envious or jealous gods, while the Devas are known as gods or divine beings. Although the Asuras and Devas live much longer than human beings do, they are, in the end, equally mortal and so are not gods as understood in the West. In the version of just five realms, the Asuras are lumped together with the Devas; then there is only *one* divine realm. The lower half of the wheel contains the three lower assignments – this time from right to left:

$$\text{Hungry ghosts,} \quad \text{hell beings,} \quad \text{animals.} \tag{14.3b}$$

Here, too, hell does not last forever (although it is just as full of frightful torments as its Western counterpart). According to Buddhist belief, *greed, hatred* and *delusion* are what keeps us on the wheel and lead to rebirth. Each of these poisons (or fires) is associated with one of the lower realms, which leads Tatz & Kent (1993, p.30) to the following assignments:

$$\text{Hungry ghosts:} \quad \text{greed,} \qquad \text{core of } vata: \quad V^+ \quad \{\text{metal}\}; \tag{14.4a}$$

$$\text{Hell beings:} \qquad \text{hatred,} \qquad \text{core of } pitta: \quad P^+ \quad \{\text{wood}\}; \tag{14.4b}$$

$$\text{Animals:} \qquad \text{delusion,} \quad \text{core of } kapha: \quad K^+ \quad \{\text{water}\}; \tag{14.4c}$$

(cf. Figure 9.1). This assignment is substantiated by further evidence (Tatz & Kent 1993, p.74f). Animals primarily live in the oceans (*water* as assigned element). The hungry ghosts are constantly hungry and thirsty (craving) but are unable to eat because their mouths are tiny and unable to drink because water instantly turns to fire in their mouths (ambivalence of vata, or rather never getting enough). Thus, the three lower realms are linked to the dosha centres (this time really interpreted as poisons). The dosha transitions, then, are reserved for the higher realms. The information in (Tatz & Kent 1993, pp.26-32) greatly facilitates this assignment, cf. also Epstein (2000, Ch. 1). The gods are in the happiest state (continuous joy). Since in TCM joy appears as an emotion of {fire} and thus is the only emotion of the elements, the realm of the gods falls on the vata/pitta border, i.e. to K^-. The Asuras and {flora} play a comparable role in the ambiguity of the number of elements (five or six). Just as the Asuras are sometimes lumped together with the Devas, {flora} is at times considered part of {fire}, sometimes as ministerial fire set apart from the (imperial) fire. The relationship emperor/minister also fits in well with god/demigod. This yields the assignment of Asuras to {flora}. The human being, then, remains for {earth}. Here we find a parallel regarding the 'middle' position. Being in human form is considered the most beneficial form with regard to spiritual development. Only human beings feel the urge to overcome their current condition due to the unusual mixture of pleasant and unpleasant experiences. Overall, this results in:

Asuras:	transitional region K/V:	P^-	{flora};	(14.5a)
Devas:	transitional region V/P:	K^-	{fire};	(14.5b)
Humans:	transitional region P/K:	V^-	{earth}.	(14.5c)

The special position of flora also follows from its paradoxical role. The following characterisation fits in very well here (Tatz & Kent 1993, p.79, italic accentuations by me):

"One who is always *devious* and *deceptive*,
But nonetheless does *not do harm* unto others,
One who enjoys *strife* but remains *generous*,
Will become ruler of the *Asuras*."

In this way, the wisdom contained in the wheel of life can be linked not only with the Far Eastern methods of healing but also with Western psychotherapy.

14.2. The Jewish Tradition: The Three Axes of Tension

In the following, we shall compare our intercultural model within the frame of the simple circle representation with two other traditions: the Jewish (Kabbalah) from the Near East and the Germanic (runes) from Europe; see also Kratky (2000c, Ch. 1). Before we delve into this, let us first summarise a few essential aspects of this model, which represents the diversity of human modes of behaviour. Three basic types fall into two poles each, resulting in a total of six characteristics ('elements'), which can be interpreted easily when arranged in a circle. The eight Chinese trigrams allude to the fact that there are still other dimensions (see Kratky 2000a, Ch.3). Six of these can be equated with the elements while the additional two trigrams, 'heaven' (absolute yang, +) and 'earth' (absolute yin, –), are usually added to the elements {metal} and {earth}. These two elements are considered the representatives of 'heaven' and 'earth' in the circle of elements. The pairs {fire}/ {water} and {wood}/ {flora} are in a yang/yin relationship; the same is true, of course, for 'heaven'/ 'earth'. What is unclear is the polarity of {metal}/{earth}. {Earth} is neutral, but the assignment of {metal} is ambiguous (Ch.7.2). If we regard it as yin – as is common in TCM – then {metal}/{earth} is in a yin/yang relationship. Then their polarity is opposite that of 'heaven'/ 'earth', whose earthly representatives they really are. We shall come back to this.

The elements of a pair are located in opposite positions on the circle and form an axis (Figure 7.3). An analogous representation with three *axes of tension* can be found in the Kabbalah, the Jewish mystic tradition (Benedikt 1986, to the right of p. 128): the *axes of love, of intuition* and *of will*, which are also characterised as *fixed, cardinal* and *mutable*. There is much similarity between the two systems and the axes can accordingly be correlated to one another (see Table 14.2).

Table 14.2a. Meridians (bottom, through the leg, see Table 7.2a&b), supplemented by the trigram 'earth', as well as their correlations to the Kabbalah, (see Benedikt 1986, Ch.II8)

Meridian (bottom)	Back	Front	& Trigram	Middle
Element Influence	**Water** Cold	**Earth** Dampness	& 'Earth'	**Wood** Wind (gusty)
Axis of Tension	Love (fixed)	Intuition (cardinal)		Will (mutable)
Pole: Characteristic	Cold	Dark	& 'Darkness'	Colourful
Pole: Colour	Blue	Violet	& Black	Red
Pole: Relationship	Take	Implement		Do
Pole: Other Associations:	Body, values	Service, sacrifice		Movement, living, ego, deed

Table 14.2b. Meridians (top, through the arm, see Table 7.2a&b), supplemented by the trigram 'heaven', as well as their correlations to the Kabbalah, (see Benedikt 1986, Ch.II8)

Meridian (top)	Back	Front	& Trigram	Middle
Element Influence	**Fire** Heat	**Metal** Dryness	& 'Heaven'	**Flora** Stillness (draught)
Axis of Tension	Love (fixed)	Intuition (cardinal)		Will (mutable)
Pole: Characteristic	Warm	Bright	& 'Light'	colourless
Pole: Colour	Orange	Yellow	& White	Green
Pole: Relationship	Give	Consider		Let
Pole: Other Associations:	Joy, e-motion	Insight, idea, mind		Wholeness, paradox

Now let us look at the correlations. According to Table 14.2 the *axis of love* has the same polarity *cold/warm* as the corresponding TCM axis {water}/{fire}, where the active, giving part of the emotion corresponds to *joy* – as does {fire} in TCM. This axis formally relates to the polarity *give/take*, which ultimately must be balanced. Love is only one (positive) example of this. The *axis of intuition* is characterised by a double assignment – just like the vertical TCM axis. First, it is about the polarity *potential/actual* or *consider/implement*. The realm of *ideas* (as an example for potentiality) is now also the representative of *light* ('heaven'), the realm of *service* (as an example for implementation) the representative of *darkness* ('earth').

This leaves the mutable *axis of will* as a correlation to the TCM axis {wood}/ {flora}. This fits in with the statements by Terrades (1996, p.48f), who sees the pair {wood}/{flora} as a *joint* and thus connects it with *movement*. It refers to the polarity *doing/ letting* (Table 14.2). The pole of the axis characterised by *movement, life, ego, deed* immediately brings to mind {wood}, which then interestingly assigns the opposite pole, {flora}, to the characteristics *paradox* and *wholeness*. A more precise list of the characteristics listed by Benedikt (1986, p. 128 on the right) is:

Flora: shaping, harmony, growth, paradox, wholeness | LETTING, colourless, green;   (14.6a)

Wood: movement, self-will, living, structure, ego, deed | DOING, colourful, red.   (14.6b)

Flora emphasises *connection*, wood *separation*. It automatically brings to mind the bond the embryo makes with the mother-to-be as opposed to the power of self-assertion in the 'raw reality' towards mid-life, which also corresponds to the assigned ages of life (see Ch. 8.4). However, the polarity ALLOWING – DOING is less trivial than it appears at first glance. What at first seems *passive* as opposed to *active* in *flora* becomes more encompassing through the terms *paradox* and *wholeness*. The Chinese term *wuwei* – actively doing nothing or participating observation – is comparable: one even lets go of *letting go*. The *gate of life (mingmen)* connected to flora also has something connecting *and* something separating in its nature: it closes the cycle of life and at the same time represents a barrier, which, however, can presumably be overcome during altered states of consciousness (Ch. 11.4). The *orgasm* ('the little death') needs to be mentioned here as well. It is the result of an action that is connected with *doing* as well as with *allowing and letting go*. It leads to the *phenomena of the dissolution of boundaries, dissolution of the ego*. Furthermore PC, the inner meridian of flora, is also called Circulation/*sex*, and *plant* (seed) is often symbolically connected with *sexuality* (see Szabó 1985, p. 53).

We now arrive at Figure 14.1. Compared with Benedikt (1986, p. 128 on the right), left and right are interchanged. Thereby, the axes are ordered in such a way as to make possible a comparison with our usual circle representation. Everything is clear for the axes of love and will with respect to polarity: *giving* and *doing* are active compared to *letting* (allowing) and *taking in* (perceiving) and thus in relation yang (+) to yin (–). The signs are specified at those words that are listed within the circle. These words, too, substantiate the classification: *warm* versus *cold* is obvious and for *colourful* versus *colourless* (14.6a&b) helps, from which we conclude that *colourful* refers to the colour *red*. In any case, the polarity of these two axes corresponds to the two axes of TCM. Only for the vertical *axis of intuition* – corresponding to the more complex relationships at {metal} and {earth} – things are not quite as clear. It concerns the relationship *potential/actual*. The active aspect of *actualisation* should be *yang*, the characteristic *dark* (as representative of '*darkness*'), however, points to *yin*. This then results in one opposite polarity just as in TCM.

Heaven, as well as *earth*, has a double meaning. This leads to thinking about the spiritual or divine heaven as 'above', for example, although God is everywhere (and nowhere). This double meaning can also be found in other languages. In TCM as well as in the Kabbalah, the vertical axis is the *representative* for another dimension, which cannot be projected into the two-dimensional plane of drawing without losing information. The *top* of the illustration also represents the *world above* ('above earth'), the *bottom* the *world below* ('below the earth'). The central region is the human realm ('on earth'). The division into different levels or worlds (upper, middle, lower world), which corresponds to a symbolic cosmology, can also be found in many shamanic traditions. The Chinese threefold partition, heaven – human being – earth, also fits in well here (see Kratky 2000a, Figure 2). The fact that the circle representation, which at first I merely chose to make things more manageable, lends itself to multiple interpretations is not surprising, for it is based on entire sequences by analogy of TCM and Ayurveda. To my amazement, this representation has developed a life of its own and can also be used as a cosmology (see below).

Let us get back to the vertical axis in Figure 14.1. We can now look at the characteristics light and dark from a different perspective. Light is 'above', dark 'below'. However, the heavens (sky) are only light (blue) when the sun (yellow) shines. The night sky on the other hand is dark and, from space, even the daytime sky is violet to black. On the other hand, there is also glowing magma below the earth's surface, which comes to the surface as lava after a volcanic eruption and only turns black as it cools off. Similar observations can be made concerning some (partly extinct) professions: the charcoal maker, the smith, the stoker of a steam engine or the chimney sweep. As a result of working with fire they are soot-blackened, 'dark figures'. In hell, supposedly, there are great fires as well. Lucifer, incidentally, translates to *carrier of light*. The word hell comes from *hel*, the Germanic realm of the dead. The German word 'hell' means light, but the etymological meaning of *hel* is the exact opposite (hidden, i.e. dark). Thus, both heaven and earth have to do with light and darkness.

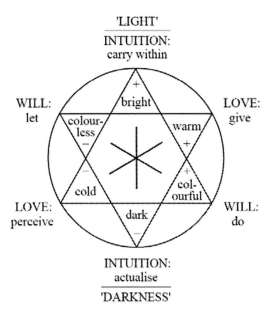

Figure 14.1. Characterisation of the three axes of tension. In addition to the circle representation, the centres as well as the dosha transitions are connected to form triangles, which then form the Star of David.

A few words need to be said concerning the *assignment of colours* in the Kabbalah (see Table 14.2). The axis of intuition (light – dark) is given the colours yellow – violet, the axis of love (warm – cold) shows the colours orange – blue (warmest and coldest colour) and the axis of will (colourful – colourless) red – green, see (14.6a&b). Red is seen – not only in the Kabbalah – as *the* typical colour ('colourful'), while the green of *flora* is considered 'colourless'. One could also speak of a 'colourless colour', see Benedikt (1986, p.128 & the corresponding figure). In any case, it expresses the paradox of flora pretty well. Recall the difficulties regarding the classification of the tastes *astringent* and *neutral* (*bland*), see Ch. 7.2. In this case, too, the assignment of the 'tasteless taste' fits in well with *flora* as a unification of opposites. Last but not least, the axes in Figure 14.1 are not drawn all the way through, in order to allow another interpretation, namely the combination of the dosha centres and transitions into two triangles offset with respect to each other. This results in the Star of David (or Solomon's seal, hexagram). As already mentioned there are also comparable mandalas in the Far East, where the interfacing triangles are interpreted as masculine and feminine. However, the assignment is not consistent. According to the polarities of Figure 14.1, yang (+) is predominant in the triangle pointing up (dosha centres), yin (–) in the triangle pointing down (transitions).

14.3. The Germanic Tradition:
In the Realm of Letters

This leads us to the Germanic tradition (Figure 14.2). A corresponding cosmology can be found in Szabó (1985, pp. 47 & 63), which is surprisingly similar to the Jewish tradition. To start with, we need to consider Figure 7.3 (concerning the horizontal axis, see Figure 7.2). The circle is now replaced or augmented by a hexagon. The vertical axis is formed by *air* (top) and *earth* (bottom). The horizontal stands for *water* (left) and *fire* (right). Furthermore, both split into an *upper* and *lower* water (fog, spring) and fire (lightning, volcano), respectively. The left region (water) is seen as feminine, the right (fire) as masculine, which fits in well with TCM. Comparing bottom/top another thing catches one's eye: The *lower* water (spring) and the *upper* fire (lightning) located on the same axis correspond to the usual terms, the *upper* water (fog, sometimes also brought into connection with ice) and the *lower* fire (volcano) are, however, unusual forms of water and fire. This axis also goes beyond the usual four elements in Germanic cosmology. Fog and ice represent the gaseous and solid forms of water, not the usual liquid phase ('spring'). Volcano, on the other hand, represents a liquid fire (via the lava during a volcanic eruption). This represents the paradox again alluded to in the Kabbalah – this time with regard to the whole axis: it connects the dry water with the liquid (damp) fire.

Furthermore, the choice of interpretation as a two- or three-dimensional representation once more presents itself. First, Figure 14.2 relates to the human level (Midgard, the middle garden). *Air* points upwards to Asgard, where the crystal palace of the gods (Asen, with Odin as Father of all) is located. *Earth* points downward to Utgard, where *hel* is located, the world of those dead who did not fall in battle. Here the dark goddess, Hel, rules. Thus, heaven is attributed more to masculine, hel more to feminine qualities. The ambivalence of this axis, which we have already encountered in TCM and the Kabbalah, now mirrors in the division of genders in the earthly representatives: the elves (feminine) live in the air, the dwarves (whom we imagine to be masculine) are at work below the surface of the earth. The connection between the three levels is made by the *world tree*: the world ash tree, Yggdrasil. It is located in Midgard and extends downward to Utgard and upward to Asgard. In other traditions, there are different means that connect the various levels symbolically and 'hold the world together': the *tree of life* (which also appears in the Kabbalah – cf. Benedikt 2003), the upright, the central axis or the shaman himself.

Combinations of the lines (line segments) of Figure 14.2 yield, incidentally, the 18 runes of the Vikings, which are not just letters but also represent words and are related to a chain of associations. We shall look at U, H, N, I & E (2nd, 7th, 8th & 17th rune – see the corresponding chapters in Szabó 1985). I (sign: |, name: IS) is the vertical axis (axis of *intuition* in the Kabbalah) and stands, among other things, for 'I' and the number 1. In English, both are still today represented by a vertical line. All signs considered now contain this axis. N (sign: ⅄, name: NOT) contains in addition the axis of will and means need (misery). On the other hand, E (sign: ⅄, name: EH) contains the axis of love in addition to the vertical axis and means law. H (sign: ✳, name: HAGAL) consists of all three axes and thus encompasses everything and brings to mind the triple heater *SJ*. This rune is completely symmetrical and can be obtained by superimposing N and E. It means crystal (or ice) and refers to the crystal palace of the Father of the gods, Odin (Hagal and Odin corresponding to each another). Finally we arrive at U (sign: ⋂, name: UR), which means primordial source. This rune looks a little different: apart from the vertical axis, there are two more lines with a sharp bend exactly at the position of flora.

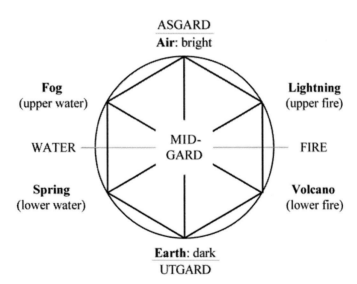

Figure 14.2. Illustration of Germanic cosmology.
Axes as in the circle representation and in Figure 14.1.

The EH and the NOT runes are closely connected, the EH rune being the result of 'turning around' the NOT rune (more precisely, EH and NOT runes are horizontally flipped versions of each other). According to Szabó, N can be connected with *chaos*, E with *order*. Great need (German 'Not'), e.g. anarchy, can be *turned around* by law, the *law* is then *needed*. **E** also has to do with marriage. In Sanskrit there is a parallel to the word *yoga* (yoke, harness, *connect*). A less successful lasting bond (connection) is also called a yoke of marriage. Whether successful or not, the axis of love has formally to do with *give* and *take*, love is only *one* contextual example. But the balance of give and take is a central shamanic law. If you want something from the gods, you have to offer them – at least symbolically – something in return. The connection to EH (law) is evident here. Let us take a closer look at the rune **N**: it stands for **n**eed and death, additionally for **n**ight and **n**egation in general. It looks as though the skewed axis **n**egates the vertical axis. Some relations (German and Italian expressions in parentheses) are:

I:	|	one (ein)	one (einer)	I (ich);	eight (acht, otto);	(14.7a)
N:	⼽	**n**o (nein)	**n**one	**n**ot (nicht);	**n**ight (Nacht, **n**otte).	(14.7b)

The **n**egating effect of **N** is still present. Words with a similar sound but different meanings in several languages could go back to one single rune such as the NOT rune (Ger. Not = **n**eed, Engl. **n**ot, Ital. **n**otte = **n**ight). 'Night' is a special case: *Nott* was not only the personified **n**ight of the Teutons, but also – as *not* – the **n**egation of **n**ight, resulting in *eight*. The similarity of **N** with the common Germanic DAG rune (*day*), which looks like the number 8, also points to this. It also is the 8th rune. What looks like a play on words and numbers had a deeper meaning for the Teutons (the terms *new* and *nine* relate another story, which we shall come back to). Thus, **N** does **n**ot just express **n**egation but also the collapse of opposites or switching into the opposite: day and night, life and death, respect and disrespect. In connection with *homoeopathy,* Hadulla & Appell (1993, p. 212) talk about the *double meaning of primal words*. In this context they mention the Latin word *sacer*, which means *holy* but also *accursed*. In the same way, yin and yang can change into each other.

The thoughts on NOT bring to mind the double meaning of LETTING at {flora}, (14.6a), which also stands for *paradox*. In addition, the relation to life and death fits in with the axis {flora}/{wood}: {flora} stands for conception, pregnancy, birth and death and {wood} for the flourishing mid-life. According to (9.3a) {wood} and {flora} are characterised by *fullness* and *emptiness* of energy. Living life to the fullest and falling into the night of death are fitting associations. At the moment of death, one can feel *all alone* or, contrariwise, *all one* or *at one* with God. It takes place between {flora} and {wood} but also within {flora}. In any case, it seems that we could also call the axis {flora}/{wood} the *axis of life*. Further considerations about the axes can be found in Kratky (2000c, Ch. 1). Ch. 2 of this paper also delves into the colours of the elements in the various systems. We have only addressed this issue with regard to the Kabbalah but further information can be found in Ch. 9.3.

Now we turn to the runes **H** and **U**. HAGAL (sign: ✳) also stands for the triad **h**ealed, **h**oly and **w**hole. As *hail,* it is the union of the opposites *fire* and *water*. If the balance of the three axes is disturbed, illness arises (the connection to *SJ* is thus substantiated). In addition, the rune *UR* (sign: ⼌, meaning *primordial source*) is also relevant in this context. Szabó (1985, pp. 75ff) says of this rune that **U** promises *healing* by befriending the symptoms of the illness. Penetration to the primordial so**ur**ce of wisdom, where an almost unlimited energy, vitality and *healing power* are available, is crucial. In primeval times all antagonisms collapse. Following on from Szabó's statement, we can say that psora as basic illness is connected to the following terms (see Ch.8.1): root cause, root of all evil, original sin. In this context, we established in Ch.11.4 that the deeper cause of illness lies in the problem of crossing flora alive. Flora, which is also associated with SJ, has already been brought into play because of the shape of the letter **U**. The Chinese counterpart to UR, incidentally, is *yuan*. Yuanyin and yuanyang are the *original* yin and yang, which form the source qi (*yuanqi*) connected to the gate of life, *mingmen,* (that is, *flora*). It can be regulated via the yuan source points (!), where SJ plays a special role (see Maciocia 1994, p.46f & pp.359-361).

There are several systems of runes. Szabó (1985, pp.17-20) mentions them but concentrates – as we have noted – on the 18 runes of the Vikings. A comparison of several runic systems can also be found in Aswynn (1991, pp.237-243). There the 33 Anglo-Saxon runes play a central role, which enables a delightful comparison. Especially interesting is the different role **HAGAL**, now called **HAGALAZ** or **HEIGL**, plays (pp.61-64 in Aswynn). The deified Heigl at first has a negative and destructive role (compare the damage caused by hail) and is associated with the netherworld (*hel*). There is a correlation to Mother **H**olle of the fairy tales and it also reminds us of **H**olland = the Netherlands, where part of the land lies 'under water'. Furthermore, there is also an alternative, 'integrated' form of Heigl, which means strong protection, e.g. from thunderstorms (simile principle!). In this context it is interesting to point out that 'hail' can also refer to a salutation (originally meaning salvation!).

In conclusion, we shall pick up again on the double meaning of primal words and go far beyond the runes. Fester (1981) investigated the similarities of the languages accessible to him and got involved in lengthy 'archaeological' studies and in research into old names of places and fields, whose origin often lies in the distant past. The worldwide similarities he found led him to propose a language system that we shall introduce briefly. According to Fester, the great majority of words can be traced back to the following six archetypal words (Fester 1981, pp.33-39):

$$\text{BA,} \quad \text{KALL,} \quad \text{TAG,} \quad \text{TAL,} \quad \text{OS,} \quad \text{ACQ.} \tag{14.8a}$$

This sequence shows the sequence of emergence associated with a narrowing of the breadth of meaning. Before we continue with Fester, let us think about what this means. We can hypothesise that behind this are various world views which have developed over thousands of years. According to Table 2.2, it is obvious to consider P4-3-2-1 as sequence of perspectives. The continued narrowing of the breadth of meaning, on the other hand, brings to mind the life spiral, where the outward spiral in a clockwise direction shows a decreasing integration of the doshas. So we can put forward the hypothesis that the sequence of the primal words corresponds to the outward spiral from flora to flora and thus to the Indo-Tibetan elements and/or the meridians assigned to them in (8.11a&b).

$$\langle\text{Ether}\rangle, \quad \langle\text{Air}\rangle, \quad \langle\text{Fire}\rangle, \quad \langle\text{Agni}\rangle, \quad \langle\text{Earth}\rangle, \quad \langle\text{Water}\rangle. \tag{14.8b}$$
$$\text{SJ,} \quad \text{LI,} \quad \text{SI,} \quad \text{LR,} \quad \text{SP,} \quad \text{KI.} \tag{14.8c}$$

Accordingly, the sequence of the first four elements also corresponds to the sequence of world views previously mentioned; see Ch.7.2, (7.5a-c).

The first word, **BA**, can in principle mean anything but primarily concerns the essential things of life. So, the triad father – mother – child is **BA**, and therefore **PAPA**, **MAMA** and **BABY** (note that *P*, *M* and *B* are essentially interchangeable). This similarity is mirrored, for example, in Sanskrit, where *P* and *M* have almost the same written characters. The vowels are even more unstable and can be changed easily. In general, there is a shift from *A* via *O* and *U* to *E* and finally *I*. In Sanskrit *A* dominates, in many modern European languages *E*, which, however, in English is often pronounced like the German *I*. A good match for the first archetypal word is ⟨ether⟩, which permeates everything (Qusar et al. 1997, p. 7), and also the symbiotic meta-perspective MP4 of *SJ* (Ch. 8.4).

The second word, **KALL**, corresponds to the element ⟨air⟩, which also has an 'earthy' component in the meridian *LI*. This is also the region of 'on the one hand – on the other' (P3), where thesis and antithesis have their place (vata can be hot or cold, damp or dry). **KALL** means, among other things, **NAKED** (**BLEAK**), **CAVE** and **VAULT**. Due to the interchangeability of *K* with *C*, *CK* and *V*, these words are all **KALL** words. **NAKED** indicates a **LACK** – a bare mountain is especially susceptible to the external climatic conditions (yin deficiency in vata). A **VAULT** can be under the earth, but it can also mean the **welkin** (vault of heaven, Lat. **COELUM**); thus, heaven and earth find their place here. The same is true for cold and hot: **COLD**, **CALOR** (heat). The double meaning of the primal words discussed earlier comes to bear here; it also fits in well with vata. There are also combinations of the two word stems, as can be seen in the actor's name Lauren **Bacall**. My own forename, **Karl**, also is **KALL** (*R* and *L* are also interchangeable, and in Germany **Karl** is sometimes called **Kalle**).

The other words will only be addressed briefly. Fester does not discuss them in detail either. TAG has, among other things, to do with loftiness, tongue and heat but also with the English word DAY (German 'TAG'). Compare ⟨fire⟩ but also tongue as the organ associated with the Chinese{fire}. TAL (DALE, valley), on the other hand, is below, a cleft, earth. This fits in with the volcano (runes), also the trigram thunder for {wood} ('the thunder emerging from earth'). The element is ⟨agni⟩, according to (14.8b). OS is an orifice of the body, also source and sea. The dampness of ⟨earth⟩ is a factor here. ACQ, the last word, really has just one meaning: drinkable water (Lat. AQUA). The assigned element is ⟨water⟩. So it seems as though the elements and the six archetypal words have a strong inner connection. There is yet a great deal to be explored.

14.4. (Pre-)Islamic Enneagram: In the Realm of Numbers

Our journey now brings us to the *enneagram*, a typology of uncertain origin, which is connected with Islam and the lore of the Sufis (Rohr & Ebert 1991, p. 10). It concerns a characterisation of nine states of the soul or modes of behaviour with a spiritual background. Rohr & Ebert studied the enneagram (*ennea*, Greek = nine) and interpreted it from the Christian perspective. The page numbers in the following paragraphs refer to their book. In order to describe the nine types, the authors draw on analogies (colours, animals, countries, etc.). Interestingly, this is, in principle, a threefold system of 'primary energies', each of which branches out again in a fractal-like manner into a further three branches. The nine types are numbered in the following manner (p. 40f):

HEART	(social, open):	**2, 3,** 4	(cf. vata: affection)	(14.9a)
HEAD	(self-preserving, withdrawn):	5, **6,** 7	(cf. kapha: ego delusion)	(14.9b)
GUT	(sexual, hostile):	8, **9,** 1	(cf. pitta: hatred, antipathy)	(14.9c)

The names of the three primal energies can – again – easily lead to confusion. Nonetheless, we have made a tentative assignment to the doshas (see their characterisation in Ch. 14.1). More precise assignments of the nine types are given in Table 14.3. The root sins can, in this scheme, be transformed by the corresponding virtue (p. 39). In Western tradition, we are used to hearing about seven deadly sins, but here we find nine root sins. This theme of 7 and 9 can be found in several contexts (see Kratky 2000a, Ch. 3). Depending on the interpretation, there are sevenfold and ninefold *cosmologies* (Eliade 1994, pp. 263-7) in shamanic societies, especially in North and Central Asia, including some geographic overlaps. The additional root sins in the enneagram are *deceit* (**3**) and *fear* (**6**). In Rohr & Ebert there is an interesting statement that one is incapable of recognising one's own sins and that deceit and fear are actually *the* deadly sins of our society (pp. 87 & 131). What's more, fear is not normally recognised as a sin.

Table 14.3. The 9 enneagram types according to Rohr & Ebert (1991)

Type	Self-image	Temptation	Root Sin	Gift / Fruit of the Spirit
2	I am helpful	Help	Pride	Humility
3	I am successful	Efficiency	Deceit	Honesty
4	I am unique	Authenticity	Envy	Balance
5	I am perceptive	Knowledge	Greed	Objectivity
6	I am loyal	Security	Fear	Courage
7	I am happy	Idealism	Gluttony	Sobriety
8	I am strong	Justice	Shamelessness	Innocence
9	I am content	Self-abasement	Sloth	Action
1	I am right	Perfection	Anger	Serenity

Again all types have their good and bad sides. Depending on how it is expressed, each type exists in unredeemed, normal and redeemed forms (pp. 211ff). Figure 14.3 shows a circle representation of the nine types according to pp. 40 & 216. It is the usual diagram of the enneagram; the directions, therefore, do not necessarily agree with my circle or disc representations. What first catches the eye is that **3**, **6** and **9** are the respective centres of the three regions. However, this does not mean that they are especially typical for the corresponding basic energies. They are rather those types in which the respective energy is *blocked*. For example, **9** (the centre for GUT) is especially peace-loving. The other two types of each region are different forms of its basic energy, while no type embodies the energy in pure form. Perhaps this is because something like that never or seldom occurs in real life. Another explanation is given by the dynamics of the types (again cf. Figure 14.3).

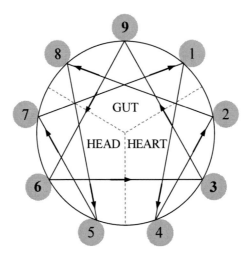

Figure 14.3. Enneagram: The three basic energies as well as the nine types and their dynamics.

The lines connecting the types and the arrows indicate the relationships of the types to each other. A first glance reveals that **3**, **6** and **9** form a feedback loop separated from the other six types, which, in turn, are also connected by a feedback loop. The direction of the arrows specifies growing disintegration (away from redemption), the reverse direction growing integration (towards redemption). For example, a normal **3** wants to develop positively. Apart from the direct goal of becoming a redeemed **3**, there is the possibility of absorbing characteristics from **6** (the point of solace for **3,** in the reverse direction of the arrows). Then the path continues as if by itself in the direction of redemption. Conversely, orientation in **9** (the stress point for **3**) means a false solace, which ultimately leads downhill. It is plain that every type is a solace as well as a stress point – for the two neighbours in the polygonal path, depending on the direction. Altogether, a 6- and a 3-cycle result. If the 'pure' three types exist at all, then, presumably, they are immutable. They are then three separate fixed points, which are no longer interesting in an enneagram oriented in spiritual development. In the system reduced from nine to seven types, **3** and **6** drop out as has been mentioned. Then only one 6-cycle remains and the 3-cycle reduces to type **9**, which thus turns into a fixed point.

If we translate the above system from psychological states to those of health and illness and identify the types with the meridians, we find some interesting associations with results established in previous chapters, especially in 11.4, where the enneagram was first mentioned. There, we spoke about cyclic illness dynamics: dynamics I (6-cycle) and II (3-cycle). Furthermore, there are three meridians not involved in any dynamics: HT, ST and PC. They were then also named as unstable fixed points, which is the reason why we do not commonly run across them. ST apparently is the 'typical' representative of GUT energy, but what about

HT and PC? Since PC is at times also called Master of the Heart, the heart appears in PC and HT but in different ways (Klinghardt 1996, p.212f as well as Kratky 2002): In *PC* we find the physical heart (connected with the circulation), in *HT* the emotional or spiritual heart – what we mean when we describe someone as good-hearted. The latter, apparently, is a pure expression of the HEART energy of the enneagram, which, for this reason, is not represented in the nine types. PC stands for the inner preservation of life and thus for the pure HEAD energy (the key word being self-preserving).

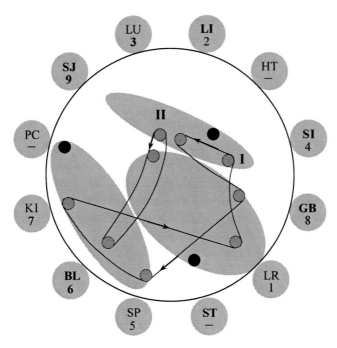

Figure 14.4. Assignment of the meridians to the enneagram types.

In Figure 14.4 the assignment of all twelve meridians is given, based on Figure 11.3. The 6-cycle even shows the (skewed and twisted) form of the corresponding enneagram cycle, Figure 14.3. The 3-cycle, however, is not as 'nicely' interlinked with it as in Figure 14.3. Clear-cut assignment to the meridians follows first for the 3-cycle by taking the root sins into account (Table 14.3). **3** is associated with *deceit*. We spoke about phantom pregnancy and theatrical talent, and about impostors and swindlers in connection with the ambivalent nature of {metal}. This fits in with **3** being characterised as an *actor* in the enneagram. Since LU is part of the 3-cycle in metal, **3** is assigned to *LU*. Furthermore, fear is typical of {water} according to TCM, therefore **6** is assigned to *BL*. **9** then automatically falls on *SJ*. This also makes sense, since the Tibetan type 'stillness' can be found in the region of SJ (see Ch.10.2). Moreover, within the frame of the *dynamics of stillness* in Ayurveda, *SJ* is the pole of pausing (**G** from AGNI or **K** from Rk Veda, see Ch.14.1).

For the 6-cycle we shall attribute the 'diabolic rage' (type 1) to *LR*, the site of Huter's disharmonious disposition (opposite the harmonious disposition at *SJ*), see Ch.10.2. The other assignments follow automatically. In fact, the meridians belonging to an enneagram energy (including *the one* not assigned to a number) do all lie in the same region, earmarked by the grey ellipses in Figure 14.4. Largely they are also located in the postulated doshas (14.9a-c). However, one irritant remains: types 2 and 4 should be interchanged so that everything fits perfectly. Type-2 people are *helpers*, who should be attributed to {fire} (*give love*, Table 14.2 & Figure 14.2). *Pride* as a mortal sin also fits in, it is in the realm of the Devas of the Buddhist realms of existence). Type-4 people are sensitive artists pertaining to creativity and sensitivity of {metal}. However, we have already determined that the sequence of falling ill with *SI* before *LI* does not correspond to Gienow's dynamics of miasms, which, by comparison, is reversed here. This, then, constitutes a second independent confirmation questioning the validity of the TCM sequence at the beginning of an illness progression. In addition, the onset of illness at *LI* instead of *SI* would also be in vata, which would fit in better with Ayurveda overall. Moreover, Ayurveda teaches that although illness typically has its onset in vata, it can start anywhere. The generalisation alluded to here can be recognised in the enneagram (see Figure 14.4): the cycles are indicated but the start and end points are not emphasised.

In this context, it is interesting to note that there is another relationship between 7 and 9 which refers to the 6-cycle and which is often indicated in the enneagram. The fraction 1/7 as a periodic decimal number corresponds exactly to the sequence of the 6-cycle. This is also true for the other fractions 2/7 to 6/7. They just start with another enneagram type. The usual sequence of dynamics I begins with type 4 corresponding to the fraction 3/7:

$$1/7 = 0.14285714\ldots, \quad 2/7 = 0.28571428\ldots, \quad 3/7 = 0.42857142\ldots,$$
$$4/7 = 0.57142857\ldots, \quad 5/7 = 0.71428571\ldots, \quad 6/7 = 0.85714285\ldots. \tag{14.10}$$

Two further points should be made:

a) There are other number systems associated with character types (see, for example, Millman 2000). This spiritual system of the 'life number' points again to the positive and negative sides of a type. The numbering is different from the enneagram. The attempt at a 'translation' should be a delightful task. Unlike in the enneagram, one's type is found by using one's date of birth and the letters of one's name, each letter having its own value. In other typologies, too, one encounters this combination of the wisdom they convey and the mechanical manner in which a certain type is assigned to an individual.

b) In Anthroposophy, a division of the circle representation into nine sections can also be found (see Ch. 10.1). This encompasses all meridians, and the regions of the dosha centres contain two meridians each. As a result, a special role is assigned to the meridians *PC, ST* and *HT*: They do not change their character with zooming in, they are compared to fixed points. This is now mirrored in the fact that they are not involved in any cycle.

14.5. The Final Question: How Spiritual Is Europe?

At the end of our journey, we return to Europe and ask the question: What about our own roots? We have a spiritual and medical tradition spanning many thousands of years, but it seems to be permanently at risk and requires saviours from outside Europe. Our Greek/ Roman cultural inheritance was largely lost in the first millennium after Christ and was reintroduced via a detour through Arabia. For the last few centuries we have regarded the Hippocratic medicine system as a mere oddity, but it reached the Indian subcontinent via Persia and today enjoys full recognition there as Unani. There were plenty of medieval mystics, but we prefer to search for ideals in other cultures. Paracelsus is mentioned again and again, but there is not all that much we can do with him, although his spagyric or al-chemical approach gives a first hint at how the path for Europe could be. With this approach, he attempted to study alchemy critically and apply its usable components to further investiga-tion. The natural sciences ultimately had a comparable concern, but they took a different turn and ended up in chemistry. The entire development of modern science is oriented in objectiv-ity and clarity (perspective P1) and attempts to avoid subjectivity (P2) as well as dependence on interpretation (P3).

P2 and P3 are connected to the axes {water} – {fire} and {earth} – {metal}, P1 to the axis of life {wood} – {flora}, especially {wood} (battle, separation). For purposes of comparison, we need to say a few words on the spagyric approach (from Ancient Greek 'spao' = I tear away, separate & 'ageiro' = I connect, unite): This art of separation and purification con-cerns itself primarily with a particular method of producing remedies. The combination of separation and merging is associated with P1 & P4, which means it involves the whole axis of life. Since P1 in extremis ultimately topples into P4, where among other things the union of opposites can be found, a spiritual path for Europe is foreshadowed. This seems now in complete contradiction to the political development, for example, which goes in the direction of secularisation by the separation of Church and state, and, in this way, builds a barrier against the Islamic countries, for instance. Looking at the development of the EU, however, one can draw a quite different conclusion: The attempt to construct an edifice located in the field of tension between federal state and federation of states is the perfect 'spagyric ap-proach'. That the side effect of this difficult endeavour is expressed in hatred of foreigners (P1 comes through) is regrettable but, presumably, is only a transitional stage until equilib-rium has been established.

In Zundel & Loomans (1994), Bauhofer (1997) and Fuchs & Kobler-Fumasoli (2002), interesting statements about the area of overlap between science – spirituality – religion can be found, which again point to the axis of life. Bauhofer (1997, pp. 65-70) sees parallels between Ayurveda and the natural sciences. Both attempt to reduce the diversity of nature to fewer and fewer principles and to lead complicated matters back to simple matters. Since there is only one truth, Bauhofer believes that it would benefit modern medicine if it were to rediscover Ayurvedic principles. The difference lies in the path taken: Vedic experiment in the laboratory of consciousness in comparison to the natural sciences, which utilise rationale, logic and mathematics. Ultimately, the same truth is expressed, just in different words.

At this point, we shall refer the reader to Gleditsch (1991), who suggests an integration of various somato-psychological approaches from East and West in her book, which incorporates spiritual/religious, psychological and medical aspects. What is remarkable here is the in-depth treatment she also gives to European traditions. Before we get involved with Zundel & Loomans (1994), we shall also mention a comparable book by Walch (2002) that addresses transpersonal psychology and holotropic breathing. This may further be compared with Fischer (2003) as well as Galuska (2004). Spirituality in various contexts is considered by Wilber(2007). Finally, a validation of spiritual healing can be found in Benor (2002).

There are several contributions in Zundel & Loomans (1994) which are of special interest here: Zundel's introduction and the articles of Grof and Wilber. The introduction tells us (on pp. 16-20) that there are many spiritual paths to enlightenment but one consistent highest goal: unio mystica = becoming one with the primal purpose of being. This necessitates speaking in metaphors, negations and paradoxes. Mystic experiences are similar all over the world and connect with the ancient images of man and his surroundings, the 'philosophia perennis' (religion behind the religions). There is little love lost between philosophia per-ennis and psychology. An approach is possible through transpersonal psychology and psy-chotherapy. On pp. 33-37, we are told that in the USA transpersonal psychology is an aware-ness psychology. James (1896; see Taylor 1984 & 1996) had already studied the altered and extraordinary states of consciousness which interlink psychology and spirituality. Wilber put everything in order and distinguishes three (or, more precisely, nine) phases:

Prerational,	prepersonal phase:	mother goddesses, magical/mystical experience	(14.11a)
Rational,	personal phase:	male gods, rationality is central, subjugates nature	(14.11b)
Transrational,	transpersonal phase:	the primal purpose for being has been achieved at last	(14.11c)

Grof's contribution addresses NOSC (non-ordinary states of consciousness), which he equates with the holotropic states of consciousness that he investigated. They clearly point to P4 and include spiritual and mystic experiences, psychological death and rebirth, transper-sonal phenomena, and being at one with others. The use of NOSC is the newest development of Western psychotherapy but, at the same time, the most ancient form of healing (pp. 159-164). The problem in the field of psychotherapy lies in a lack of agreement and competitive-ness between schools. The work with holotropic states offers an alternative, a way out of the confusion. Moreover, spirituality must be distinguished from religion. Two trans-biographic fields are especially important: the perinatal (the link to the beginning and end of life, birth and death) and the transpersonal. In NOSC that which is most important in terms of psycho-dynamics is brought forth from the unconscious automatically. The schools show no agree-ment here; NOSC go around this problem and eliminate subjectivity. The inevitable selection of relevant problems directs the process spontaneously to the perinatal and transpersonal levels of the psyche. In transpersonal experiences, merging with other individuals is possible (pp. 171-178). This is a good way to describe P4 and {flora}.

In conclusion, the article by Wilber distinguishes spirituality and mysticism from common religion. Direct experience takes place in the laboratory of consciousness in the former case, whereas in the latter one falls back on myths. Statements made by mystics are the same the world over but there are some clear differences between religions. As a result, mysticism is no longer seen as dark and private but rather something scientific (pp. 293-297). In this statement, Wilber is saying practically the same thing as Bauhofer. Last but not least, on pp. 301-318, he introduces the nine stages of development which we have already mentioned, see (14.11a-c). These go in the direction of higher and higher integration and enable an interesting comparison with the life spiral I propose (from PC to SJ). The beginning and the end at first glance appear to be the same, but they differ fundamentally: An infant cannot distinguish between subject and object, but for a mystic, subject and object collapse into a greater identity. The stages are connected to corresponding world views. Wilber concludes by suggesting that the science of the external world unified with the science of the internal world is the true encounter of East and West.

Europe's task, then, could be to stay with the axis of life but extend it to {flora}/ P4, complementing external experiments through the no less universally valid internal experiments. This path was already foreordained in Greek Antiquity. For more information on this subject, the reader is referred to the book by Berner-Hürbin (1997), which also addresses the intercultural principles that govern medicine. A final quote from pp. 174ff refers to the goal of avoiding duality by means of unifying *dry water* and *damp fire*. What at first sounds absurd appears plausible in light of Ch. 14.3: Dry water corresponds to {flora}, damp fire ultimately refers to {wood} – which brings us back to the axis of life.

References

The page references and quotations refer to the editions that were originally used by the author. If the quoted book is not written in English but there exists an English translation, then the most recent one is additionally shown (*EE*: English edition). If there is a new edition in the original language, this is also referred to (*NE*: new edition, indented). If only the year of publication has changed, *NE* is indicated with the name(s) of the author(s) or editor(s) and the new year of publication.

Achterberg J. (1989), *Die heilende Kraft der Imagination. Heilung durch Gedankenkraft. Grundlagen und Methoden einer neuen Medizin.* Scherz, Bern, Switzerland.

EE: Achterberg J. (2002), *Imagery in Healing: Shamanism and Modern Medicine.* Shambhala, Boston, MA, USA.

Aerni F. (2000), *Lehrbuch der Menschenkenntnis. Einführung in die Huter'sche Psychophysiognomik und Kallisophie.* Carl-Huter-Verlag, Waldshut-Tiengen, Germany.

NE: Aerni F. (2003)

Aihara C. (1992), *Die Hohe Kunst des makrobiotischen Kochens – Ryori-Do. Mit Rezepten speziell für die vier Jahreszeiten und einem kompletten Menüplan für das ganze Jahr.* Mahajiva, Holthausen, Germany.

NE: Aihara C. (1993)

Aniscenko V.S. & A. Neiman (Eds., 1998a), *Proceedings of the International Conference on Nonlinear Dynamics and Chaos: Applications in Physics, Biology and Medicine, Part 1.* International Journal of Bifurcation and Chaos in Applied Sciences and Engineering 8_4.

Aniscenko V.S. & A. Neiman (Eds., 1998b), *Proceedings of the International Conference on Nonlinear Dynamics and Chaos: Applications in Physics, Biology and Medicine, Part 2.* International Journal of Bifurcation and Chaos in Applied Sciences and Engineering 8_5.

Arhem P., C. Blomberg & H. Liljenström (Eds., 2000), *Disorder versus Order in Brain Function. Essays in Theoretical Neurobiology.* World Scientific, Singapore.

Asshauer E. (1993), *Heilkunst vom Dach der Welt. Tibets sanfte Medizin.* Herder, Freiburg, Germany.

NE: Asshauer E. (1999)

Aswynn F. (1991), *Die Blätter von Yggdrasil. Runen, Götter, Magie. Nordische Mythologie & Weibliche Mysterien.* Ananael, Vienna, Austria.

NE: Aswynn F. (2001)

EE: Aswynn F. (1994), *Leaves of Yggdrasil: A Synthesis of Runes. Gods, Magic, Feminine Mysteries, and Folklore.* Llewellyn Publications, St.Paul, MN, USA.

Baatz U. (1989), *Ich – Seele – Augen. Zur Wahrnehmungspsychologie im 19. Jahrhundert.* In: J. Clair, C. Pichler & W. Pircher, Wunderblock. Eine Geschichte der modernen Seele. Katalog zur Ausstellung der Wiener Festwochen. Löcker, Vienna, Austria (S.357-378).

Badelt F. (1983), *Chinesische Klassik aus ärztlicher Sicht. Die Bedeutung altchinesischer Funktionsmodelle für unsere heutige Medizin.* Haug, Heidelberg, Germany.

Bäumer B. (1996), *Primal Elements – Mahabhuta. Kalatattvakosa Vol. III.* Indira Ghandi National Centre for the Arts, New Delhi, India.
NE: Bäumer B. (1998)

Bäurle R. (1988), *Körpertypen. Vom Typentrauma zum Traumtypen.* Simon+ Leutner, Berlin, Germany.
NE: Bäurle R. (2001)

Bahr F.R. (1981), *Ohr-Akupunktur. Neue Waffe gegen viele Leiden.* Fischer TBV, Frankfurt am Main, Germany.

Barbi M. & S. Chillemi (Eds., 1999), *Chaos and Noise in Biology and Medicine.* World Scientific, Singapore.

Barnsley M.F. & L.P. Hurd (1993), *Fractal Image Compression.* AK Peters, Wellesley, MA, USA.

Bauhofer U. (1997), *Aufbruch zur Stille. Maharishi Ayur-Ved, eine leise Medizin für eine laute Zeit.* Lübbe, Bergisch Gladbach, Germany.
NE: Bauhofer U. (2002)

Baumgart G. (1995), *Von Akupunktur bis Zelltherapie. Komplementär-Medizin zum Nachschlagen.* Ueberreuter, Vienna, Austria.

Beck D.E. & C.C. Cowan (1996), *Spiral Dynamics. Mastering Values, Leadership, and Change.* Blackwell Business, Cambridge, MA, USA.

Benedikt H.E. (1986), *Die Kabbala als jüdisch-christlicher Einweihungsweg. 1. Farbe, Zahl, Ton und Wort als Tore zu Seele und Geist.* Bauer, Freiburg, Germany.
NE: Benedikt H.E. (2003), *Die Kabbala als jüdisch-christlicher Einweihungsweg. 1. Farbe, Zahl, Ton und Wort als Tore zu Seele und Geist.* Ludwig, Munich, Germany.

Benedikt H.E. (2003), *Die Kabbala als jüdisch-christlicher Einweihungsweg. 2. Der Lebensbaum: Spiegel des Kosmos und des Menschen.* Ludwig, Munich, Germany.

Benor D. (2002), *Spiritual Healing. Scientific Validation of a Healing Revolution. Professional Supplement.* Vision Publications, Southfield, MI, USA.

Bergé P., Y. Pomeau & C. Vidal (1986), *Order within Chaos. Towards a Deterministic Approach to Turbulence.* Hermann, Paris, France.
NE: Bergé P., Y. Pomeau & C. Vidal (1987), *Order within Chaos. Towards a Deterministic Approach to Turbulence.* Wiley, Hoboken, NJ, USA.

Bergsmann O. (1994), *Bioelektrische Phänomene und Regulation in der Komplementärmedizin. Eine Einführung.* Facultas, Vienna, Austria.

Berner-Hürbin A. (1997), *Hippokrates und die Heilenergie. Alte und neue Modelle für eine holistische Therapeutik.* Schwabe, Basel, Switzerland.

Bettschart R., G. Glaeske, K. Langbein, R. Saller & C. Skalnik (1996), *Bittere Naturmedizin. Wirkung und Bewertung der alternativen Behandlungsmethode, Diagnoseverfahren und Arzneimittel.* Bertelsmann Club, Rheda Wiedenbrück, Germany.

Bialas V. (1998), *Vom Himmelsmythos zum Weltgesetz. Eine Kulturgeschichte der Astronomie.* Ibera, Vienna, Austria.

Böse R. & G. Schiepek (1989), *Systemische Theorie und Therapie. Ein Handwörterbuch.* Asanger, Heidelberg, Germany.
     NE: Böse R. & G. Schiepek (2000)

von Bonin D., M. Frühwirth, P. Heusser & M. Moser (2001), *Wirkungen der Therapeutischen Sprachgestaltung auf Herzfrequenz-Variabilität und Befinden.* Forsch Komplementärmed Klass Naturheilkd *8:* 144-160.

Brandl-Nebehay (Hrsg., 1998), *Systemische Familientherapie. Grundlagen, Methoden und aktuelle Trends.* Facultas, Vienna, Austria.

Briggs J. & F.D. Peat (1990), *Die Entdeckung des Chaos. Eine Reise durch die Chaos-Theorie.* Hanser, Munich, Germany.

Briggs J. & F.D. Peat (1998), *Turbulent Mirror. An Illustrated Guide to Chaos Theory and the Science of Wholeness.* Harper & Row, New York, NY, USA.

Brückner K.-H. (Hrsg., 1999), *Die heilende Kraft veränderter Bewußtseinszustände. Transpersonale Psychotherapie und Atemarbeit.* Österreichischer Arbeitskreis für transpersonale Psychologie und Psychotherapie, Klosterneuburg, Austria.

Busch P. (2002), *Elementare Regelungstechnik.* Vogel, Würzburg, Germany.

Calabrese E.J. (2008), *Hormesis: why it is important to toxicology and toxicologists.* Environ Toxicol Chem *27*: 1451-1474.

Chopra D. (1993), *Die Körperseele. Grundlagen und praktische Übungen der indischen Medizin.* Droemer Knaur, Munich, Germany.
     NE: Chopra D. (2001)

Chopra D. (2001), *Perfect Health: The Complete Mind/Body Guide.* Harmony Books, New York, NY, USA.

Clair J., C. Pichler & W. Pircher (1989), *Wunderblock. Eine Geschichte der modernen Seele. Katalog zur Ausstellung der Wiener Festwochen.* Löcker, Vienna, Austria.

Connelly D.M. (1995), *Traditionelle Akupunktur: das Gesetz der fünf Elemente.* Endrich, Heidelberg, Germany.
     NE: Connelly D.M. (2002)

EE: Connelly D.M. (1994), *Traditional Acupuncture: The Law of the Five Elements.* The Centre for Traditional Acupuncture, Columbia, MD, USA.

Coveney P. & R. Highfield (1994), *Anti-Chaos. Der Pfeil der Zeit in der Selbstorganisation des Lebens.* Rowohlt, Reinbek bei Hamburg, Germany.

Coyle-Demetriou M. & Demetriou A. (2007), *Integrating Complementary and Conventional Medicine.* Radcliff Publ., Oxford, UK.

Crutchfield J.P. (1984), *Space-Time Dynamics in Video Feedback.* Physica *10D*, 229-245.

Crutchfield J.P. (1987), *Chaotica. 1. Space-Time Dynamics in Video-Feedback. Chaotic Attractors of Driven Oscillators.* The visual mathematics library. Aerial Press, Santa Cruz, CA, USA.

Darras J.C., P. de Vernejoul & P. Albarede (1987), *Visualisation isotopique des méridiens d'acupuncture*. Cahiers des Biothérapie *95*: 12-22.

Dash B. (1980): *Fundamentals of Ayurvedic Medicine*. Bansal & Co, Delhi, India.
NE: Dash B. (1999), *Fundamentals of Ayurvedic Medicine*. Konark Publishers, New Delhi, India.

D'Adamo P.J. (1997), *Eat Right for Your Type: The Individualized Diet Solution to Staying Healthy, Living Longer & Achieving Your Ideal Weight*. Penguin Putnam Inc., New York, NY, USA.

Dellmour F. (1992), *Homöopathie*. Facultas, Vienna, Austria.

Dellmour F. (1994), *Zur Situation der homöopathischen Arzneimittel (2)*. Homöopathie in Österreich 5_2: 4-11.

Diamond. J. (2000), *The Clinical Practice of Complementary, Alternative, and Western Medicine*. CRC Press, Boca Raton, FL, USA.

Diamond. J. (2001), *Holism and Beyond: The Essence of Holistic Medicine*. Enhancement Books, Ridgefield, CT, USA.

Dillard J. & T. Ziporyn (1999), *Alternative Medicine for Dummies*. John Wiley & Sons Inc., Hoboken, NJ, USA.

Doepp M. (1998), *Diagnostik mit einem neuen biophysikalischen Meßverfahren*. Erfahrungsheilkunde 10_{11}: 821-830.

Doerper Reckeweg M. & P. Maschke (1996), *Sechs Phasen zwischen gesund und krank: Das Leben des Begründers der Homotoxikologie Hans-Heinrich Reckeweg*. Forum-Medizin Verlagsgesellschaft, Gräfelfing, Germany.

Dorcsi M., H. Gyürky & I. Rumpold (1991), *Handbuch der Homöopathie*. Orac, Vienna, Austria.
NE: Dorcsi M. (2002), *Handbuch der Homöopathie. Geschichte, Theorie, Praxis*. Bassermann, Niederhausen, Germany.

Dossey L. (1995). *Heilende Worte. Die Kraft der Gebete und die Macht der Medizin*. Martin, Südergellersen, Germany.

Dossey L. (1993), *Healing Words: The Power of Prayer and the Practice of Medicine*. Harper, San Francisco, CA, USA.

Ebert H. (1992), *Homöosiniatrie. Die Komplementarität von Homöopathie und Akupunktur in neuer und erweiterter Form*. Haug, Heidelberg, Germany.

Eliade M. (1994), *Schamanismus und archaische Ekstasetechnik*. Suhrkamp, Frankfurt am Main, Germany.
NE: Eliade M. (2001)

Eliade M. (1972), *Shamanism: Archaic Techniques of Ecstasy*. Princeton University Press, Princeton, NJ, USA.

Endler P.C. (1998), *Expedition Homöopathieforschung. Ein altes Heilsystem wird plausibel*. Maudrich, Vienna, Austria.

Endler P.C. (2003), *Homeopathy Research – An Expedition Report: An Old Healing System Gains Plausibility*. Edition@inter-uni.net, Graz, Austria.

Endler P.C & J. Schulte (Eds., 1994), *Ultra High Dilution. Physiology and Physics*. Kluwer, Dordrecht, The Netherlands.

Endler P.C. & J. Schulte (Hrsg., 1996), *Homöopathie – Bioresonanztherapie. Physiologische und physikalische Voraussetzungen – Grundlagenforschung.* Maudrich, Vienna, Austria.

Endler P.C. & A. Stacher (Hrsg., 1997), *Niederenergetische Bioinformation. Physiologische und Physikalische Grundlagen für Bioresonanz und Homöopathie.* Facultas, Vienna, Austria.

Engler I. (1989), *Information durch elektromagnetisches Feld.* In: I. Engler (Hrsg.), Wasser. Polarisationsphänomen, Informationsträger, Lebens-Heilmittel. Sommer, Teningen, Germany (S.101-106).

Enne M. (2000), *Die elektrische Aktivität des menschlichen Gehirns vom Neuron zum EEG.* Diploma thesis, Vienna, Austria.

Epstein M. (2000), *Gedanken ohne den Denker. Das Wechselspiel von Buddhismus und Psychotherapie.* Fischer, Frankfurt am Main, Germany.

Epstein M. (1996), *Thoughts Without a Thinker. Psychotherapy from a Buddhist Perspective.* Basic Books, New York, NY, USA.

Eschenbach U.G. (1996), *Der Ich-Komplex und sein Arbeitsteam. Topographie der Selbstentfaltung.* Bonz, Leinfelden-Echterdingen, Germany.

Farrington E.A. (2002a), *The Comparative Materia Medica.* B. Jain Publishers, New Delhi, India.

Farrington E.A. (2002b), *Clinical Materia Medica.* B. Jain Publishers, New Delhi, India.

Faust J. (Hrsg., 1993), 1. A. Masi-Elizalde, *Überarbeitung der Lehre, Materia Medica und Technik der Homöopathie.* 2. S. Preis, *Seminar zur Sicht der Homöopathie nach Dr. Masi-Elizalde.* Sylvia Faust, Höhr, Germany.

Federspiel K. (1996), *Die Andere Medizin. Nutzen und Risiken sanfter Heilmethoden.* Stiftung Warentest, Stuttgart, Germany.

Federspiel K. & I. Lackinger Karger (1996), *Kursbuch Seele. Was tun bei psychischen Problemen? 120 Psychotherapien auf dem Prüfstand.* Kiepenheuer & Witsch, Cologne, Germany.

Fester R. (1981), *Urwörter der Menschheit. Eine Archäologie der Sprache.* Kösel, Munich, Germany.

Fintelmann V. (2000), *Intuitive Medizin. Einführung in eine anthroposophisch ergänzte Medizin.* Hippokrates, Stuttgart, Germany.

Fisch G. (1994), *Die Traditionelle Chinesische Medizin. Orientierungs- und Lehrbuch.* Wenderoth, Kassel, Germany.

Fischer K.H. (Hrsg., 2003), *Heimkehr der Seele. Psychotherapie und Spiritualität.* edition pro mente, Linz, Austria.

Focks C. & N. Hillenbrand (Hrsg., 1997), *Leitfaden Traditionelle Chinesische Medizin. Schwerpunkt Akupunktur. Methoden, Diagnostik, Therapie.* G. Fischer, Ulm, Germany. *NE:* Focks C. & N. Hillenbrand (Hrsg., 2003)

Freeman L. (Ed., 2004), *Mosby's Complementary & Alternative Medicine: A Research-Based Approach.* Mosby, St.Louis, MO, USA.

Freund J.A. & T. Pöschel (Eds., 2001), *Stochastic Processes in Physics, Chemistry, and Biology.* Springer, Berlin, Germany.

Früh S. (Hrsg., 1998), *Der Kult der Drei Heiligen Frauen. Märchen, Sagen und Brauch.* edition amalia, Bern, Switzerland.

Fuchs B. & N. Kobler-Fumasoli (Hrsg., 2002), *Hilft der Glaube? Heilung auf dem Schnittpunkt zwischen Theologie und Medizin*. LIT, Münster, Germany.

Galuska J. (Hrsg., 2004), *Den Horizont erweitern. Die transpersonale Dimension in der Psychotherapie*. Leutner, Berlin, Germany.

Gawlik W. (1990), *Arzneimittelbild und Persönlichkeitsportrait. Konstitutionsmittel in der Homöopathie*. Hippokrates, Stuttgart, Germany.
NE: Gawlik W. (2002)

Gedeon W. (Hrsg., 2000), *Eigenbluttherapie und andere autologe Verfahren. Ein Lehrbuch für die ärztliche Praxis*. Haug, Heidelberg, Germany.

Geyer G. & A. Stacher (Hrsg., 1992), *Chronobiologie und ihre Bedeutung für die Therapie. Behandlung nach Tageszeit*. Facultas, Vienna, Austria.

Gienow P. (2000), *Homöopathische Miasmen: Die Psora. Ein Lern- und Praxisbuch*. Sonntag, Stuttgart, Germany.

Gienow P. (2003), *Homöopathische Miasmen: Die Sykose. Ein Lern- und Praxisbuch*. Sonntag, Stuttgart, Germany.

Girke M. (1994), *Krankheit und Heilung. Ein Beitrag aus der anthroposophischen Medizin*. In: R.G. Appell (Hrsg.), Homöopathie 150 Jahre nach Hahnemann. Standpunkte und Perspektiven. Haug, Heidelberg, Germany (S.195-222).

Glass L. & M.C. Mackey (1988), *From Clocks to Chaos. The Rhythms of Life*. Princeton University Press, Princeton, NJ, USA.

Gleditsch A. (1991), *Vom Bewußtsein zum Gewißsein. Hinführung zu einem somatopsychischen Menschenbild. Opal, Augsburg*, Germany.

Gleditsch J. (1988a), *Differenzierte Schmerztherapie aufgrund der Akupunktur-Systematik*. Akupunktur – Theorie und Praxis *16*$_2$: 71-82.

Gleditsch J. (1988b), *Reflexzonen und Somatotopien als Schlüssel zu einer Gesamtschau des Menschen*. WBV Biologisch-medizinische Verlagsgesellschaft, Schorndorf, Germany.
NE: Gleditsch J. (2005), *Reflexzonen und Somatotopien. Vom Mikrosystem zu einer Gesamtschau des Menschen*. Urban & Fischer / Elsevier, Munich, Germany.

Gleditsch J. (2001), *Akupunktur und Psychosomatik*. In: A. Stacher & W. Marktl (Hrsg.), Ganzheitsmedizin in der Zukunft. Bericht des 1. Zukunftssymposiums der Wiener Internationalen Akademie für Ganzheitsmedizin. Facultas, Vienna, Austria (S.111-116).

Gleditsch J. & H.P. Ogal (2002), *MAPS – MikroAkuPunktSysteme. Grundlagen und Praxis der somatotopischen Therapie*. Hippokrates, Stuttgart, Germany.

Goldbeter A. (1997), *Biochemical Oscillations and Cellular Rhythms. The Molecular Bases of Periodic and Chaotic Behaviour*. Cambridge University Press, Cambridge, UK.

Granet M. (1993), *Das chinesische Denken. Inhalt – Form – Charakter*. Suhrkamp, Frankfurt am Main, Germany.
NE: Granet M. (2000)

Grawe K., R. Donati & F. Bernauer (1998), *Psychotherapy in Transition: From Speculation to Science*. Hogrefe & Huber, Cambridge, MA, USA.

Grof S. (1994), *Das Heilungspotential außergewöhnlicher Bewußtseinszustände. Beobachtungen aus der psychedelischen und holotropen Therapie* In: E. Zundel & P. Loomans (Hrsg.), Psychotherapie und religiöse Erfahrung. Konzepte und Methoden transpersonaler Psychotherapie. Herder, Freiburg, Germany (S.159-204).

Gruber W. & K.W. Kratky (2002), *Verhaltensweisen von Schamanen und psychosozialer Streß*. In: Pritz A. & T. Wenzel (Hrsg., 2002), Weltkongreß Psychotherapie. Mythos – Traum – Wirklichkeit. Ausgewählte Beiträge des 2. Weltkongresses für Psychotherapie. Facultas, Vienna, Austria.(S.247-266).

Haas E. (1992), *Staying Healthy with Nutrition: The Complete Guide to Diet & Nutritional Medicine*. Celestial Arts, Berkeley, CA, USA.
NE: Haas E. & B. Levin (2006).

Hadulla M. & R.G. Appell (1993), *Der Doppelaspekt von Aurum in Psychotherapie und Homöopathie*. In: R.G. Appell (Hrsg.), Homöopathie, Psychotherapie & Psychiatrie. Hahnemanns weiterwirkender Impuls. Haug, Heidelberg, Germany (S.207-218).

Hänggi P. (2001), *Stochastische Resonanz. Rauschen macht sensibel*. Physikalische Blätter *57*: 15-16.

Hanzl G.S. (2002), *Das neue medizinische Paradigma. Theorie und Praxis eines erweiterten wissenschaftlichen Konzepts*. Haug, Heidelberg, Germany.

Heine H. (1997), *Lehrbuch der biologischen Medizin. Grundregulation und Extrazelluläre Matrix. Grundlagen und Systematik*. Hippokrates, Stuttgart, Germany.

Heise T. (1996), *Chinas Medizin bei uns. Einführendes Lehrbuch zur traditionellen chinesischen Medizin*. WVB – Verlag für Wissenschaft und Bildung, Berlin, Germany.
NE: Heise T. (1999)

Herbert D.E. (Ed., 1996), *Chaos and the Changing Nature of Science and Medicine: an Introduction*. AIP Press, Woodbury, New York, NY, USA.

Hertzer D. (1996), *Das Mawangdui-Yijing. Text und Deutung*. Diederichs, Munich, Germany.

Heusser-Buchs U. (2002), *Gedanken zu Chinas Heilkunst in Ursprung und Gegenwart. Spiritualität in der Traditionellen Chinesischen Medizin (TCM)*. In: B. Fuchs & N. Kobler-Fumasoli (Hrsg.), Hilft der Glaube? Heilung auf dem Schnittpunkt zwischen Theologie und Medizin. LIT, Münster, Germany (pp.3-34).

Heyartz S. (1996), *Kinesiologie. Überprüfung kinesiologischer Grundaspekte*. Diplomarbeit, Munich, Germany.

Hildebrandt G., M. Moser & M. Lehofer (1998), *Chronobiologie und Chronomedizin. Biologische Rhythmen. Medizinische Konsequenzen*. Hippokrates, Stuttgart, Germany.

Hofkirchner W. (2001), *The Hidden Ontology: Real World Evolutionary Systems Concept as Key to Information Science*. Emergence *3₃*: 22-41.

Hsu E. (1999), *The Transmission of Chinese Medicine*. Cambridge University Press, Cambridge, UK.

Hütter A., J. Perger & T. Hug (Hrsg., 1992), *Paradigmenvielfalt und Wissensintegration. Beiträge zur Postmoderne im Umkreis von Jean-Francois Lyotard*. Passagen, Vienna, Austria.

Huntington S.P. (2002), *The Clash of Civilizations and the Remaking of World Order*. Free Press, Glasgow, UK.

Jarmey C. & G. Mojay (1995), *Das große Shiatsu-Handbuch. Alles über Theorie, Praxis und therapeutische Methoden der japanischen Heilmassage*. Barth/ Scherz, Bern, Switzerland.

NE: Jarmey C. & G. Mojay (1996), *Das große Shiatsu-Handbuch. Alles über Theorie, Praxis und therapeutische Methoden der japanischen Heilmassage.* Econ-Taschenbuchverlag, Düsseldorf, Germany.

Jarmey C. & G. Mojay (2000), *Shiatsu: The Complete Guide.* Thorsons Publishers, London, UK.

Jonas W.B. & J.S. Levin (Eds., 1999), *Essentials of Complementary and Alternative Medicine.* Lippincott Williams & Wilkins, Philadelphia, PA, USA.

Jonas W.B. (Ed., 2004), *Mosby's Dictionary of Complementary and Alternative Medicine.* Mosby, St.Louis, MO, USA.

Kaptchuk T.J. (1996), *Das große Buch der Chinesischen Medizin. Die Medizin von Yin und Yang in Theorie und Praxis.* Heyne, Munich, Germany.
NE: Kaptchuk T.J. (2002)

Kaptchuk T.J. (2000), *The Web that Has no Weaver: Understanding Chinese Medicine.* Mc Graw-Hill Companies, New York, NY, USA.

Kastrinidis P. (1994), *Die Daseinsanalytische Psychotherapie und das Transpersonale nach L. Binswanger und M. Boss.* In: E. Zundel & P. Loomans (Hrsg.), Psychotherapie und religiöse Erfahrung. Konzepte und Methoden transpersonaler Psychotherapie. Herder, Freiburg, Germany (S.105-136).

King S.K. (1998), *Der Weg des Abenteurers. Eine Beschreibung des hawaiianischen Schamanismus.* Lüchow, Freiburg, Germany.

King S.K. (2001), *Sehen ist Glauben. Die vier Welten eines hawaiianischen Schamanen.* Lüchow, Freiburg, Germany.

Klinghardt D. (1996), *Lehrbuch der Psycho-Kinesiologie. Ein neuer Weg in der psychosomatischen Medizin.* Bauer, Freiburg, Germany.

Kluge, F. (2002), *Etymologisches Wörterbuch der deutschen Sprache.* de Gruyter, Berlin.

Kobau C. (1993), *Bodybalance. Intuitiv kreatives Körperbewußtsein.* Kobau, Klagenfurt, Austria.
NE: Dahlke R., A.L. Rossaint, C. Kobau, & L. Tandl (2006), *Bodybalance. Intuitiv kreatives Körperbewusstsein.* Kobau, Klagenfurt, Austria.

Kobau C., H. Heine & R. Dahlke (1996), *Ganzheitliche und naturheilkundlich orientierte Zahnmedizin. Eine Verbindung westlichen und östlichen Wissens.* Kobau, Klagenfurt, Austria.

Krämer D. (1991), *Neue Therapien mit Bach-Blüten 1. Beziehung der Blüten untereinander.* Ansata, Interlaken, Switzerland.
NE: Krämer D. (2001), *Neue Therapien mit Bach-Blüten 1. Beziehungen der Blüten untereinander.* Ludwig, Munich, Germany.

Krämer D. (1994), *Neue Therapien mit Bach-Blüten3. Akupunkturmeridiane und Bach-Blüten.* Ansata, Interlaken, Switzerland.

Kratky K.W. (1989), *Vom linearen zum systemischen Denken.* In: K.W. Kratky & E.M. Bonet (Hrsg.), Systemtheorie und Reduktionismus. Österreichische Staatsdruckerei, Vienna, Austria (S.11-32).

Kratky K.W. (1990), *Der Paradigmenwechsel von der Fremd- zur Selbstorganisation.* In: K.W. Kratky & F. Wallner (Hrsg.), Grundprinzipien der Selbstorganisation. Wissenschaftliche Buchgesellschaft, Darmstadt, Germany (S.3-17).

Kratky K.W. (1992), *Chaos and disorder*. In: W. Tschacher, G. Schiepek & E.J. Brunner (Eds.), Self-Organization and Clinical Psychology. Empirical Approaches to Synergetics in Psychology. Springer, Berlin, Germany (pp.89-101).

Kratky K.W. (1993), *The Generalized Simile Principle as a Joint Framework of Allopathy and Homoeopathy*. In: C. Bornoroni (Ed.), OMEOMED 92. Proceedings Book. Editrice Compositori, Bologna, Italy (pp.49-54).

Kratky K.W. (1994), *Moderne Naturwissenschaft und Homöopathie – Offenere Einstellung durch neue Entwicklungen?* In: R.G. Appell (Hrsg.), Homöopathie 150 Jahre nach Hahnemann. Standpunkte und Perspektiven. Haug, Heidelberg, Germany (S.90-125).

Kratky K.W. & T.J. Milavec (1994), *Besteht ein qualitativer Unterschied zwischen Hochpotenz und reinem Lösungsmittel?* In: O. Bergsmann (Hrsg.), Struktur und Funktion des Wassers im Organismus. Facultas, Vienna, Austria (S.40-56).

Kratky K.W. (1995a), *Chaos: Influence of Finite Computer Accuracy*. In: J. Tran Thanh Van, P. Bergé, R. Conte & D. Dubois (Eds.), Chaos and Complexity. Editions Frontières, Gif-sur-Yvette, France (pp.253-254).

Kratky K.W. (1995b), *Systems Thinking, Systems Control, and Systems Regulation*. In: G.E. Lasker (Ed.), Advances in Systems Studies, Volume II. The International Institute of Advances Studies in Systems Research and Cybernetics, Windsor, Ontario, Canada (pp.11-15).

Kratky K.W. (1996a), *Analysis and Control of Chaotic Systems – Two Sides of the Same Coin?* In: J. Ramaekers (Ed.), Proceedings of the 14th International Congress on Cybernetics. Association Internationale de Cybernetique, Namur, Belgium (pp.548-553).

Kratky K.W. (1996b), *Interaktivität, Rückkopplung und Chaossteuerung*. In: P.C. Endler & J. Schulte (Hrsg.), Homöopathie – Bioresonanztherapie. Physiologische und physikalische Voraussetzungen – Grundlagenforschung. Maudrich, Vienna, Austria (S.57-63).

Kratky K.W. (1996c), *Elements and Tempers – Thinking in Analogies among the Old Greeks, in India and China*. In: G.E. Lasker, H. Koizumi & M. Okuyama (Eds.), Proceedings of the Focus Symposium on Health, Healing and Medicine, Vol. II. The International Institute for Advanced Studies in Systems Research and Cybernetics, Windsor, Ontario, Canada (pp.21-25).

Kratky K.W. (1996d), *Traditional Chinese Medicine, Ayurveda and Bach flowers: common principles*. In: G.E. Lasker, H. Koizumi & M. Okuyama (Eds.), Proceedings of the Focus Symposium on Health, Healing and Medicine, Vol. II. The International Institute for Advanced Studies in Systems Research and Cybernetics, Windsor, Ontario, Canada (pp.26-30).

Kratky K.W. (1997a), *Bachblüten – Homöopathie – Ayurveda: Gemeinsame Prinzipien und Beziehung zur Psychosomatik*. In: U. Kropiunigg & A. Stacher (Hrsg.), Ganzheitsmedizin und Psychoneuroimmunologie. Vierter Wiener Dialog. Facultas, Vienna, Austria (S.334-341).

Kratky K.W. (1997b), *Human Typology and its Relevance for Health and Healing – Static Aspects*. In: G.E. Lasker, H. Koizumi & M. Okuyama (Eds.), Proceedings of the Focus Symposium on Health, Healing and Medicine, Vol. III. The International Institute for Advanced Studies in Systems Research and Cybernetics, Windsor, Ontario, Canada (pp.32-37).

Kratky K.W. (1997c), *Human Typology and its Relevance for Health and Healing – Dynamic Aspects*. In: G.E. Lasker, H. Koizumi & M. Okuyama (Eds.), Proceedings of the Focus Symposium on Health, Healing and Medicine, Vol. III. The International Institute for Advanced Studies in Systems Research and Cybernetics, Windsor, Ontario, Canada (pp.38-43).

Kratky K.W. (1998a), *Comparison of Different Dilutions of the Same Substance*. In: C. Taddei-Ferretti & P. Marotta (Eds.), High Dilution Effects in Cells and Integrated Systems. World Scientific, Singapore (pp.95-106).

Kratky K.W. (1998b), *Wie kann eine Verständigung zwischen verschiedenen Disziplinen und Weltbildern gelingen?* Zeitschrift für Hochschuldidaktik 22_3: 69-88.

Kratky K.W. (1998c), *Interactivity, Feedback and Chaos Control*. In: J. Schulte & P.C. Endler (Eds.), Fundamental Research in Ultra High Dilution and Homoeopathy. Kluwer, Dordrecht, The Netherlands (pp.117-125).

Kratky K.W. (2000a), *Lebenspforte und chinesische Elemente. I. Räumliche Anordnung*. Ethnopsychologische Mitteilungen *9*: 82-108.

Kratky K.W. (2000b), *Lebenspforte und chinesische Elemente. II. Zyklische Abfolge*. Ethnopsychologische Mitteilungen *9*: 160-196.

Kratky K.W. (2000c), *Lebenspforte und chinesische Elemente. III. Spiegelung in anderen Traditionen*. Ethnopsychologische Mitteilungen *9*: 197-235.

Kratky K.W. (2002), *Die drei Prinzipien in östlichen und westlichen Heilsystemen*. In: A. Stacher & W. Marktl (Hrsg.), Ganzheitsmedizin in der Zukunft II. Facultas, Vienna, Austria (S.22-44).

Kratky K.W. (2003a), *Komplementäre Medizinsysteme. Vergleich und Integration*. Ibera/European University Press, Vienna, Austria.

Kratky K.W. (2003b), *Comparative and Integrative Medicine. I. From Different Views to a Common Essence*. In: G.E. Lasker & A. Aydin (Eds.), Health, Healing and Medicine, Vol. IX. The International Institute for Advanced Studies in Systems Research and Cybernetics, Windsor, Canada (pp.27-32).

Kratky K.W. (2003c), *Comparative and Integrative Medicine. II. Health Geometry and Life Spiral*. In: G.E. Lasker & A. Aydin (Eds.), Health, Healing and Medicine, Vol. IX. The International Institute for Advanced Studies in Systems Research and Cybernetics, Windsor, Canada (pp.33-38).

Kratky K.W. (2004), *Homöopathie und Wasserstruktur: ein physikalisches Modell (Homeopathy and Structure of Water: A Physical Model)*. Forsch Komplementärmed Klass Naturheilkd (Research in Complementary and Classical Natural Medicine) *11*: 24-32.

Kratky K.W. (2005a), *The Development of Chinese Medicine from a Cross-Cultural Point of View*. In: G.E. Lasker & K.W. Kratky (Eds.): Health, Healing and Medicine, Vol. XI. Comparative and Integrative Medicine. The International Institute for Advanced Studies in Systems Research and Cybernetics, Windsor, Canada (pp.49-60).

Kratky K.W. (2005b), *Chronobiology and Cross-Cultural Medicine: Cyclic Processes during a Day, a Year, and a Lifetime*. In: G.E. Lasker & K.W. Kratky (Eds.), Health, Healing and Medicine, Vol. XI. Comparative and Integrative Medicine. The International Institute for Advanced Studies in Systems Research and Cybernetics, Windsor, Canada (pp.61-76).

Kratky K.W. (2006a), *Rhythmen, Übergänge und Lebensspirale (Teil 1)*. CO'MED 2/2006; 138-140.

Kratky K.W. (2006b), *Rhythmen, Übergänge und Lebensspirale (Teil 2)*. CO'MED 3/2006; 118-121.

Kriz J. (1997), *Systemtheorie. Eine Einführung für Psychotherapeuten, Psychologen und Mediziner*. Facultas, Vienna, Austria.
NE: Kriz J. (1999), *Systemtheorie für Psychotherapeuten, Psychologen und Mediziner. Eine Einführung*. UTB, Stuttgart, Germany.

Kropiunigg U. & A. Stacher (Hrsg., 1997), *Ganzheitsmedizin und Psychoneuroimmunologie. Vierter Wiener Dialog*. Facultas, Vienna, Austria.

Kubiena G. (1995), *Kleine Klassik für die Akupunktur. Eine einfache Einführung in die Grundlagen der Traditionellen Chinesischen Medizin*. Maudrich, Vienna, Austria.
NE: Kubiena G. (2000)

Kubny M. (1995), *Qi – Lebenskraftkonzepte in China. Definitionen, Theorien und Grundlagen*. Haug, Heidelberg, Germany.
NE: Kubny M. (2002)

Kuhn T.S. (1997), *The Structure of Scientific Revolutions*. University of Chicago Press, Chicago, IL, USA.

Kutter E. (2003), *Der Kult der drei Jungfrauen. Eine Kraftquelle weiblicher Spiritualität neu entdeckt*. Kösel, Munich, Germany.

Lack M. (1996), *Myostatiktest und Aussage über die Aktualität des Befundes*. Hausarzt *10/96*: 40-42.

Lack M. (1997), *Bioresonanz – theoretische Vorstellungen und praktische Erfahrungen am Beispiel der dualen Biosignalmodulation unter Verwendung des K-MED-Systems*. Arzt & Praxis *51₇₆₄*: 146-148.

Laskar J., F. Joutel & P. Robutel (1993), *Stabilization of the Earth's Obliquity by the Moon*. Nature *361*: 615-617.

Lasker G.E. & K.W. Kratky (Eds., 2005), *Health, Healing and Medicine, Vol. XI. Comparative and Integrative Medicine*. The International Institute for Advanced Studies in Systems Research and Cybernetics, Windsor, Canada.

Laudan R. (2000), Birth of the Modern Diet. *Scientific American. 283₂*: 76-81.

Lecar M., F.A. Franklin, M.J. Holman & N.W. Murray (2001), *Chaos in the Solar System*. Annual Review in Astronomy and Astrophysics *39*: 581-631.

Lehnertz K., C.E. Elger, J. Arnhold & P. Grassberger (Eds., 2000), *Workshop on: Chaos in Brain?* World Scientific, Singapore.

Lemmer B. (2004), *Chronopharmakologie. Tagesrhythmen und Arzneimittelwirkung*. Wissenschaftliche Verlagsgesellschaft, Stuttgart, Germany.

Lemmer B. (Ed., 1996), *From the Biological Clock to Chronopharmacology*. medpharm, Stuttgart, Germany.

Leven R.W., B.-P. Koch & B. Pompe (1994), *Chaos in dissipativen Systemen*. Akademie-Verlag, Berlin, Germany.

Linde K. (1991), *Dosisabhängige Umkehreffekte. Eine differenzierende Literaturbetrachtung*. Dissertation, Munich, Germany.

Litscher G. & Z.H. Cho (Eds., 2000), *Computer-Controlled Acupuncture*. Pabst, Lengerich, Germany.

Litscher G. (2001), *High-Tech Akupunktur. Computergestützte Objektivierungstechniken der Akupunktur*. Pabst, Lengerich, Germany.

Litscher G. & D. Schikora (Hrsg., 2003), *LASERneedle®-Akupunktur. Wissenschaft und Praxis*. Pabst, Lengerich, Germany.

Lo V. (2002), *Spirit of Stone: Technical Considerations in the Treatment of the Jade Body*. Bulletin of SOAS 65_1: 99-128 (School of Oriental and African Studies, UK).

Locker A. (1999), *"Was dich schlägt, wird dich heilen". Reifung und Verklärung des Menschen durch (geheilt / ungeheiltes) Leid. Ein Anwendungsfall Transklassischer System-Theorie*. In: G. Dörner, K.-D. Hüllemann, G. Tembrock, K.-Fr. Wessel & K.S. Zänker (Hrsg), Menschenbilder in der Medizin – Medizin in den Menschenbildern. Kleine, Bielefeld, Germany (pp. 288-317).

Lorenz E.N. (1963), Deterministic Nonperiodic Flow. *J. Atmos. Sci. 20*: 130-141.

Ludwig W. (1994), *SIT – System-Informations-Therapie. Schwingungsmedizin in Theorie und Praxis*. Spitta, Balingen, Germany.

Ludwig W. (1999), *Informative Medizin. Krankheits-Ursachen/Behandlung ohne Chemie*. Verlag für Ganzheitsmedizin, Essen, Germany.

Machleidt W., L. Gutjahr & A. Mügge (1989), *Grundgefühle. Phänomenologie, Psychodynamik, EEG-Spektralanalytik*. Springer, Berlin, Germany.

Machleidt W. (1995), *Vater und Tochter. Gefühlslandschaften einer Beziehung*. Deutscher Studien Verlag, Weinheim, Germany.
NE: Machleidt W. (2002)

Maciocia G. (1994), *Die Grundlagen der Chinesischen Medizin. Ein Lehrbuch für Akupunkteure und Arzneimitteltherapeuten*. Verlag für TCM Dr. Wühr, Kötzting, Germany.
NE: Maciocia G. (2002)

Maciocia G. (2002), *Foundations of Chinese Medicine A Comprehensive Text for Acupuncturists and Herbalists*. Churchill Livingstone, London, UK.

Maheshwarananda P.S. (2000), *Yoga im täglichen Leben. Das System*. Ibera/ European University Press, Vienna, Austria.

Mandelbrot B.B. (1987), *The Fractal Geometry of Nature*. Freeman, New York, NY, USA.

Matthiessen P.F., B. Rosslenbroich & S. Schmidt (1994), *Unkonventionelle Medizinische Richtungen. Bestandsaufnahme zur Forschungssituation*. Bundesministerium für Forschung und Technologie, Bonn, Germany.

Matthiessen P.F. (2002), *Perspektivität und Paradigmenpluralismus in der Medizin*. In: B. Fuchs & N. Kobler-Fumasoli (Hrsg.), Hilft der Glaube? Heilung auf dem Schnittpunkt zwischen Theologie und Medizin. LIT, Münster, Germany (pp.3-34).

Melchart D. & H. Wagner (Hrsg., 1993), *Naturheilverfahren. Grundlagen einer autoregulativen Medizin*. Schattauer, Stuttgart, Germany.
NE: Melchart D. & R. Brenke (Hrsg., 2002), *Naturheilverfahren. Leitfaden für die ärztliche Aus-, Fort- und Weiterbildung*. Schattauer, Stuttgart, Germany.

Meng A. (1997), *Die Basistheorie der Akupunktur und der Traditionellen Chinesischen Medizin. Eine Physiologie der TCM für den westlichen Mediziner*. Maudrich, Wien.

Meyer F. (1988), *Gso-Ba Rig-Pa. Le Systeme Medical Tibetain*. C.N.R.S., Paris, France.

NE: Meyer F. (2002)

Micozzi M.S. (Ed., 1999), *Current Review of Complementary Medicine.* Current Medicine, Philadelphia, PA, USA.

Micozzi M.S. (Ed., 2001), *Fundamentals of Complementary and Alternative Medicine.* Churchill Livingstone, New York, NY, USA.

Milavec T.J., K.W. Kratky & F.J. Badelt (1994), *Altchinesische Systeme als Netzwerk (Network Aspects of Old Chinese patterns).* Forsch Komplementärmed (Research in Complementary Medicine) *1*: 87-99.

Millman D. (2000), *The Life You Were Born to Live.* Fine Communications, New York, NY, USA.

Mittwede M. (1998), *Der Ayurveda. Von den Wurzeln zur Medizin heute.* Haug, Heidelberg, Germany.

Morfill G. & H. Scheingraber (1991), *Chaos ist überall... und es funktioniert. Eine neue Weltsicht.* Ullstein, Frankfurt am Main, Germany.

NE: Morfill G. & H. Scheingraber (1993)

Morrison J.H. (1995), *Ayurveda. Ein Weg zu Gesundheit und Lebensfreude. Wie wir das Wissen der traditionellen indischen Medizin nutzen können.* TRIAS, Stuttgart, Germany.

Morrison J.H. (2001), *The Book of Ayurveda. A Guide to Personal Wellbeing.* Gaia Books, London, UK.

Moser M. & L. Schwarz (1994), *Phänomene des Potenzierens und der Kreislauf des Wassers.* In: O. Bergsmann (Hrsg.), Struktur und Funktion des Wassers im Organismus. Versuch einer Standortbestimmung. Facultas, Vienna, Austria (S.57-69).

Moser M., L. Dorfer, F. Muhry, D. Messerschmidt, M. Frühwirth & F. Bayr (1998), *Untersuchungen zur Physiologie des Nogier-Reflexes.* Akupunktur/ Aurikulomedizin *2*/1998: 3-13.

Moser M., M. Frühwirth, D. von Bonin, D. Cysarz, R. Penter, C. Heckmann & G. Hildebrandt (1999), *Das autonome Bild als Methode zur Darstellung der Rhythmen des menschlichen Herzschlags.* In: P. Heusser (Hrsg.), *Akademische Forschung in der Anthroposophischen Medizin. Beispiel Hygiogenese: Natur- und geisteswissenschaftliche Zugänge zur Selbstheilungskraft des Menschen.* Lang, Bern, Switzerland (S.207-223).

Moser M., Frühwirth M. & T. Kenner (2008), *The symphony of life. Importance, interactions, and visualization of biological rhythms.* IEEE Eng Med Biol Mag *27*: 29-37.

Moss F. (1994), *Stochastic Resonance. From the Ice Ages to the Monkey's Ear.* In: G.H. Weiss (Ed.), Contemporary Problems in Statistical Physics. SIAM, Philadelphia, PA, USA (pp.205-253).

Müller M. (2000), *Das Gesicht als Spiegel der Gesundheit. Visuelle Diagnostik.* Ehrenwirth, Munich, Germany.

NE: Müller M. (2000)

Nadkarni A.K. (Ed., 2000), *Dr. K.M. Nadkarni's Indian materia medica: with Ayurvedic, Unani-Tibbi, Siddha, allopathic, homeopathic, naturopathic & home remedies, appendices & indexes. Vols. 1, 2.* Popular Prakashan, Bombay, India.

Netzhammer M. (2000), *Heilen mit Arsen und Quecksilber.* DAO 3/2000, S.59-62.

Nogier P. & B. Bricot (1978), *Die RAC-Registrierung.* Deutsche Zeitschrift für Akupunktur 5/1978: 127-130.

Norretranders T. (1997), *Spüre die Welt. Die Wissenschaft des Bewußtseins*. Rowohlt, Reinbek bei Hamburg, Germany.
NE: Norretranders T. (2000)

Oberbaum M. & J. Cambar (1994), *Hormesis: dose-dependent reverse effects of low and very low doses*. In: P.C. Endler & J. Schulte (Eds.), Ultra High Dilution. Physiology and Physics. Kluwer, Dordrecht, The Netherlands (pp.5-18).

Oberbaum M., I. Yaniv, Y. Ben-Gal, J. Stein, N. Ben-Zvi, L.S. Freedman & D. Branski (2001), *A Randomized, Controlled Clinical Trial of the Homeopathic Medication TRAUMEEL S® in the Treatment of Chemotherapy-Induced Stomatitis in Children Undergoing Stem Cell Transplantation*. Cancer 92_3: 684-690.

Ortega S. (2000), *Die Miasmenlehre Hahnemanns. Diagnose, Therapie und Prognose der chronischen Krankheiten*. Haug, Heidelberg, Germany.

Paik H.S. & D.J. Yoo (1979), *Grundlagen der Pulsologie und neue klinische elektronische Pulsographie*. Forschungsgemeinschaft für Euro-Asiatische Medizin, Uetersen, Germany.

Payrhuber D. (1997), *Dimensionen der homöopathischen Medizin*. Eigenverlag, Salzburg, Austria.

Peitgen H.-O. & P.H. Richter (2000), *The Beauty of Fractals. Images of Complex Dynamical Systems*. Springer, Berlin, Germany.

Pelletier K.R. (2002), *The Best Alternative Medicine*. Fireside, Simon & Schuster, New York, NY, USA.

Pichler E. (1996), *Die Homöopathie ist eine Regulationstherapie und Interzellulärtherapie*. Homöopathie in Österreich 7_1, S.29-32.

Pietschmann H. (1993), *Paradigmenwechsel und Paradigmenvielfalt*. In: A. Stacher & O. Bergsmann (Hrsg.), Grundlagen für eine integrative Ganzheitsmedizin. Facultas, Vienna, Austria (S.29-37).

Pietschmann H. (2002), *Eris & Eirene. Eine Anleitung zum Umgang mit Widersprüchen und Konflikten*. Ibera, Vienna, Austria.

Pischinger A. (2004), *Das System der Grundregulation. Grundlagen einer ganzheitsbiologischen Medizin*. Haug, Heidelberg, Germany.

Porkert M. (1992), *Die chinesische Medizin*. Econ, Düsseldorf, Germany.

Porter R. (2000), *Die Kunst des Heilens. Eine medizinische Geschichte der Menschheit von der Antike bis heute*. Spektrum Akademischer Verlag, Heidelberg, Germany.
NE: Porter R. (2003)

Porter R. (2003), *The Greatest Benefit to Mankind. A Medical History of Humanity*. Fontana Press, London, UK.

Pschyrembel W. (2000), *Pschyrembel Wörterbuch Naturheilkunde und alternative Heilverfahren mit Homöopathie, Psychotherapie und Ernährungsmedizin*. de Gruyter, Berlin, Germany.
NE: Pschyrembel W. (2001), *Pschyrembel Wörterbuch Naturheilkunde und alternative Heilverfahren*. Gondrom, Bindlach, Germany.

Pudel V. & J. Westenhöfer (2003), *Ernährungspsychologie. Eine Einführung*. Hogrefe, Göttingen, Germany.

Pyragas K. (1992), *Continuous Control of Chaos by Self-Controlling Feedback*. Physics Letters *A170*: 421-428.

Pyragas K. (2006), *Delayed Feedback Control of Chaos*. Phil. Trans. R. Soc *A364*: 2309-2334.

Qusar N. & J.-C. Sergent (1997), *Tibetische Medizin und Ernährung*. Droemer Knaur, Munich, Germany.

    NE: Qusar N. & J.-C. Sergent (2001)

Qusar N., T. Paljor, T. Dakpa & L. Tsultrim (1997), *Fundamentals of Tibetan Medicine according to the Rgyud-Bzhi*. Men-Tsee-Khang, Dharamsala, India.

    NE: Qusar N., T. Paljor, T. Dakpa & L. Tsultrim (2001)

Ranade S. (1994), *Ayurveda – Wesen und Methodik*. Haug, Heidelberg, Germany.

    NE: Ranade S. (2004)

Ranade S. (1992), *Natural Healing through Ayurveda*. Morson Publishing, Salt Lake City, UT, USA.

Rastogie D.P. et al. (1993), *Evaluation of Homeopathic Therapy in 129 Asymptomatic HIV Carriers*. British Homoeopathic Journal 82_1: 4-8.

Reckeweg H.H. (1978), *Homotoxikologie*. Aurelia, Baden-Baden, Germany.

    NE: Reckeweg H.H. (1993)

EE: Reckeweg H.H. (1989), *Homotoxicology*. Menaco Publishing Company, Albuquerque, NM, USA.

Redfern P.H. & B. Lemmer (1998*), Physiology and Pharmacology of Biological Rhythms*. Springer, Berlin, Germany.

Reibold E., W. Just, J. Becker & H. Benner (1999), *Stochastic Resonance without Noise*. In: M. Ding, W. Ditto, L. Pecora, M. Spano & S. Vohra (Eds.), Proceedings of the 4th Experimental Chaos Conference. World Scientific, Singapore (pp.229-234).

Reichle F. (Hrsg., 1997), *Das Wissen vom Heilen. Tibetische Medizin*. Haupt, Bern, Switzerland.

    NE: Reichle F. (Hrsg., 2003), *Das Wissen vom Heilen. Tibetische Medizin*. Oesch, Zürich, Switzerland.

Reisser P., D. Mabe & R. Velarde (2001), *Examining Alternative Medicine: An Inside Look at the Benefits & Risks*. InterVarsity Press, Downers Grove, IL, USA.

Reuter U. & R. Oettmeier (2001), *Biologische Krebsbehandlung heute oder Sag JA zum Leben! Wegweiser für Betroffene, Angehörige und zur Vorbeugung*. ProLeben, Greiz, Germany.

Rhyner H.-H (2001), *Das Praxis Handbuch Ayurveda. Gesund leben, sanft heilen*. Urania, Neuhausen, Switzerland.

Richter K. & H. Becke (1989), *Akupunktur. Tradition – Theorie – Praxis*. VEB Verlag Volk und Gesundheit, Berlin, Germany.

    NE: Richter K. & H. Becke (Hrsg., 1995), *Akupunktur. Tradition – Theorie – Praxis*. Ullstein Mosby, Berlin, Germany.

Risch G. (1998), *Homöopathik. Die Heilmethode Hahnemanns*. Pflaum, Munich, Germany.

Robert R. (2001), *Das Ende des Schmetterlingseffekt*s. Spektrum der Wissenschaft *11*/2001: 66-75.

Rohr R. & A. Ebert (1991), *Das Enneagramm. Die 9 Gesichter der Seele*. Claudius, Munich, Germany.

NE: Rohr R. & A. Ebert (2004)

Rohr R. & A. Ebert (2001), *The Enneagram. A Christian Perspective.* Crossroad Publishing Company, New York, NY, USA.

Rosenthal C. (2000), *Kingdoms Understanding in Homeopathy. A New Research.* Homoeophatic Links *13₁*: 42-46.

Rossaint A.L. (2002), *Ganzheitliche Zahnheilkunde in physischer, psychischer und metaphysischer Schau.* Haug, Heidelberg, Germany.

Rossaint A.L. (2005), *Medizinische Kinesiologie, Physio-Energetik und Ganzheitliche (Zahn-)-Heilkunde.* VAK, Kirchzarten bei Freiburg, Germany.

Ruelle D. (1993), *Chance and Chaos.* Penguin Books, London, UK.

Sachs R. (1997), *Tibetisches Ayurveda. Gesundheit zum Leben.* Ariston, Kreuzlingen, Switzerland.

   NE: Sachs R. (2001), *Tibetisches Ayurveda. Gesundheit zum Leben.* Bechtermünz, Augsburg, Germany.

Sachs R. (2000), *Health for Life. Secrets of Tibetan Ayurveda.* Clear Light Publishers, Santa Fe, NM, USA.

Sankaran R. (1997), *The Soul of Remedies.* Homoeopathic Medical Publishers, Mumbai, India.

Sankaran R. (1999), *The Substance of Homoeopathy.* Homoeopathic Medical Publishers, Mumbai, India.

Sankaran R. (2002), *An Insight into Plants. Vols. 1 & 2.* Homoeopathic Medical Publishers, Mumbai, India.

Sankaran R. (2005), *The Sensation in Homoeopathy.* Homoeopathic Medical Publishers, Mumbai, India.

Sargant W. (1958), *Der Kampf um die Seele. Eine Physiologie der Konversion.* Piper, Munich, Germany.

Sargant W. (1997), *Battle for the Mind: A Physiology of Conversion and Brainwashing.* Marlor Press Inc., Saint Paul, MN, USA.

Sathaye B.V. & S.N. Nadkarni (2000), *Die fünf Elemente. Körperphysiologie nach Ayurved.* CO'MED 6/2000: 86-88.

Schamanek A. & K.W. Kratky (1994), *Die Logistische Abbildung: Auswirkungen der endlichen Rechengenauigkei*t. In: H. Bremer, S. Habermeier & S. Wladarsch (Hrsg.), Chaos und Strukturbildung. Faktum, Technische Universität München, Munich, Germany (S.157-164).

de Schepper L. (2003), *Homeopathy and the Periodic Table.* Full of Life Publishing, Santa Fé, NM, USA.

Schlitz M., T. Amorok & M.S. Micozzi (2004), *Consciousness And Healing: Integral Approaches To Mind-body Medicine.* Elsevier/Mosby, St.Louis, MO, USA.

Schlote K.-H. (Hrsg., 2002), *Chronologie der Naturwissenschaften. Der Weg der Mathematik und der Naturwissenschaften von den Anfängen in das 21. Jahrhundert.* Harri Deutsch, Frankfurt am Main, Germany.

Schmidt R.F., G. Thews & F. Lang (Hrsg., 2000), *Physiologie des Menschen.* Springer, Berlin, Germany.

Schmidt R.F., G. Thews & F. Lang (Hrsg., 1989), *Human Physiology.* Springer, Berlin, Germany.

Schmiedel V. & M. Augustin (1997), *Handbuch Naturheilkunde. Methoden, Anwendung, Selbstbehandlung.* Haug, Heidelberg, Germany.

Scholten J. (1997), *Homöopathie und die Elemente.* Alonnissos, Utrecht, The Netherlands. *NE:* Scholten J. (2004).

Scholten J. (2000), *Homoeopathy and the Elements.* Alonnissos, Utrecht, The Netherlands.

Scholten J. (2000), *Homoeopathy and Minerals.* Alonnissos, Utrecht, The Netherlands.

Scholten J. (2001), *Minerals in Plants.* Alonnissos, Utrecht, The Netherlands.

Scholten J. (2002), *Minerals in Plants 2.* Alonnissos, Utrecht, The Netherlands.

Schramm E. (1992), *Biologische Testmedizin, ein Beitrag zur Elektrodiagnostik. In:* O. Bergsmann (Hrsg.), Elektrodiagnostik. Facultas, Vienna, Austria (S.63-68).

Schrott E. (1994), *Ayurveda für jeden Tag. Die sanfte Heilweise für vollkommene Gesundheit und Wohlbefinden.* Mosaik, Munich, Germany. *NE:* Schrott E. (2003)

Schulte J. & P.C. Endler (Eds., 1998), *Fundamental Research in Ultra High Dilution and Homoeopathy.* Kluwer, Dordrecht, The Netherlands (pp.117-125).

Schuster H.G. (Ed., 1999), *Handbook of Chaos Control.* Wiley-VCH, Weinheim.

Schwarz G. (1988), *Philosophie der Krankheit: die Heilungsäquivalenztheorie. In:* Wiener Dialog über Ganzheitsmedizin. Dokumentation. Jugend & Volk, Vienna, Austria (S.67-73).

Schwarz A.A. & R.P. Schweppe (1998), *Praxisbuch Tibetische Medizin. Ganzheitlich behandeln durch Ernährung, Massagen, Meditation und tibetische Arzneimittel.* Ludwig, Munich, Germany.

Sernetz M. (2000), *Die fraktale Geometrie des Lebendigen.* Spektrum der Wissenschaft Juli 2000: 72-79.

Simon F.B. & C. Rech-Simon (2002), *Zirkuläres Fragen. Systemische Therapie in Fallbeispielen: ein Lernbuch.* Carl-Auer-Systeme, Heidelberg, Germany.

Smith C.W. & P.C. Endler (1994), *Resonance Phenomena of an Ultra High Dilution of Thyroxine – Preliminary Results.* In: P.C. Endler & J. Schulte (Eds.), Ultra High Dilution. Physiology and Physics. Kluwer, Dordrecht, The Netherlands (pp.203-207).

Sokal A. & J. Bricmont (2001), *Fashionable Nonsense. Postmodern Intellectuals' Abuse of Science.* Saint Martin's Press, New York, NY, USA.

Song L.Z.Y.X., A.E.R. Schwartz & L.G.S. Russek (1998), *Heart-Focused Attention and Heart-Brain Synchronization: Energetic and Physiological Mechanisms.* Alternative Therapies in Health and Medicine 4_5: 44-62.

Sponsel R. (1995), *Handbuch integrativer psychologischer Psychotherapie. Zur Theorie und Praxis der schulen- und methodenübergreifenden psychologischen Psychotherapie. Ein Beitrag zur Entmythologisierung der Psychotherapieschulen.* EIC, Erlangen, Germany.

Stacher A. (1996), *Warum fehlt der Dialog zwischen Schulmedizin und Komplementärmedizin.* GAMED 4/1996, S.8-12.

Sternberg R.J. (1999), *Thinking Styles.* Cambridge University Press, Cambridge, UK.

Sukul N.C. (1998), *Interaction of a High Dilution of Agaricus Muscarius L with Dopamine Agonists and Antagonists in Modulating Catalepsy of Mice*. In: C. Taddei-Ferretti & P. Marotta (Eds.), High Dilution Effects in Cells and Integrated Systems. World Scientific, Singapore (pp.193-199).

Szabó Z. (1985), *Buch der Runen. Das westliche Orakel*. Droemer Knaur, Munich, Germany.

NE: Szabó Z. (2000), *Buch der Runen. Götter, Lebensbaum und Runenkosmos*. Neue Erde, Saarbrücken, Germany.

Taddei-Ferretti C. & P. Marotta (Eds., 1998), *High Dilution Effects on Cells and Integrated Systems*. World Scientific, Singapore.

Tatz M. & J. Kent (1993), *Reise ins Nirvana. Das tibetische Orakelspiel von Karma und Wiedergeburt*. Hugendubel, Munich, Germany.

Tatz M. & J. Kent (1978), *Rebirth. Tibetan Game of Liberation*. Rider & Company, London, UK.

Tatzky B., A. Trökes & J. Pinter-Neise (1995), *Theorie und Praxis des Hatha-Yoga. Ein Leitfaden zur Erfahrung der Energie*. Via Nova, Petersberg, Germany.

NE: Tatzky B., A. Trökes & J. Pinter-Neise (1998)

Taylor E. (Ed., 1984), *William James on Exceptional Mental States. The 1896 Lowell Lectures*. University of Massachusetts Press, Amherst, MA, USA.

Taylor E. (1996), *William James on Consciousness beyond the Margin*. Princeton University Press, Princeton, NJ, USA.

Terrades G. (1996), *Menschentyp und Heilmethoden. Einführung in die chinesische Medizin*. Ariston, Kreuzlingen, Switzerland.

Tian L. & A. Lachner (2006), *Wortschatz Chinesische Medizin. Die Sprache der TCM – verstehen, begreifen, korrekt aussprechen*. Elsevier Urban & Fischer, München.

Toifl K. (1995), *Chaos im Kopf. Chaostheorie – ein nichtlinearer Weg für Medizin und Wissenschaft*. Maudrich, Vienna, Austria.

Touitou Y. (Ed., 1998), *Biological Clocks. Mechanisms and Applications*. Elsevier, Amsterdam, Netherlands.

Treugut H., C. Görner, R. Lüdtke & V. Burghardt (1998), *Reliabilität der energetischen Meridianmessung mit Prognos A*. Forschende Komplementärmedizin 5: 284-289.

Trumble W.R., L. Brown & A. Stevenson (Eds., 2003), *Shorter Oxford English Dictionary*. Oxford University Press, Oxford, UK.

Tschuschke V., C. Heckrath & W. Tress (2001), *Zwischen Konfusion und Makulatur. Zum Wert der Berner Psychotherapie-Studie von Grawe, Donati und Bernauer*. Vandenhoeck & Ruprecht, Göttingen, Germany.

Überall A. (2000), *Spiritualität des Heilens. Christus Medicus – Buddha Shakyamuni*. Ibera, Vienna, Austria.

NE: Überall A. (2001)

Ulmer-Janes E. (1998), *Die Magie kehrt zurück. Vom bewußten Gestalten der Realität*. Ibera, Vienna, Austria.

NE: Ulmer-Janes E. (2001)

Unschuld P.U. (2002), *Medicine in China. Historical Artifacts and Images*. Prestel, Munich, Germany.

Unschuld P.U. (2003), *Huang Di Nei Jing Su Wen. Nature, Knowledge, Imagery in an Ancient Chinese Medical Text.* University of California Press, Berkeley, CA, USA.

de Vernejoul P., P. Albarède & J.C. Darras (1985), *Etude des méridiens d'acupuncture par les traceurs radioactifs.* Bull Acad Natl Med *169*: 1071-1075.

Vester F. (2002), *Die Kunst vernetzt zu denken Ideen und Werkzeuge für einen neuen Umgang mit Komplexität. Ein Bericht an den Club of Rome.* dtv, Munich, Germany.
NE: Vester F. (2003)

Voll R. (1976), *20 Jahre Elektroakupunktur-Diagnostik und Elektroakupunktur-Therapie mit niederfrequenten Stromimpulsen nach Voll.* Medizinisch-literarische Verlagsgesellschaft, Uelzen, Germany.

Walch S. (2002), *Dimensionen der menschlichen Seele. Transpersonale Psychologie und holotropes Atmen.* Walter, Düsseldorf, Germany.

Warnke U. (1999), *Die geheime Macht der Psyche. Quantenphilosophie – die Renaissance der Urmedizin.* Popular Academic Verlags-Gesellschaft, Saarbrücken, Germany.

Waterstone R. (1996), *Indien. Religion und Riten. Götter und Kosmos. Meditation und die Kunst des Yoga.* Bertelsmann Club, Rheda-Wiedenbrück, für die Buchgemeinschaft Donauland, Kremayr & Scheriau, Vienna, Austria.
NE: Waterstone R. (2001), *Indien. Götter und Kosmos, Karma und Erleuchtung, Meditation und Yoga.* Taschen, Cologne, Germany.

Waterstone R. (2002), *India. The Cultural Companion.* Duncan Baird, London, UK.

Waterstone R. (2002), *India. Belief and Ritual, the Gods and the Cosmos, Meditation and the Yogic Arts.* Thorsons Publishers, London, UK.

Wehr M. (2002), *Der Schmetterlingsdefekt. Turbulenzen in der Chaostheorie.* Klett-Cotta, Stuttgart, Germany.

Weil A. (1995), *Spontanheilung. Die Heilung kommt von innen.* Bertelsmann, Munich, Germany.
NE: Weil A. (1996)
Weil A. (2000), *Spontaneous Healing. How to Discover and Enhance Your Body's Natural Ability to Maintain and Heal Itself.* Ballantine Books, New York, NY, USA.

Weinschenk F. (2002), *Miasmen, haben sie Bedeutung in der täglichen Praxis?* Homöopathie in Österreich *13*$_2$, S.3.

Weisshuhn T.E.R. (1997), *Das schwarze Loch der Homöopathie.* Homöopathie-Zeitschrift I/97, S.24-37.

Wenzel G. (1999), *Qigong. Quelle der Lebenskraft.* Edition Tau, Bad Sauerbrunn, Austria.

West B.J. (1990), *Fractal Physiology and Chaos in Medicine.* World Scientific, Singapore.

van Wijk R. (1998), *Pressure-Induced Electrical Skin Conductivity as a Sensitive Mean for the Detection by Human-Human Interaction of Subtle Bodily Changes.* In: C. Taddei-Ferretti & P. Marotta (Eds.), High Dilution Effects on Cells and Integrated Systems. Proceedings of the International School of Biophysics; Casamicciola, Napoli, Italy, 23-28 October 1995. World Scientific, Singapore (pp.273-282).

van Wijk R. & F.A.C. Wiegant (1994), *Physiological Effects of Homoeopathic Medicines in Closed Phials; a Critical Evaluation.* In: P.C. Endler & J. Schulte (Eds.), Ultra High Dilution. Physiology and Physics. Kluwer, Dordrecht, The Netherlands (pp.81-95).

Wilber K. (1994), *Esoterische Religion, Bewußtseinsentwicklung und Psychotherapie*. In: E. Zundel & P. Loomans (Hrsg.), Psychotherapie und religiöse Erfahrung. Konzepte und Methoden transpersonaler Psychotherapie. Herder, Freiburg, Germany (S.291-318).

Wilber K. (2000), *Integral Psychology. Consciousness, Spirit , Psychology, Therapy*. Shambhala, Boston, MA, USA.

Wilber K. (2001), *A Theory of Everything. An Integral Vision for Business, Politics, Science and Spirituality*. Shambhala, Boston, MA, USA.

Wilber K. (2007) *Integral Spirituality: A Startling New Role for Religion in the Modern and Postmodern World*. Shambhala, Boston, MA, USA.

Wilhelm R. (Übers., 1973): *I Ging. Texte und Materialien*. Diederichs, Munich, Germany.
NE: Wilhelm R. (Übers., 1998): *I Ging. Texte und Materialien*. Bertelsmann-Club, Rheda-Wiedenbrück, Germany.

Wiseman N. & Y. Feng (1998), *A Practical Dictionary of Chinese Medicine*. Paradigm Publications, Brookline, MA, USA.

Worg R. (1993), *Deterministisches Chaos. Wege in die nichtlineare Dynamik*. BI Wissenschaftsverlag, Mannheim, Germany.

Yoo T.W. (1994), *Lecture on Koryo Hand Therapy (Korean Hand Acupuncture)*. Eum Yang Maek Jin Publishing, Seoul, Republic of Korea.

Zagriadskii W.A. (1996), *Wissenschaftliche Grundlage der Elektroakupunkturdiagnostik und -therapie. Russische Raumfahrttechnologie*. Akademie der Medizinisch-Technischen Wissenschaften Rußlands, Moscow, Russia.

Zagriadskii W.A., V. Zlokasov, A. Rozanov & J. Bistrov (Hrsg., 1996), *Computergestützte Elektropunktur-Diagnostik. Russische Raumfahrttechnologie für die prophylaktische Medizin*. Akademie der Medizinisch-Technischen Wissenschaften Rußlands, Moscow, Russia.

van der Zee H. (2001), *Miasms in Labour. A Revision of the Homoeopathic Theory of the Miasms – a Process towards Health*. Stichting Allonissos, Utrecht, the Netherlands.

Zundel E. (1994), *Einleitung*. In: E. Zundel & P. Loomans (Hrsg.), Psychotherapie und religiöse Erfahrung. Konzepte und Methoden transpersonaler Psychotherapie. Herder, Freiburg, Germany (S.9-38).

Zundel E. & P. Loomans (Hrsg., 1994), *Psychotherapie und religiöse Erfahrung. Konzepte und Methoden transpersonaler Psychotherapie*. Herder, Freiburg, Germany.
NE: Zundel E. & P. Loomans (Hrsg., 2002).

About the Book

Brief Description

For almost all of us the question of health and illness is essential but although a considerable amount of relevant literature is available, the confusion concerning this subject matter still seems to grow. In general people tend to trust no less than their own personal approach, while alternate positions find themselves either ignored or opposed. This book chooses a different path as it investigates not only the potentiality of communication among the various disciplines but also considers four basic views or perspectives as interpretations of reality. In the process it becomes apparent that classical science and more recent developments, like chaos theory, no longer speak the same language. Furthermore, several well-known modes of healing are compared (like orthodox medicine and homoeopathy from the West and Indian, Tibetan and Chinese medicine from the East) whereby – in addition to the natural differences – surprising parallels emerge, above all assertions concerning fundamental reactions of the human organism. This comparison leads to an integration of common results regarding the various medicine systems, which can be illustrated (health disc, life spiral) as well. Thus, the basis for the translation of insights and findings from one medicine system to another has successfully been established. Therefore, the utilisation of the knowledge of one mode of healing in other therapeutic systems proves to be possible. The proposed model also creates the groundwork for translating discoveries in one medicine system to another, which makes utilising them possible.

Target Audience

- Health professionals who are interested in an overview
- Those interested in basic questions and interlinked knowledge, especially in the area of medicine
- Those dissatisfied with the current divisions and specialisations ('expert knowledge')

Motivation for Reading this Book

- Deepening one's understanding of the meaning of the terms *healthy* and *ill.*
- Gaining an overall view of the jungle of therapeutic methods.
- Discovering a common basis of these approaches.

Mode of Illustration

- The 'multimedia' approach (aside from the text: illustrations, tables, formulae) provides understanding also via parallel tracks – according to individual preferences.
- The topic of the book is presented in a plain and comprehensible language. Formulae are only necessary in a few chapters and are explained in full. More demanding formulae are included in the more advanced sections, which are available to those with a greater thirst for knowledge. These more in-depth sections can be skipped without losing the thread.

A Short Biography of the Author

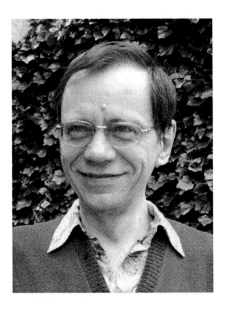

Karl W. Kratky, born in 1948 in Vienna, married, two children and three grandchildren.

PhD, Professor at the Faculty of Physics, University of Vienna. Since 1987 increasing interdisciplinary activity (keywords: systems research, self-organisation, chaos, complexity). 1989-1991 publisher of three books in this area, 1991 organiser of a summer seminar concerning systemic thinking. Since 1992 shifting of focus towards medicine (comparison and integration of medicine systems as well as their corresponding world views); 1992 vice president of the homoeopathy congress 'OMEOMED 92' (Urbino, Italy).

Focal points in research and teaching: physics and medicine, Asian methods of healing, homoeopathy, ethno-therapies and intercultural connections. Lectures and seminars about complementary medicine at the University of Vienna since 1997. Organizer of the symposium 'Comparative and Integrative Medicine' at the International Conferences on Systems Research, Informatics and Cybernetics 2004 and 2006 in Baden-Baden, Germany.

The author belongs to the team of the Interuniversity College for Health and Development, Graz / Castle of Seggau, Austria, where he is also a lecturer at the European Master's

Degree Programme for Integrated Health Sciences. The present book has been developed in connection with this programme. He is also a lecturer at the Academy for Traditional European Medicine (Windischgarsten, Austria).

The author is not only a member of the board of the scientific association 'Dynamics – Complexity – Human Systems' (Vienna, Austria) but also of the scientific advisory board of the Journal 'Research in Complementary Medicine' (Karger), the International Viennese Academy of Complementary Medicine and the Institute for Ethno-Music Therapy (Rosenau, Austria), where he is also a lecturer. He is a reviewer of the Journals 'Evidence Based Complementary and Alternative Medicine' and the above-mentioned 'Research in Complementary Medicine'. Furthermore he is a Fellow at the IIAS (International Institute for Advanced Studies in Systems Research and Cybernetics, Tecumseh, Ontario, Canada).

Index

B

C

F

I

J

K

L

S

T